The Pilon Tibial Fracture
Classification, Surgical Techniques, Results

PD Dr. Med. Dr. h.c. Urs F.A. Heim
Gumligen, Switzerland

W.B. SAUNDERS COMPANY
A Division of Harcourt Brace & Company
Philadelphia London Toronto Montreal Sydney Tokyo

W.B. SAUNDERS COMPANY
A Division of
Harcourt Brace & Company

The Curtis Center
Independence Square West
Philadelphia, Pennsylvania 19106

Library of Congress Cataloging-in-Publication Data

Heim, Urs

[Pilon-tibial-Fraktur. English]

The pilon tibial fracture: classification, surgical techniques, results / Urs F.A. Heim.—1st ed.

    p.   cm.

Includes bibliographical references and index.

ISBN 0–7216–5658–7

1. Tibia—Fractures.   I. Title.

[DNLM: 1. Tibial Fractures—surgery.   2. Tibial Fractures—classification.   WE 870 H467p 1906a]

RD560.H4413   1996

615.8′22—dc20
DNLM/DLC   94–36597

THE PILON TIBIAL FRACTURE:
CLASSIFICATION, SURGICAL TECHNIQUES, RESULTS   ISBN 0–7216–5658–7

Printed in the United States of America.

Last digit is the print number: 9   8   7   6   5   4   3   2   1

Contributors

Translator

Dr. Birgit Studtmann
Betzendorf, Germany

Contributors

André Gächter, Prof. Dr.med.
Director, Department of Orthopaedics and Trauma, Klinik Kantonsspital St.
  Gallen, St. Gallen, Switzerland
Corrective Surgery after Malunion in Pilon Fractures

Magdalena Müller-Gerbl, PD Dr.med.
Anatomical Anstalt, Munich, Germany
*Functional Anatomy of the Ankle Joint; Clinical Consequences of the
  Anatomy*

Reinhard Putz, Prof. Dr.med.
Ordinarius für Anatomie, Lehrstuhl I, Anatomische Anstalt, Munich,
  Germany
Functional Anatomy of the Ankle Joint

Thomas Rüedi, Prof. Dr.med.
Chief of Surgery, Surgical Clinic, Kantonsspital Chur, Chur, Switzerland
Pilon Fractures: What's New?

Artist

Klaus Oberli
Technical Illustrator, Bern, Switzerland

Foreword

The Pilon Tibial Fracture, written by Urs Heim, represents Professor Heim's lifelong intense interest in these complex injuries and is an encyclopedic treatise on all aspects of the pilon tibial fracture.

The book contains an extremely detailed discussion of the anatomy of the region and an original description of the failure mechanisms of cancellous bone, which Heim has based on his studies, new careful observations, and his rare grasp of the biomechanics of this region. An understanding of these mechanisms will provide the reader excellent insight into the different fracture patterns that are produced as a result of axial compressive loads and bending forces. These are the forces most often responsible for the pilon fractures and which distinguish these fractures from malleolar fractures, which are mostly the result of torsion.

Professor Heim has been interested in the problems of fracture classification for many years, particularly in the classification of fractures of this segment. He has decided to accept the principles of classification established in the *Comprehensive Classification of Fractures of the Long Bones,* to which he contributed the concept of the "rule of squares," which makes it possible to establish a clear definition of the end segment of any long bones. The pilon fractures are therefore classified on the basis of their morphologic complexity in an ascending order of severity into types A, B, and C and their corresponding groups and subgroups.

Professor Heim has had personal experience with almost every fracture pattern in this region. This is clear from the very detailed and personal descriptions of the surgical techniques and each step of the internal fixation of the different fractures. His astute observations have made it possible for him to warn the reader of all the pitfalls in all phases of treatment and give a clear description of how to avoid them.

Despite the strong emphasis on the mechanical aspects of the internal fixation of these fractures, Professor Heim does not lose sight of the most commonly encountered problems in treatment, namely, problems with the soft tissue envelope. He provides the reader with a clear explanation as to why the soft tissues of the distal tibia differ so much from the tissues surrounding the malleoli, and why pilon fractures are so different from ankle fractures in their soft tissue response to injury. He also lays down guidelines to the evaluation of the soft tissue envelope and to the staging of treatment, which if followed will certainly lead to a decrease in the incidence of soft tissue and bony complications.

This fine book is a synthesis of many years of astute observations coupled with a wealth of clinical experience. It is the product of meticulous classification and documentation of all of the collected clinical material, which was then painstakingly analyzed and interpreted with a rare insight into the biological and biomechanical problems of the different fracture patterns of this segment. The work is definitely a feast for the connoisseur and a most valuable reference volume for all those entrusted with the care of these difficult injuries.

JOSEPH SCHATZKER, M.D.

Preface
to the German Edition

The idea to write a monograph about tibial pilon fractures had existed for many years. The necessary preparations for this endeavor continued step by step. The data on the many patients operated on by the author between 1959 and 1983 formed the basis of this work. In cooperation with Th. Rüedi, a first classification was worked out in the years 1979 and 1980 [128, 169] and this was used for AO documentation purposes.

During the preliminary work on the third edition of *Periphere Osteosynthesen* [72], I was again reminded of the unsolved problems regarding the classification of these fractures. At the same time, I also started to work with Professor M.E. Müller on the *Classification AO des Fractures* [132]. Our objective was to define and classify all fractures of terminal segments of long bones according to a uniform scheme, but this had to be based on strictly clinical points of view. The subsequent review of the preliminary studies of 1979 showed that data from my personal experience would be insufficient to meet all aspects for a comprehensive work. The majority of my cases had been operated on by a single surgeon and the injuries had resulted from skiing accidents. Meanwhile, the pattern of accidents had changed.

If a monograph of general validity was to be written, a larger, collaborative study that included more patients was required. My change of residence to Bern brought the opportunity to increase the cooperation with the AO Documentation Centre, in particular with its former head Privat-Dozent (PD) Dr. R. Zehnder, who unfortunately died too early. With this book, we wish to keep his memory alive, both as an expert and a friend. We are indebted to him for the eight years he worked in our group, achieving major contributions to improve the understanding of traumatology in the context of the AO.

The objective to complete this study in 1988 could not be realized because of a series of unexpected obligations. The year 1988 was the pilon-jubilee year: 25 years earlier, in 1963, Gay and Evrard [46] had published the first comprehensive publication, nearly a monograph. Again and again, one has to admire the painstaking care and precision of the authors (both now retired) who did pioneering work in their time. Their extraordinary perception and the analysis of their case material remain remarkable. The impact of their studies continues to be felt in the whole of the French-speaking world.

In 1963, the first AO book, *Technik der operativen Frakturenbehandlung* [129], was also published. In this book, M. Allgöwer described the basic principles and the details of internal fixation for fractures of the distal tibia. These have not lost their validity even today.

Except for the 1968 codification of the AO tactics [172], nothing more than case reports have appeared on this subject and there were no fundamentally new concepts or ideas. A comprehensive description of this subject was lacking, presenting many diagnostic and therapeutic problems. To close this gap was a venture, and to tackle the task alone an impossible undertaking. I am indebted to numerous friends of our AO circle for their suggestions and advice, in particular to the contributors of special sections: Mrs. PD Dr. M. Müller-Gerbl, and PD Dr. A Gächter, PD Dr. F. Hefti, and Professor Th. Rüedi. With combined efforts, a coherent analysis could be presented.

We owe special thanks to our illustrator, K. Oberli, who has worked on our team for many years as a friend. Once again he knew how to master unusual difficulties and emphasize the essential points in black and white. Our secretaries, Mrs. J. Tschanz and Mrs. I. Küenzi, have accomplished an enormous task with great patience. We also wish to thank the Springer-Verlag for accepting this hardly gratifying subject matter and for its perfect presentation.

This book is dedicated to the surgeon engaged in traumatology who rarely comes across such fractures. It is intended both to encourage him to deal with the complicated matter and to remind him of the need for caution. Management of a complex tibial pilon fracture certainly involves great responsibilities.

In their early beginnings 30 years ago, the AO group of the hospitals at Chur, St. Gallen, and Interlaken embarked on the operative treatment of tibial pilon fractures. Therefore, we would like to continue with some personal remarks:

In the early months of 1960, the surgical team at the hospital in Chur, headed at the time by Dr. M. Allgöwer, became aware of the peculiarities of this fracture, which typically presented as a consequence of skiing accidents. We immediately realized that these injuries required surgical treatment, but the technical difficulties inherent in the operative reconstruction were often underestimated. Despite our "blind" commitment as traumatologists, our enthusiasm was often struck by harsh surprises. Too often we found ourselves in full operation, when progress stopped and despair was felt. On the other hand, there was overwhelming joy in the successes of joint reconstruction and the amazingly good functional results, providing a constant stimulus.

The younger surgeons then started to develop a sort of hate–love relationship toward the tibial pilon fracture, which proved to be lifelong. These apparently contradictory feelings were shared by our masters, revealed by the racy anecdotes they surprise us with still today, telling about incidents and patients in those early days.

During the twenty years I worked as head of a surgical clinic I operated on numerous tibial pilon fractures [30, 67]. Yet the turmoil of feelings toward this injury never calmed down. A simultaneous mixture of anticipation and anxiety was felt each time a patient was admitted, examined, and prepared for operation. Before the intervention, hours would be spent, consumed with investigations, consideration of x-ray films, tactical reflections, and doubtful questions. The preoperative tension that took over the whole team did not ease until after the operation, when the patient, in an atmosphere of silent devotion shared by all the staff, was taken away from the operating table and placed in bed.

It is as if a club of ''The Pilons'' had formed. It is not so much a subspecialty of trauma surgery as a small group of friends, who, at occasional discussion rounds, exchange opinions on the unsolved problems of this injury with meaningful looks of bittersweet feelings. Names need not be named. The reader will come across them at every step in the text and in the references. I am delighted that as the senior of this circle I have been able to write this book, and wish to express my gratitude.

PD Dr. Med. Dr. h.c. URS HEIM

Preface
to the English Edition

The publication of this book in English was an undertaking that unfortunately could not be realized without delay after publication of the German edition. I wish to express my appreciation to the W.B. Saunders Company in Philadelphia for their efforts to bring out the English edition in an extended version.

I am very thankful to Birgit Studtmann, M.D., for the excellent translation and to Mrs. Sandra Schoch-Lehnherr for the secretarial work. Once again, our friend Mr. Klaus Oberli prepared all the new artwork.

I am also indebted to Professors A. Leutenegger and Th. Rüedi, of Chur, for permission to present their exceptional cases in Figures 199, 200, and 201.

Four years have passed since the German edition was published. Preparation of the English edition required revision, update, and expansion of both text and figures, but also provided the opportunity to include the most recent opinions and latest publications. This book therefore may be considered a revised second edition of the German version.

The sections and illustrations are arranged according to didactic aspects of the cases. We hope practical needs will be better met with this presentation.

This book is dedicated to the surgeon embarking on repair of the fresh injury. Fractures of the tibial pilon have always been rare injuries—a fact that is clearly reflected by the number of cases in individual publications, and a fact that limits the knowledge and experience of most surgeons. The authors continue to believe that good functional results may be achieved even in the majority of severe injuries, provided these are recognized early and adequately managed. With this book we hope to contribute to this aim.

PD Dr. Med. Dr. h.c. URS HEIM

Contents

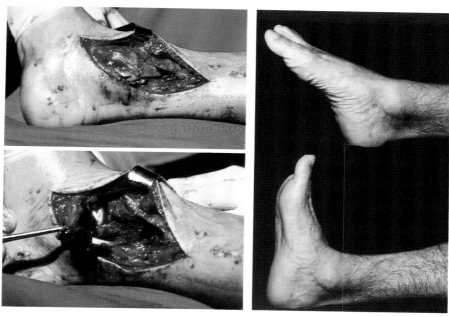

Color Figure 199. Internal fixation of a depression fracture with small screws only in a 29-year-old construction worker who sustained a closed fracture without concomitant injuries after falling from a 6-m-high scaffolding. Because of swelling and early blister formation, traction was applied primarily and internal fixation performed 8 days later. Active mobilization was started on day 6. The patient was discharged from hospital on day 20 with a crutch to allow partial weightbearing. Partial rehabilitation as a construction worker was gained after 18 weeks, full rehabilitation at 20 weeks. **B.** An atypical, posteromedial incision is made; the fracture line comes into view; cortical fenestration is carried out. **C.** Intraoperative view: the fragments and the depression are clearly recognizable; the medial malleolus is retracted distally. Posteriorly, the tendon of the posterior tibial muscle is visible. **G.** At 3 years, there was full dorsiflexion and plantarflexion.

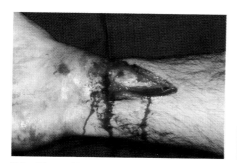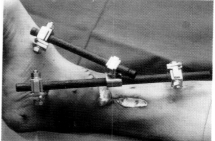

Color Figure 200. A. This 42-year-old man fell from a scaffolding and sustained a second-degree open right pilon fracture (C2.2-type morphology). **D.** External fixator bridging the talus, the calcaneus, and the tibial shaft. Partial adaptation of the wound.

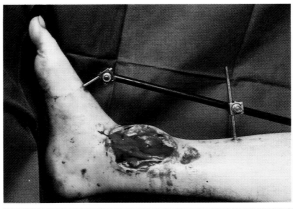

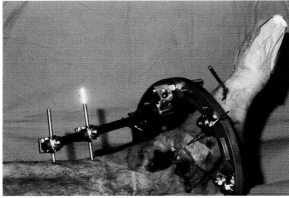

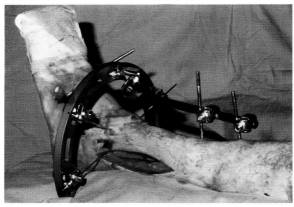

Color Figure 201. A 33-year-old patient ran into a car and sustained a third-degree, open and very soiled pilon fracture of the left leg (C2.2-type morphology). **C.** An emergency operation was performed 2 hours after the accident under antibiotic cover. **E, F.** ORIF at day 13: fixation of the fibula with a 3.5-mm titanium LCDCP. Transfixation of the articular fragments with two Kirschner wires fixed in a half-frame prototype and connected to the Schanz screws in the tibial shaft with carbon fiber bars. Iliac cancellous bone graft into the huge metaphyseal defect. No complications. The fixator was removed at 3 months.

- *Chapter 1*

The Lower Segment of the Tibia

1. FUNCTIONAL ANATOMY OF THE ANKLE JOINT

M. Müller-Gerbl and R. Putz

1.1. General Considerations

The ankle joint and the talocalcaneonavicular joint, together with their ligaments and the eight muscle tendons reaching across them, represent a defined functional unit. These joints must somehow adjust the inertial mass of the human body to the supporting surface. When walking, at least one foot—or part of a foot—is at any one moment resting on the ground while the ankle must in turn support and balance the total body weight. The cinematic sequence of the movements shows that at each phase of progression a considerable load must be transmitted through the components of the joint [35, 82, 193].

The tibia and fibula are of comparable length, but the distal end of the fibula is about 1 cm lower. It is so firmly bound to the tibia by the interosseous membrane and other firm ligaments that it produces a stable crutch—the ''malleolar fork''—for the trochlear articular surface of the talus (Fig. 1). The central region of the malleolar fork, or mortise, which is principally responsible for the transmission of axial load, was designated the *pilon tibial* (tibial pilon) by Destot in 1911 [37].

Because of some similarities, we also discuss the distal radius in this study.

1.2. The Bones of the Ankle Joint

Tibia

The tibia articulates with the trochlear surface of the talus through a rectangular inferior facet with irregular edges (Figs. 2–5). Its anterior and posterior borders diverge laterally, so that the medial part of the facet is narrower than the lateral part. The articular facet shows a slightly concave shape with a blunt sagittal ridge in the middle. This ridge is hard to identify in macerated bone, but in the presence of cartilage it is easily recognized. The ridge and the flat depressions on either side of the facet are differently curved in the sagittal plane. The radius of curvature of the ridge is about 24 mm and that of the surfaces is about 20 mm. This produces a concavity 4 to 5 mm in depth in the macerated specimen. According to Schmidt [179], the sagittal width attains about 28 mm. The anterior transverse measurement is about 30 mm [179]. The articular surface of the tibia blends with the articular facet of the medial malleolus at an angle of about 110 degrees. The latter is directed in a sagittal position to the long axis of the foot. The longitudinal extension of its articular surface measures about 13 mm, and in the sagittal plane, it reaches a width of approximately 24 mm.

In the middle of the diaphysis, the tibia is approximately triangular in cross section (Fig. 6). As it passes into the metaphysis, the apices become rounded. In the sectional view, the tibia resembles a compressed half-moon with the flat side facing posteriorly. Adjacent to the joint, the section broadens out into a nearly rectangular trapezoid with the shortest side laterally.

Fibula

The articular facet of the lateral malleolus shows a central curvature (see Figs. 2–5). The proximal sagittal portion forms an angle of 90 degrees with the inferior articular surface of the tibia, but curves outward below to increase this angle to 120 degrees. The articular surface does not reach the tip of the malleolus, being separated from it by a notch that is continued upward and backward as a furrow for ligamentous insertion. The vertical length of the facet is about 23 mm and the width up to 18 mm [179].

Structure of the Malleolar Fork

The above measurements indicate that the malleolar fork has an upper internal width of about 47 mm and, according to Schmidt [179], an external diameter of about 67 mm. The vertical difference between the distal ends of the two malleoli, which measures approximately 12.6 mm [179], is of particular importance to the radiologist.

The proximal part of the articular facet of the fibula fits into a corresponding facet in the fibular notch on the tibia (see Fig. 3), but there is no complete contact. The fibular notch, or incisura fibularis tibiae, is slightly concave and about 23 mm wide [179].

Radius

In the transverse plane, the carpal articular surface of the radius presents a flattened ellipse, which is sharply delimited by the ulna (see Fig. 2). It is well known to overhang somewhat posteriorly, and presents a sagittal ridge toward the ulnar side, rather similar to the corresponding articular surface of the tibia. Unlike the tibia, however, the two articular facets of the joint are not simply curved in the sagittal plane, but resemble shallow depressions. The radial articular surface merges smoothly into the tip of the radial styloid. The maximum sagittal width averages 18.1 mm; the transverse length reaches up to 29.2 mm [90, 180].

A transverse section through the radial diaphysis approximates an isosceles triangle. At the transition with the metaphysis, the transverse section forms a regular ellipse. Near the joint it gradually assumes the shape of an elongated rectangle with a slight prominence posteriorly (posterior tubercle).

Talus

The articular surface of the talus measures about 34 mm in the sagittal plane (see Figs. 2 and 3). At approximately 30 mm, the breadth is widest in the middle part. Anteriorly the bony border measures roughly the same, but posteriorly it tapers to about 21 mm [156, 157, 179].

The facet for the lateral malleolus is nearly vertical in the long axis of the foot, and it makes a sharp rectangular border with the superior surface. Its height is 25 mm, and in the sagittal plane it measures 27 mm [179].

The facet for the medial malleolus makes an obtuse angle with the superior surface. It is usually described as "comma-shaped." Its depth is about 14 mm, and its length is about 28 mm [179] in the sagittal plane.

The articular surface of the talar trochlea shows a flat groove in the sagittal direction, which corresponds to the elevation of the inferior articular surface of the tibia. The medial border of the superior surface tends to be higher than the lateral one, and the term *talus profile quotient* is used to describe its slight concavity in the frontal plane (Fig. 7). According to Riede et al. [162, 163], the ratio changes during life from 0.1 in young persons to 0.01 in the elderly.

1.3. Subchondral Mineralization

The density of subchondral bone is regularly distributed in the larger joints and provides information about the individual adaptation to the mechanical conditions prevailing at that particular location. By means of computed tomography (CT osteoabsorptiometry), objective and reproducible measurements may be obtained from living subjects [135, 139] (Fig. 8). Enlargement of the relevant details on the resulting CT data sets or CT sections will then allow the recording of the zones of subchondral mineralization in each section through the joint in terms of isodensities, and their subdivision into regions of different density representing steps on the Hounsfield density scale. Appropriate coloring allows better recognition of regions of equal density. An image analyzing system is finally used to apply the density contours to the surface of each joint. The demonstration of the surface projection thus obtained (Fig. 9) provides very precise information on the distribution of mineralization in each individual joint, and consequently, on the actual qualitative stresses.

Tibia and Fibula

The region of greatest mineralization is found where the inferior articular facet of the tibia merges into that of the medial malleolus (Fig. 10). Further density peaks are located in the anterolateral region of the joint surface and in the center of the articular facet of the medial malleolus. An area of high density also appears in the most distal zone of the articular facet of the lateral malleolus.

Radius

The surface demonstration of the subchondral bone density of the carpal articular facet shows two areas of high density, which are centrally located in the two facets of the joint surface [124] (Fig. 11).

Talus

The distribution of subchondral mineralization in the talus varies according to the talus profile ratio (Figs. 9, 10, and 12). In type 1, density is highest in the medial part of the superior articular facet and also in the anterior section of the articular facet of the medial malleolus and in the lowest sections of the lateral malleolus. In type 2, the highest levels of density are located along the medial border. They include the adjacent medial portion of the joint surface and extend into the antero-medial third of the trochlea. A further maximum is seen at the lower border of the articular facet of the medial malleolus. The same disposition is found in type 3 where similar regions of high density extending anteriorly onto the articular facet of the medial malleolus are found along the medial border of the superior surface. In this type, the posterior aspect of the trochlea also shows an extensive area of high mineralization [138].

1.4. The Articular Cartilage

Tibia and Fibula

The thickest areas of cartilage are found at the junction between the inferior articular facet and the articular surface of the medial malleolus, in the anterolateral region, and in the distal region of the lateral joint surface. We thus find a distribution pattern similar to that of the mineralization (Fig. 13).

Radius

The relative thickness of the hyaline cartilage covering the carpal articular surface is similar to the subchondral bone density. In the two shallow depressions of the articular surface, the cartilaginous coat is a little thicker than over the dividing ridge but falls off toward the edges of the joint surface. Near the border of the ulnar notch of the radius, however, there remains a thick covering of cartilage (Fig. 14).

Talus

Although the cartilage coverings of the tali examined ($N = 8$) showed some variations, thickness generally measures up to 3 mm along the sagittally directed medial border, gradually decreasing laterally (see Fig. 13). On the medial surface, the thickness decreases distally.

The thickness of the calcified zone of the articular cartilage over the articular surfaces of the ankle joint shows a high degree of correlation with the total thickness ($r = 0.88$–0.95) [136, 137].

1.5. Architecture of the Cancellous Bone

The Malleolar Fork

The subchondral cancellous bone consists of thick, dense trabeculae oriented at right angles to the surface. Even though this applies to the articular surfaces of the malleolar fork as a whole [188], the trabecular structure is particularly dense at the junction between the inferior articular surface of the tibia and the medial malleolar facet (Fig. 15).

The trabeculae of the cancellous bone run for 2 to 3 cm from the articular surface directly in the long axis of the tibia and then turn gently away from the center of the bone toward the diaphyseal cortex. Contrary to previous representations [120], there is no acute angle between cancellous trabeculae arising from the medial and lateral regions. This is clearly revealed by contact radiographs. The cortical bone of the medial malleolus blends with that of the shaft. Diaphyseal cancellous trabeculae in combination with trabeculae adjacent to the joint form a Gothic arch–like structure, which is classically interpreted as an adaptation to bending stresses. At the base of the medial malleolus, where it passes into the tibial metaphysis, little cancellous bone is found. Akin to the circumstances found at the femoral neck, this reflects rarefaction due to bending stresses within the ankle bones [193].

The situation in the lateral malleolus is similar (Fig. 15). Here, there is also relatively dense, prominent subchondral bone, with the trabeculae running perpendicular to the joint surface. A comparatively thick outer layer of cortical bone stretches up to the tip of the malleolus. The central lucent zone and the Gothic arch–like layout of the cancellous bone toward the tip correspond more or less to the structure on the medial side and suggest bending stresses in the lateral part of the ankle.

The arrangement of the cancellous bone near the inferior tibiofibular contact zone is not easy to interpret (see Fig. 15). The neighboring trabeculae on both sides run in a longitudinal direction, and this suggests that the two bony surfaces transmit very little pressure. The cortical bone on the fibular side is somewhat more dense.

Increased density of cancellous bone, lying about 1 cm from the surface and curving around parallel to the inferior articular surface and then parallel to the medial malleolus, can often be seen on the anteroposterior (AP) radiograph. Taking into account the postulated bending stresses in the medial malleolus, we interpret this as an answer to tensile stresses.

Radius

Whereas the subchondral cancellous bone of the radius up to a width of 1.2 mm also runs exactly perpendicular to the joint surface, it differs essentially from the situation in the tibia further proximal in the metaphysis (see Fig. 15). Since the marrow cavity of the radius is somewhat narrower, the medial and lateral groups of trabeculae do not diverge, as in the tibia, but run parallel for 3 or 4 cm. They are bound together by individually variable, transversely directed trabeculae acting as tensile filaments. Unlike the orientation of the corresponding structures in the tibia, these tensile trabeculae do not project into the styloid process, but bend somewhat proximally in the lateral third to follow the earlier course of the epiphyseal plate.

Talus

Owing to its functional role as the keystone of the plantar arch, the talus displays a highly complicated bony structure (see Fig. 15). Again, the subchondral trabeculae are of variable length and run perpendicular to the joint surface. Further to the center, however, they become so intricately interwoven as to preclude a detailed analysis of their structure. Within the talar neck, a lucent region circumscribed by dense cancellous bone can be seen. In some specimens, a Gothic arch–like arrangement of the trabeculae may be observed at this site.

1.6. Ligaments

The Junction Between Tibia and Fibula

The tibia and fibula are linked by three layers of connective tissue (Fig. 16). The interosseous membrane runs steeply downward from tibia to fibula. No transverse fibers are found near the fibular notch of the tibia where the bones are in contact. The direct contact zone of the bones is mostly filled with loose connective tissue that gives rise to a synovial fold reaching down into the joint space (see Fig. 2). This space stretches for 1 cm from the articular surface and lacks a cartilaginous covering. This confirms that there is no transmission of pressure between tibia and fibula at this level.

The lateral malleolus is attached anteriorly and posteriorly to the corresponding borders of the tibia, and both ligaments (tibiofibular ligaments) deviate some 45 degrees from the horizontal axis (see Fig. 16). In other words, they continue the direction of the fibers of the interosseous membrane, but at a somewhat different angle.

With a thickness of 4 mm [179], the anterior tibiofibular ligament is weaker than the posterior ligament, which can be as thick as 6.3 mm. The latter ligament always consists of two parts: a thin plate about 1 mm thick separated by a narrow recess from an underlying 6-mm component. Splaying of the malleolar fork in the extreme position of dorsiflexion causes predominantly stretching of the posterior ligament, which may be explained by the rotation of the lateral malleolus [87, 144, 159].

Medial Ligaments

The medial ligamentous apparatus is formed by the continuous plate of the deltoid ligaments (Fig. 17). Proximally, an extension of about 2 cm embraces the tip of the medial malleolus, and superficial fibers spring tangentially from its medial surface.

The tibionavicular and tibiotalar ligaments lie widely divergent along the neck of the talus and reach below the medial facet of the trochlea. They are overlapped posteriorly by the tibiocalcaneal ligament, which passes up to the superior border of the sustentaculum tali. The posterior tibiotalar ligament lies deepest and runs posteriorly to the medial tubercle of the posterior process of the talus. These two components of the deltoid ligaments are separated by a space containing connective tissue and blood vessels.

Photographs demonstrating the ligamentous function in an anatomic specimen with intact ligaments (Fig. 17) show the tension in the anterior tibiotalar ligament in the extreme position of plantarflexion. The posterior parts of the deltoid ligament are here twisted together. In the extreme position of dorsiflexion it is apparently only the posterior tibiotalar ligament that is stretched. The tibiocalcaneal ligament is under particular tension with varus deformation.

Lateral Ligaments

The ligaments of the fibula are subdivided into three parts [108] (see Fig. 17). The anterior talofibular ligament has its origin between the anterior surface of the tip of the lateral malleolus and the edge of its articular facet. The calcaneofibular ligament, on the other hand, inserts near the lower border of the tip of the malleolus, so that the tip itself remains free. The posterior talofibular ligament is similarly attached close to the tip of the malleolus in a groove between the latter and the posterior border of the articular facet.

The anterior and posterior talofibular ligaments lie almost in the transverse plane. The anterior talofibular ligament runs slightly downward toward the proximal part of the neck of the talus, whereas the posterior talofibular ligament runs exactly from lateral to medial to reach the lateral tubercle of the posterior process of the talus. According to Draenert [40], this ligament consists of three separate parts that converge laterally and between which layers of connective tissue containing blood vessels may be found. The calcaneofibular ligament runs obliquely downward and backward toward the outer surface of the calcaneus, about 1 cm behind the peroneal trochlea.

Photographs showing the function of the ligaments clearly display the complex interaction of the three lateral ligaments (see Fig. 17). During the final phase of dorsiflexion, it is the posterior talofibular ligament that primarily comes under tension, but in the specimen it can be seen that the anterior talofibular ligament is also taut. This is due to the fact that, because of the rather more proximal position of the oblique axis of the joint, the tip of the lateral malleolus tends to rotate in the opposite direction. The calcaneofibular ligament is most under tension during the final phase of plantarflexion, when it becomes to some extent wrapped around the anterior border of the tip of the malleolus. Comparison of the anatomy of the lateral and medial ligaments leads to the conclusion that the most important task of the deltoid ligament is to limit medial movement of the foot (varus stress), which is a static function. It seems that the lateral ligaments oppose rotation of the fibula and also attenuate the end phases of dorsi- and plantarflexion.

1.7. The Joint Capsule

In the area of the malleolar fork, the medial, lateral, and posterior aspects of the joint capsule are attached close to the bone-cartilage boundary (Fig. 18). The tips of the malleoli lie outside the joint space. Anteriorly, the line of attachment at the fork is displaced a few millimeters proximal to the bone-cartilage boundary. The same applies to the talar neck, where the line of attachment may be as far as 10 mm away from the cartilage border.

The anterior part of the capsule is thin and has no ligamentous reinforcements. The collateral ligaments (see section 1.6; Figs. 16 and 17) on both sides blend with the joint capsule. Posterolaterally, the capsule is strengthened only by the posterior talofibular ligament. Posteromedially, it remains relatively thick without extraligamentous support.

Synovial Folds

The broad and obliquely running fatty synovial fold along the anterior border of the joint space is particularly impressive (see Fig. 3). This fold projects several centimeters beyond the anterior circumference of the joint and its lower part may be as thick as 5 mm. Particularly on the medial side, complex synovial folds of varying size run from the posterior surface of the capsule and reach into the joint anteriorly.

An orderly sagittal fold of synovia is lodged in the lateral corner of the joint between tibia and fibula (see section 1.2; Fig. 2). It runs proximally for about 1 cm between the two bones near the fibular notch of the tibia and thus forms the actual limit of the narrow recess found there.

Extent of the Joint Capsule

Up to now the arthrogram has provided the best method for determining the extent of a joint space. Impressive investigations carried out by Weissmann and Lazis [209, 210] have shown that the ankle joint gives rise to many extensions. On an AP film, one sees that it extends fairly regularly about 0.5 to 1.0 cm beyond the limit of its bony components. From here outward, isolated pockets extend both upward and downward, and we believe the tibiofibular recess to be the most significant among these. Its length may vary from 9 mm [179] to 15 mm [209], and in the sagittal plane it extends for about 20 mm. Fingerlike pockets, known as posterior extensions, appear posteriorly. Communications with nearby tendon sheaths may be present.

1.8. Blood Supply of the Ankle Joint

Arteries

The distal end of the tibia is normally supplied by the longitudinally running anterior tibial artery (Fig. 19). Immediately above the tibiofibular syndesmosis a perforating artery provides direct anastomosis with the peroneal artery. Posteriorly, the posterior artery follows a similar course, but lies somewhat more medial. A few centimeters above the ankle joint these two last-named arteries are connected by a communicating branch arising from the peroneal artery immediately above the syndesmosis.

The medullary spaces of the tibia and fibula, including the metaphyses and cancellous bone near the joint, are supplied by nutrient arteries that enter the bone through a nutrient foramen at about the middle of the posterior surface. The talus is supplied by several small vascular trunks that mostly enter the cancellous bone near the interosseous groove and the neck of the bone. Both malleoli are provided with an extensive arterial network lying directly on the periosteum: the malleolar medial rete and malleolar lateral rete. These are fed by connecting vessels from each of the neighboring arteries [8, 18, 97, 152, 154].

Venous Drainage

The venous drainage around the ankle joint depends on two main vessels. From the anterior side, the greater saphenous vein and its tributaries run upward and medially. The lesser saphenous vein carries the blood from the posterior and lateral aspects up to the middle of the leg. A thick network of veins is spread out around the joint, divided according to position into the rete venosum malleolare mediale and rete venosum malleolare laterale. These are connected to the rete venosum calcaneare.

Lymph Drainage

As is generally the case in the extremities, lymph drainage is concentrated on the side of the joint where the subcutaneous connective tissue is under less tension (Fig. 20). The majority of lymph vessels lie on the anteromedial aspect and tend to follow the course of the greater saphenous vein. The lymph drainage of the posterior and posterolateral regions of the joint is, by contrast, rather sparse. It follows the area of drainage of the lesser saphenous vein.

Figure 1. Tibia and fibula (sectioned in the frontal plane). Anterior aspect. *1*, Tibia. *2*, Fibula. *3*, Interosseous membrane. *4*, Tibiofibular joint. *5*, Tibiofibular syndesmosis. *6*, Lateral malleolus. *7*, Medial malleolus.

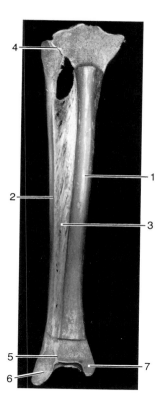

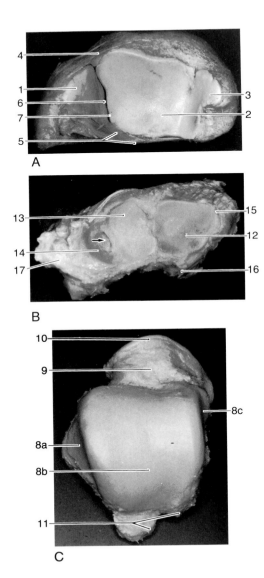

A

B

C

Figure 2. The surfaces of the ankle joint and of the distal radius. **A.** Right malleolar fork, inferior aspect. *1*, Articular facet of lateral malleolus. *2*, Anterior articular surface of tibia. *3*, Articular facet of medial malleolus. *4*, Anterior tibiofibular ligament. *5*, Posterior tibiofibular ligament. *6*, Tibiofibular synovial fold. *7*, Mouth of tibiofibular recess. **B.** Distal surface of right radius, distal aspect. *12*, Lateral part of articular surface of carpus (facet of scaphoid). *13*, Medial part of articular surface of carpus (facet of lunate). *14*, Interarticular disk (*arrow* indicates perforation). *15*, Styloid process of radius. *16*, Posterior tubercle. *17*, Styloid process of ulna. **C.** Left talus, superior aspect. *8*, Trochlea. *8a*, Facet of lateral malleolus. *8b*, Superior articular surface. *8c*, Facet of medial malleolus. *9*, Neck of talus. *10*, Head of talus. *11*, Posterior process of talus.

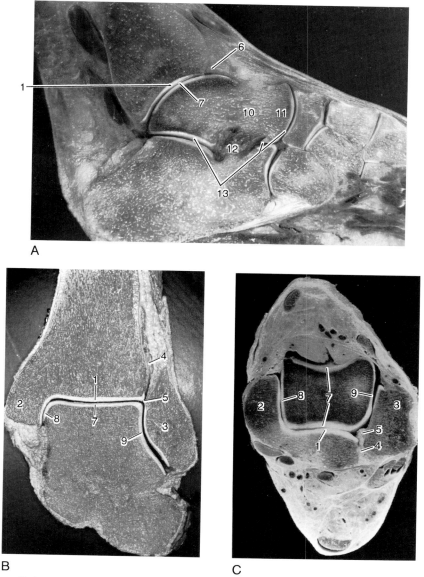

Figure 3. Anatomic sections through the foot. **A.** Sagittal section. **B.** Frontal section. **C.** Transverse section. *1,* Inferior articular facet of tibia. *2,* Medial malleolus. *3,* Lateral malleolus. *4,* Tibiofibular syndesmosis. *5,* Sagittal synovial fold. *6,* Anterior oblique synovial fold. *7,* Superior articular surface of talus. *8,* Facet of medial malleolus. *9,* Facet of lateral malleolus. *10,* Neck of talus. *11,* Head of talus. *12,* Sinus tarsi. *13,* Talocalcaneonavicular joint.

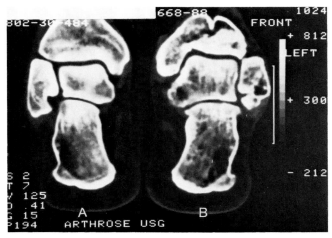

Figure 4. Axial computed tomography scan of the ankle joints. **A.** Normal proportions. **B.** Pathologic changes in the lower region of the tibia and talocalcaneal joint.

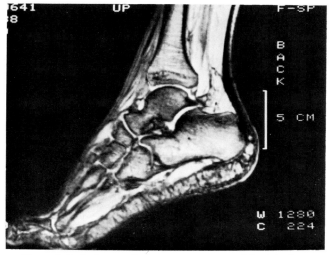

Figure 5. Sagittal magnetic resonance tomogram of the right foot.

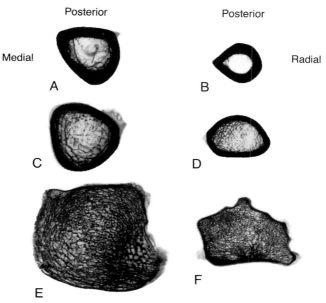

Figure 6. X-ray films of transverse sections through the tibia and radius (2-mm sections). **A, C, E.** Tibia. **B, D, F.** Radius. **A, B.** Transverse sections through the shaft. **C, D.** Transverse sections through the metaphysis. **E, F.** Transverse sections near the joint. The orientation of **C–F** corresponds to that of **A** and **B.**

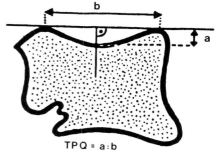

Figure 7. Determination of the frontal talus profile quotient *(TPQ)* according to Riede et al. [162] (from a frontal CT scan). *a,* depth of the trochlear groove; *b,* transverse diameter of the trochlea.

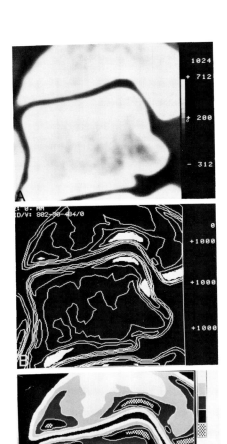

Figure 8. CT osteoabsorptiometry of the ankle joint for the determination of the distribution of subchondral mineralization in the living subject [135]. **A.** Axial CT (enlarged). **B.** Demonstration of isodensity. *White,* region of greatest density. **C.** Pseudocolor representation. Maximum, *black stippled* (density gradations, 200 Hounsfield units).

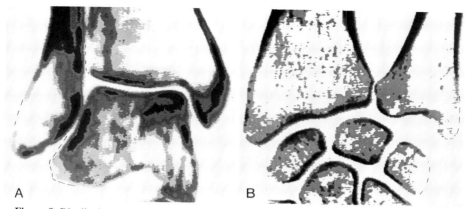

Figure 9. Distribution of subchondral mineralization in x-ray densitometry film from sections through **(A)** the ankle joint and **(B)** the wrist joint. The density gradations pass from *black* (maximum), through various stages of *gray,* to *white* (minimum).

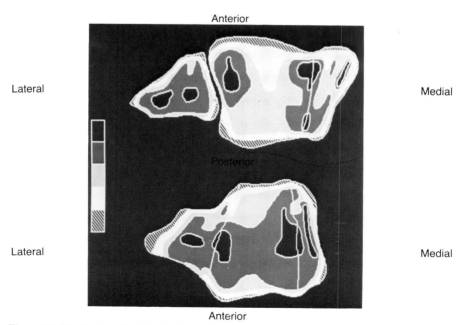

Figure 10. Distribution of subchondral mineralization in the ankle joint; the malleolar fork is rotated upward (n = 20). **Top.** Malleolar fork from below. **Bottom.** Talus from above. The regions of different density are ordered in gradations of 200 Hounsfield units. Density maxima, *black*; minima, *hatched.*

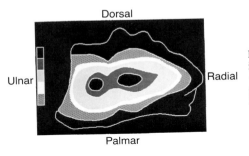

Dorsal

Ulnar

Radial

Palmar

Figure 11. Distribution of subchondral mineralization over the distal surface of the radius (n = 15). The regions of different density are ordered in gradations of 200 Hounsfield units. Density maxima, *black*; minima, hatched.

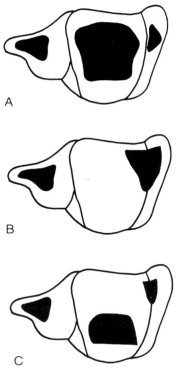

A

B

C

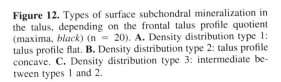

Figure 12. Types of surface subchondral mineralization in the talus, depending on the frontal talus profile quotient (maxima, *black*) (n = 20). **A.** Density distribution type 1: talus profile flat. **B.** Density distribution type 2: talus profile concave. **C.** Density distribution type 3: intermediate between types 1 and 2.

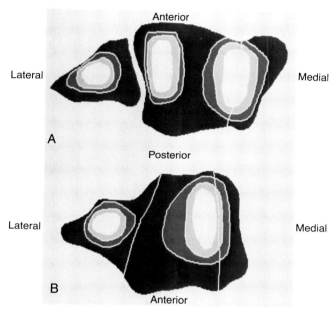

Figure 13. Surface projection of the distribution of cartilage thickness in the ankle joint with the malleolus fork rotated upward (n = 8). **A.** Malleolar fork from below. **B.** Talus from above. *White,* regions of greatest cartilage thickness.

Figure 14. Distribution of cartilage thickness over the distal surface of the radius (n = 10). Distal view. *White,* regions of greatest cartilage thickness.

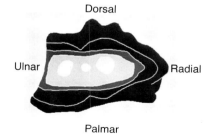

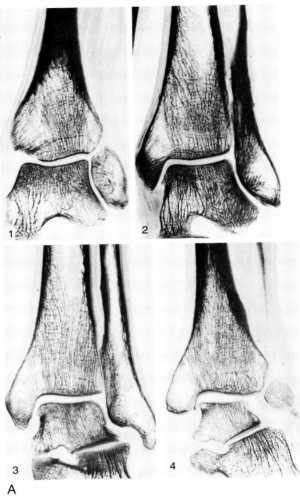

Figure 15. Architecture of the cancellous bone from the lower ends of the tibia and radius from x-ray films of anatomic section (2 mm).

    A. Frontal section through the ankle joint. *1–4*, Anterior to posterior.

    B. Sagittal sections through the ankle joint. *1–3*, Lateral to medial.

    C. Distal transverse sections through the leg bones. *1–6*, Anterior to posterior.

    D. Frontal sections through the distal region of the forearm and wrist. *1–3*, Palmar to dorsal.

    E. Frontal sections through an isolated radius. *1–4*, Palmar to dorsal.

    F. Sagittal sections through the wrist. *1–4*, Radial to ulnar.

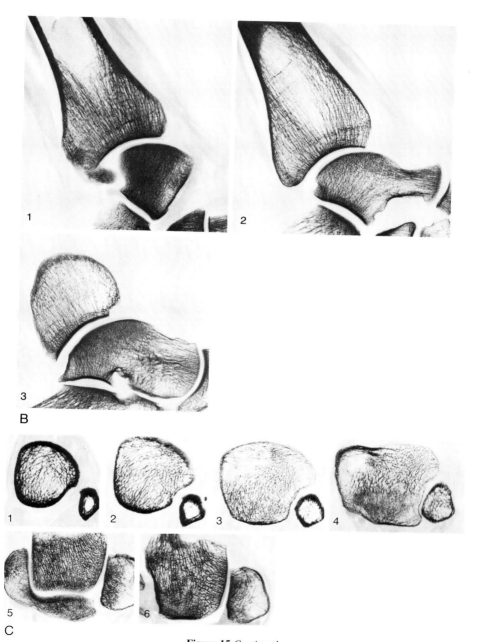

Figure 15 *Continued*

Illustration continued on following page

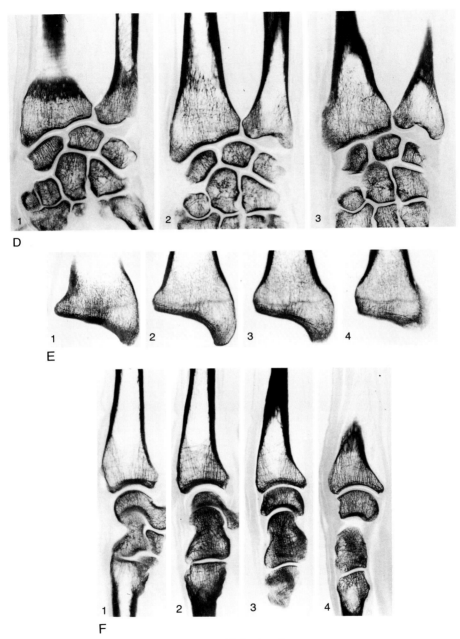

Figure 15 *Continued*

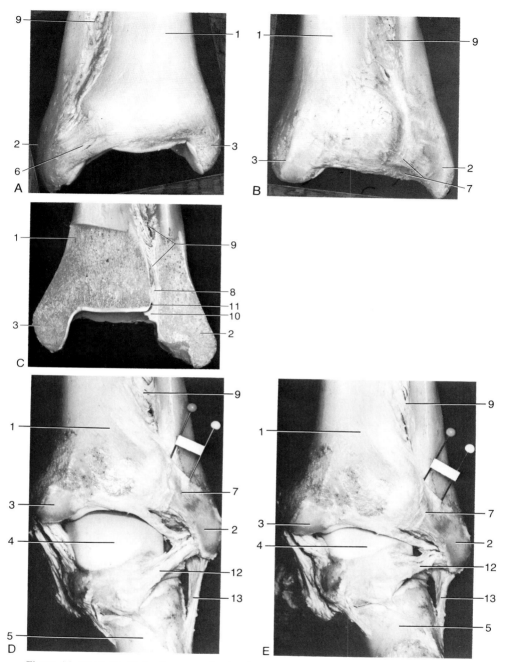

Figure 16. Distal tibiofibular ligaments. **A.** Anterior aspect. **B.** Posterior aspect. **C.** Frontal section, anterior aspect. **D, E.** Function of the posterior tibiofibular ligament, posterior view. **D.** Dorsiflexion. **E.** Plantarflexion. In extreme dorsiflexion the distance between the measuring points increases. *1,* Tibia. *2,* Lateral malleolus. *3,* Medial malleolus. *4,* Talus. *5,* Calcaneus. *6,* Anterior tibiofibular ligament. *7,* Posterior tibiofibular ligament. *8,* Tibiofibular syndesmosis. *9,* Distal part of interosseous membrane. *10,* Synovial fold. *11,* Sagittal recess. *12,* Posterior talofibular ligament. *13,* Calcaneofibular ligament.

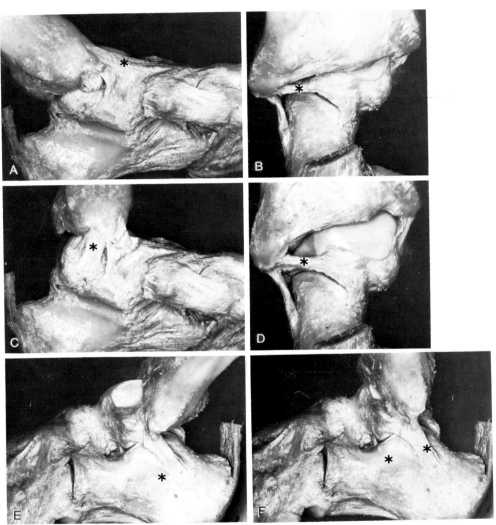

Figure 17. Function of the ligaments around the ankle joint. **A, B.** Deltoid ligament. **A.** Plantarflexion, anterior parts taut (*). **B.** Dorsiflexion, posterior parts taut (*). **C, D.** Lateral ligaments. **C.** Plantarflexion, calcaneofibular ligament taut (*). **D.** Dorsiflexion, anterior and posterior talofibular ligaments taut (*). **E, F.** State of tension of the posterior talofibular ligament (*). **E.** Plantarflexion, relaxed. **F.** Dorsiflexion, taut.

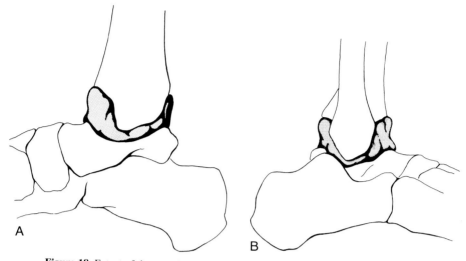

Figure 18. Extent of the capsule of the ankle joint. **A.** Medial aspect. **B.** Lateral aspect.

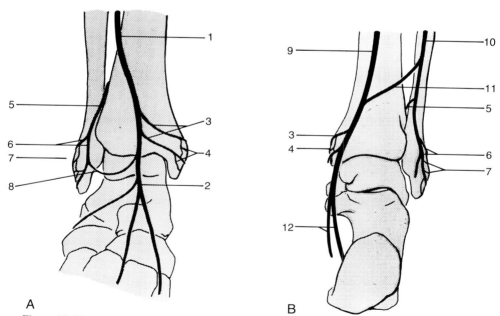

Figure 19. Blood supply of the ankle joint. **A.** Anterior aspect. **B.** Posterior aspect. *1,* Anterior tibial artery. *2,* Dorsalis pedis artery. *3,* Medial malleolar branches. *4,* Medial malleolar rete. *5,* Perforating branch of fibular artery. *6,* Lateral malleolar branches. *7,* Lateral malleolar rete. *8,* Communicating branch of fibular artery. *9,* Posterior tibial artery. *10,* Peroneal artery. *11,* Fibular circumflex branch of posterior tibial artery. *12,* Medial and lateral plantar arteries.

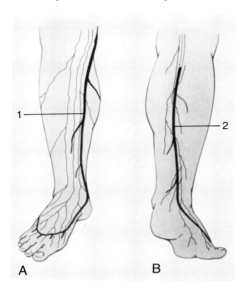

Figure 20. Lymph drainage of the ankle region. **A.** Ventromedial main tributary. **B.** Accessory dorsilateral tributaries. *1*, Greater saphenous vein. *2*, Lesser saphenous vein.

2. CLINICAL CONSEQUENCES OF THE ANATOMY

U. Heim and M. Müller-Gerbl

There are several reasons why recent histologic studies performed by means of more sophisticated methods are of surgical interest. We include the distal radius in these considerations, since fractures involving the distal radius and distal tibia bear many parallels and are often compared (Figs. 21 and 22). While the mechanisms of accident often correspond, the radial fracture in the elderly is often characterized by a fall from a low height with the hand in dorsiflexion. To cause a fracture of the weightbearing articular surface of the tibia, much higher forces are required. Only malleolar fractures, which result mainly from rotatory (shearing) forces, occur through minor forces in this anatomic region. However, in traffic accidents involving young people, we also find fracture patterns at the radius that closely resemble the pilon fracture. In this section we discuss areas that warrant special emphasis.

2.1. Cartilage Covering and Subchondral Mineralization of the Tibia (see Figs. 8 to 10).

Both findings are almost congruent. It was found that the physiologic load is not evenly distributed on the articular surface. In the frontal plane, the areas where cartilage is thickest and subchondral mineralization most pronounced are located primarily lateral and medial. This indicates that valgus and varus forces prevail among the physiologic loads acting on the distal tibia. As we explain below, collapse of these areas is frequent in pilon fractures. Meticulous and precise anatomic restoration of these depressions is therefore of utmost importance if normal function is to be regained with no or minimal arthrosis. In contrast, a particularly strengthening construction of the central or anterior and posterior marginal borders was not observed. This finding is thought to result from the broad contact engaging the concave joint surface with the talar trochlea and also from the tension band effect of the muscle tendons, which is especially pronounced in the sagittal plane (antagonists: Achilles tendon and the tendon of the anterior tibial muscle). These forces were recognized by Bandi [4] who in 1970 explained why the tension band effect of the Achilles tendon accounted for fractures with impaction mainly in the metaphysis.

The muscular tension, which is so pronounced in the sagittal plane, also explains the tendency of the talar trochlea to dislocate anteriorly or posteriorly when marginal parts of the joint surface are fractured, and the difficulties encountered when attempting to counteract these forces by nonoperative traction. The mirror image of this situation is found at the talar trochlea, at least for types 2 and 3 (see Figs. 9, 10, and 12).

The radius shows a homogeneous but transverse arrangement over the joint surface, including the styloid process. The morphologic features, cartilaginous covering, and subchondral mineralization have a completely different arrangement compared with the lower tibia.

2.2. The Cancellous Trabecular Structure in Epiphysis and Metaphysis (see Fig. 15)

In contrast to the findings of Takechi et al. [188], a parallel arrangement of trabeculae was found proximal to the joint and running perpendicular to the articular surface (Fig. 23). Further upward, the trabeculae diverge in the form of a Gothic arch and merge with the thickening cortical bone. This underscores the weightbearing function of the tibial articular surface in the long axis and also suggests how eventual impactions will evenly involve the rather extensive metaphyseal bone, either the corticocancellous or the purely cancellous area. The disposition of the fine, but very short trabeculae in the malleoli with their vertical orientation toward the articular surface (see Fig. 23) emphasizes the physiologic task of these structures, which is to stabilize the joint, but also reflects their exclusion from actual weightbearing. This holds true at least for the medial malleolus. The absence of such trabeculae between the tibia and fibula points to the preponderance of tensile forces at this site, which are absorbed by the tibiofibular plate and the elastic complex of the syndesmotic ligaments. The trochlea of the talus shows a dense, meshlike structure reflecting its pathologic function as a depressor.

A meshlike structure is also found at the radius, but the density of its arrangement is significantly lower in line with the radial function to stabilize the position of the hand. At the radius, however, we find a more pronounced angulation of the trabeculae toward the cortical bone. Obviously a balance with the softer and highly more mobile carpus has been established. Only when in extreme dorsiflexion or anteflexion will the latter depress the radial margin, and this occurs in the sagittal plane and rarely in the frontal plane. The much shorter metaphysis and the significant difference between the articular surface and the diaphyseal cross section indicate that totally different lever arm situations are found in radius and tibia. This also accounts for the fact that impactions in the radius are predominantly cortico-cancellous in nature and tend to go along with significant axial deviations.

2.3. Ligamentous Stabilization

In the sagittal plane, the differences between tibia and radius are less pronounced. Whereas at the radiocarpal joint stabilization is mainly exerted by the tendons of the distal articular chains, ligamentous stabilization is much more prominent at the ankle joint, the ligaments acting mainly to stabilize a hinge joint. The fact that the strong deltoid ligament remains intact with fractures of the distal tibia, but is often torn with malleolar fractures, is another indication of the greater vulnerability of ligaments to shearing movements than to tensile stresses.

2.4. New Findings

New findings have also been gained from investigations on the arterial blood supply, particularly the studies of Aubry and Fievé [2] (Figs. 24 and 25). Emphasis so far has been placed on the fact that deep perfusion is secured by the three arterial branches, and a precarious circulation is only found in the skin. The anastomoses between the apophyseal and the metaphyseal retia were known [12] (Fig. 26).

Recently, new details of clinical relevance regarding the distal tibia have become known [2]. In addition to the vertical arrangement (epiphysis-metaphysis-diaphysis) (Fig. 27), we must also take into account that the various layers of the leg are supplied by different sources requiring separate evaluation (skin, subcutaneous tissue, subfascial spaces, periosteum, cancellous bone [see Fig. 27]). This affects not only the type of surgical approach selected but also the surgical performance within deeper structures. In particular, we would point to the significance of the arterioles with their netlike arrangement in the anterior and posterior articular capsule. These require especially careful handling when exposing articular fragments from an anteromedial approach (Fig. 27A).

Finally, the vertical arrangement of the lymph vessels needs attention (see Fig. 20). If these are divided by transverse incisions, permanent edema of the foot may result.

Figure 21. Schematic showing differences in anatomy between the distal tibia and the distal radius. The tibia shows only a comparatively slight difference between its weight-bearing articular surface and the diaphyseal cross section. The radius with its short metaphysis displays a much more pronounced difference between the broad articular surface, including the styloid process and the slim diaphysis. Opposite to the rectangular tibial facet is the trochlea of the talus with its marked edges. Opposite to the cup-shaped radial facet are the scaphoid and lunate bones, mobile bodies with rounded edges. See also Figure 15.

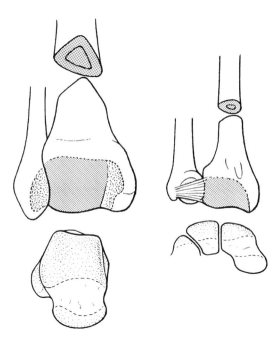

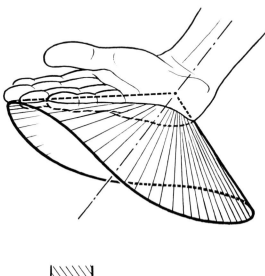

Figure 22. Schematic showing the functional differences between the tibiotalar and radiocarpal joints. Motion in the tibiotalar joint is limited and, as in every hinge joint, principally confined to one plane. The range of motion at the radiocarpal joint is complex and extensive (circumduction). [From Kapandji IA (1980). *Physiologie Articulaire. Membre supérieur,* ed 5. Paris, Maloine.]

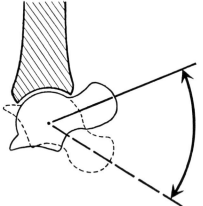

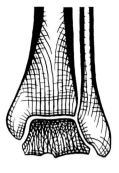 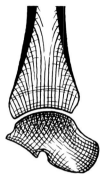

Figure 23. Comparison of the cancellous bone architecture between tibia and talus: sections in the frontal and the sagittal plane. In the tibia, the trabeculae run vertically from the weightbearing articular surface, and only after reaching the metaphysis do they change direction, taking an oblique course approaching the cortical bone. This structure emphasizes the loadbearing function of the horizontal articular portion. The concentric arrangement of the fine trabeculae of the malleoli underlines the function of the latter, which is to stabilize the joint. At the distal radius, a fine, netlike structure (see Figure 15**D, E**) prevails. The reticular structure of the talus is particularly dense.

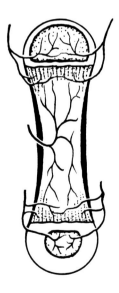 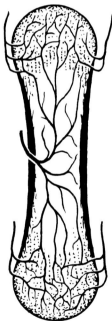

Figure 24. The arterial blood supply to the long bones according to Bloom and Fawcett [12]. *On the left,* during growth; *on the right,* adult bone. The central nutrient artery supplies the diaphysis and branches off in the metaphysis. The main metaphyseal arteries supply the central epiphysis as well as the metaphysis, and in the adult they anastomose with the rete of the nutrient artery. [From Bloom W, Fawcett DW (1962). *A Textbook of Histology.* Philadelphia, WB Saunders.]

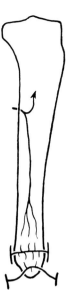

Figure 25. The arterial blood supply to the distal tibia. Besides the diaphyseal arterial rete and the metaphyseal arteries, an independent arterial blood supply area exists. [Modified from Aubry P, Fievé J (1984). Vascularisation osseuse et cutanée du quart inférieur de jambe. *Rev Chir Orthop* 70:590.]

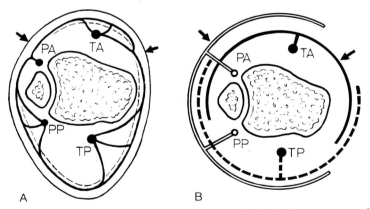

Figure 26. The arterial blood supply to the distal tibial metaphysis in the transverse section. **A.** A subfascial and subcutaneous arterial network is connected by anastomoses and supplied by the four main arteries: *PA*, anterior peroneal artery; *PP*, posterior peroneal artery; *TA*, anterior tibial artery; *TP*, posterior tibial artery. The *arrows* indicate the anteromedial and the anterolateral incisions described in Figures 151 and 156. They have the least effect on this comunicating system. Following the incision the blood supply to the entire anterior region is provided by the anterior tibial artery only. **B.** Arterial blood supply to the skin itself in the metaphyseal region: overlapping supply areas of the anterior tibial artery, the posterior tibial artery, and the two peroneal arteries. The *arrows* indicate the incisions. The critical zone is at the anteromedial side where the skin is supplied exclusively by the anterior tibial artery. [Modified from Aubry P, Fievé J (1984). Vascularisation osseuse et cutanée du quart inférieur de jambe. *Rev Chir Orthop* 70:596.]

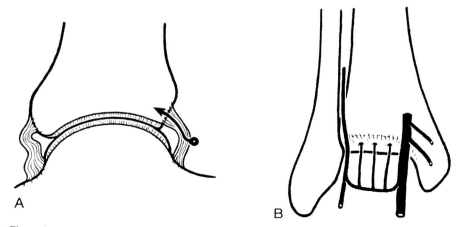

Figure 27. The arterial blood supply to the distal tibial epiphysis. **A.** Sagittal section showing entry of the vessel through the anterior (or posterior) articular capsule. **B.** Anterior view. The arterioles with their comblike arrangement commence at the arterial arch formed between the anterior tibial artery and the anterior peroneal artery. [Figure 27**B** modified from Aubry P, Fiévé J (1984). Vascularisation osseuse et cutanée du quart inférieur de jambe. *Rev Chir Orthop* 70:596.

3. DEFINITION AND DEMARCATION

Before we elaborate on classification, some definitions and explanations are required.

The distal tibial segment includes the metaphysis and epiphysis. The anatomy and the varieties found in trauma account for the fact that first of all a clear demarcation from peripheral and neighboring structures has to be made. In the region of the tibia, this concerns the upper boundary toward the diaphysis and the proportion and significance of lesions to the medial malleolus.

3.1. The Boundary Between Metaphysis and Diaphysis

The primary problem is in the lack of any anatomic or radiologic definition of the metaphyseal border. The area in which the cortical bone becomes narrower and the medullary cavity tapers off to blend with the purely cancellous bone forms a zone of varying extension at the distal tibia. This becomes evident in the frontal section (see Fig. 15). No landmarks suitable for demarcation can be visualized. In the anatomic literature, clear definitions are not provided. The metaphysis is thought to commence at the site where, at the inner table of the cortical bone, cancellous bone starts to form. This boundary cannot be recognized on a radiograph of the distal tibia. The "demarcation" then was a personal impression based on the experience of the investigator. Diaphyseal fractures displaying fracture lines also running distally were often allocated to metaphyseal fractures—a practice leading to con-

fusion. Because fractures frequently occur in this region, classification problems
were the consequence: the case data made available to us by the AO documentation
center contained about 1500 cases referred to as ''distal tibia''; in about one third
of these, the classification was incorrect. This concerned mainly diaphyseal fractures extending into the metaphysis, less often malleolar fractures. This wide error
range made it clear that even experienced traumatologists encounter problems, not
only with definitions but also in delineating and demarcating the upper limit of the
metaphysis. This is why we embarked on a more precise classification. Admittedly,
only arbitrary solutions are possible, but they must take into account the physical
and bony constitution of the individual subject. Rigid measurements taken from the
joint line would not meet this requirement. Our suggestion has been designed for
the distal tibia, but it may also be applied to other demarcations of diaphyseal and
terminal segments of long bones [61]. In 1987, the classification was adopted by
M. E. Müller [132].

3.2. Square or Inverse T Measurement

We suggested measuring the greatest width in the transverse axis near the joint of
the bone in question (in most cases, measurement is carried out in the frontal plane,
i.e., on the AP radiograph). This dimension is then transferred from the joint to the
longitudinal axis. A square or T-shaped figure is created, which, in any subject,
depending on his or her skeleton, will be of a different size (Fig. 28A). In accordance with the anatomy and the experience of the traumatologist, the application of
this square must be conceived and defined individually for each bone. Precise
measurement, however, is feasible on the original radiograph, as well as on 35-mm
photographic copies.

The landmarks for measurement at the distal tibia are one of the easily
recognizable tubercles laterally and the projection of the outer medial malleolar
surface (Fig. 28B). The first question to ask is if, and to what extent, this measurement from the x-ray film will vary with different positions of the foot and leg. This
concerns predominantly the rotational position. Postinjury radiographs are often out
of focus. They are made in the vertical position or sometimes even with the foot in
external rotation. In the ankle joint, a position of internal rotation of 20 degrees is
best suited for the recognition of the various structures.

In studies on 24 cadaver bones of different sex, race, and constitution, the
maximal breadth was measured from radiographs with the foot in various positions:
in about 20 degrees of internal rotation, in the vertical position, and in about 30
degrees of external rotation. It was shown that differences in rotation only slightly
influenced the measured distances. On average, the deviation was 2.5 mm with a
mean breadth of 53 mm (range, 49–59 mm). Depending on the degree of rotation,
we had less than 5% of deviation (Fig. 29).

This negligible difference may be explained by the anatomy, since, depending
on the direction of rotation, the anterior or posterior tubercle will form the lateral
border and may be clearly recognized. If the measurements from AP radiographs

are unclear (e.g., as a result of superimposition effects, anteversion, etc.), they may be controlled on the lateral radiograph, provided that the object-film distance is the same. Only in the case of extreme malposition is measurement impeded in both planes because of overprojection.

The findings on cadaver bones also apply to living bones. If postinjury radiographs are out of focus, measurement may be carried out later by comparison with the radiograph obtained after reduction or internal fixation. This later film is made under optimal conditions, and there is always proper focusing (Figs. 30 and 31). Slight antecurvature or recurvation does not interfere with the measurement. The same holds true for concomitant fractures of the medial malleolus. No major problems arise when a possible dislocation of the latter must be taken into account.

All this has shown the practicability of the method of measurement selected, which may be employed even with radiographs that are less than optimal.

3.3. Mechanical Center of the Fracture

A second question regards the assessment of fracture lines within the metaphysis. In order to decide whether a fracture is to be considered and classified as diaphyseal or metaphyseal, the concept of *mechanical center* must be introduced.

In simple spiral and oblique fractures (the angle to the diaphyseal axis does not fall below 30 degrees in any of the planes), the mechanical center is the center of the fracture line. In diaphyseal wedge fractures, it is in the middle of the contact area between the main fragments. Generally, this coincides with the broadest part of the wedge. In multifragmentary fractures, it is determined by the center of the comminuted area. But in fractures with a short oblique or transverse component (the area where instability is greatest), the latter will decide the determination.

Only those fractures may be referred to as metaphyseal if their center lies in the metaphysis. Determination of the latter is easy in simple fractures and long spiral fractures. Their centers, being more proximal, are occasionally referred to as diaphyseal fractures. On the other hand, we find that complex metaphyseal fractures often extend into the diaphysis, i.e., they are metaphyseal-diaphyseal, which complicates the classification. If the distal main fragment clearly belongs to the metaphysis, and its upper limit is highly oblique or almost transverse, it is generally thought to form one unit with a directly adjacent comminuted area (site of greatest instability). The same holds true for individual wedge fragments extending proximal.

Examples

Figures 28A through 35, schematic drawings and radiographs, illustrate how to determine the border between metaphysis and diaphysis and how to define the center of the fracture.

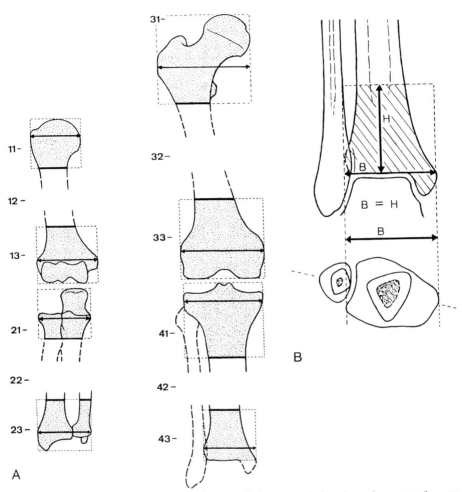

Figure 28. A. Determination of the limits of the terminal segments in long bones by means of square measurement. The greatest width of the metaphysis is projected onto the long axis. **B.** Details of this measurement applied to the distal tibia, the foot being in internal rotation of about 20 degrees: anterior view and frontal section. In the radiograph the lateral border of the tibia corresponds to the posterior margin of the fibular notch, while the medial border is the margin of the medial malleolus. [From Heim U (1987). Die Grenzziehung zwischen Diaphyse und Metaphyse mit Hilfe der Viereckmessung. *Unfallchirurg* 90:274–280.]

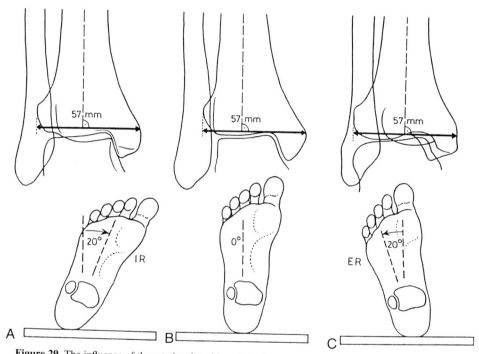

Figure 29. The influence of the rotational position of the foot on measurement of tibial breadth (contour drawings of measured radiographs). The rounded contours of the medial malleolus remain unchanged in the various positions. The posterior edge of the fibular notch forms the lateral border when the foot is held in internal rotation *(IR)* of about 20 degrees (**A**). In neutral position (**B**), one of the two tubercles is slightly more prominent. In 20 degrees of external rotation *(ER)* (**C**), the anterior edge of the fibular notch (tubercle of Tillaux Chaput) forms the boundary. The distance to be measured remains unchanged within these angles.

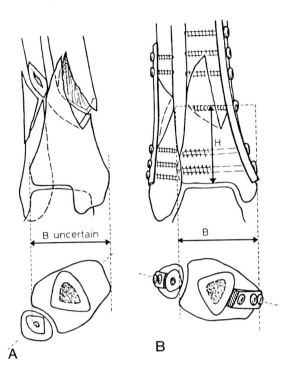

Figure 30. Measurement with the foot in extreme external rotation (contour drawing from radiographs). Extreme external rotation of the foot (**A**) is a common accident-related position of the distal lower leg. In borderline cases, control by means of postoperative radiographs becomes necessary (**B**). *B,* breadth; *H,* height.

B uncertain

B

A

B

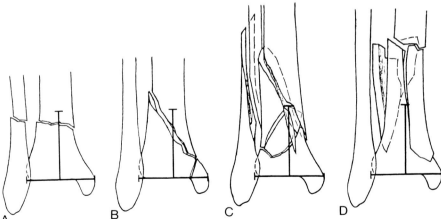

A

B

C

D

Figure 31. Examples of measurement in various fractures (contour drawings from radiographs). **A.** Transverse tibial fracture, which is metaphyseal (segment 43). **B.** Oblique fracture of the tibia. The fracture line lies mostly in the metaphysis (segment 43). The oblique fracture of the medial malleolus need not be considered. **C.** Extraarticular tibial fracture with a multifragmented wedge and fragments extending into the diaphysis. The mechanical center (center of the multifragmented area) is located in the metaphysis. The fracture is metaphyseal-diaphyseal and is part of segment 43. Some contact between the main fragments is preserved on the posteromedial side. Thus it is classified as A2. **D.** Complex fracture with a transverse component (center) located in the diaphysis. Several fragments extend distally to the metaphysis. The fracture is diaphyseal-metaphyseal and is part of segment 42.

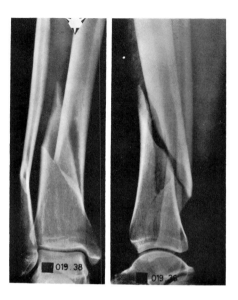

Figure 32. A long spiral fracture of the tibia in the varus position. The fracture has its center in the diaphysis (segment 42). A simple diaphyseal fracture of the fibula and a vertical fissure in the medial malleolus are not considered. Classification of this case by the surgeon as "distal tibia" was incorrect, and it was removed from our series.

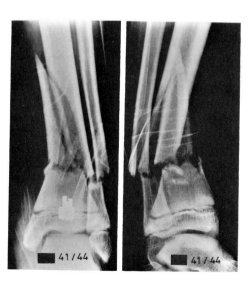

Figure 33. A transverse fracture in an adolescent. The fracture has its center (transverse component) in the metaphysis in segment 43. With a wedge, it extends into the diaphysis. Some contact between the main fragments is found posterolaterally. The fracture is classified as A2.3: supramalleolar transverse fracture of the fibula.

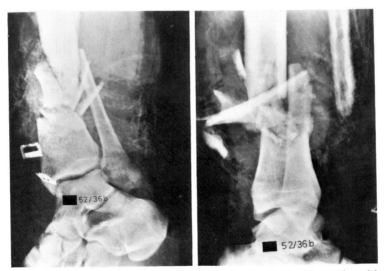

Figure 34. A complex fracture (third-degree open fracture) at the diaphyseal-metaphyseal boundary. The distal main fragment is short and rectangular; the foot is in extreme external rotation. Also, the "lateral" radiograph is out of focus. Because stabilization was performed by means of an external fixator device rather than with implants, postoperative measurement was likewise impeded (the region of the ankle being concealed behind the metal rods). The distal main fragment shows a sharp demarcation and is clearly located within the metaphysis. The transverse component of the fracture is considered a dominant feature, which is why the case is interpreted as being "distal" and is included in our series.

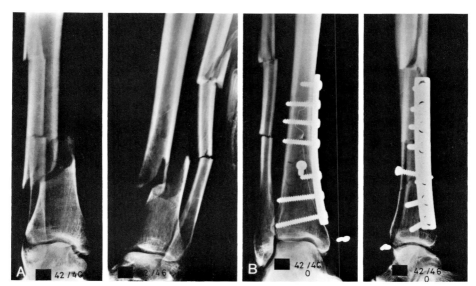

Figure 35. A short spiral fracture of the tibia at the diaphyseal-metaphyseal border; a segmental fracture of the fibula. **A.** Anteroposterior postinjury radiograph in marked external rotation precludes determination of the border. **B.** Determination of the boundary by means of the postoperative radiograph: the center of the fracture, which is also indicated by the separate interfragmentary lag screw, is located just above the boundary. The fracture is diaphyseal involving segment 42. It had been classified as "distal tibia" by the surgeon and was subsequently excluded from our series.

■ *Chapter 2*

Fractures of the Distal Tibial Segment: Analysis of the Various Injuries and Their Combinations

CLASSIFICATION OF FRACTURES OF DISTAL TIBIAL SEGMENT 43

Fractures of the terminal segments of long bones are basically divided into three types:

Type A: extraarticular metaphyseal fractures

Type B: partial articular fractures in which one part of the articular surface has maintained its anatomic connection to the diaphysis

Type C: complete articular fractures in which there is complete disruption of the anatomic connection between the articular surface and diaphysis

This scheme applies to distal tibial segment 43 while strictly observing the demarcation from the metaphysis as indicated on pp. 33 to 41.

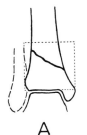 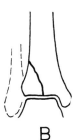 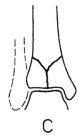

A   B   C

Figure 36. Scheme of the general division of fractures of terminal segments applied to the distal tibia according to the square measurement depicted in Figure 28**B. A,** metaphyseal fractures (within the square); **B,** partial articular fractures; **C,** complete articular fractures (complete mechanical discontinuation between the joint and diaphysis). Simplified representation in the frontal plane.

1. SURROUNDING STRUCTURES

1.1. Fractures of the Medial Malleolus

The medial malleolus serves as the marginal stabilizing element of the mortise. Its articular surface has no weightbearing function. The subchondral, fine trabecular structure is orientated toward the trochlea of the talus (see Fig. 15).

Fractures of the medial malleolus are a part of ankle fractures. They provide evidence of a bilateral lesion and indicate increased instability. Their biomechanical equivalent is given by disruption of the deltoid ligament, a finding to be referred to later in this context (see sections 1.1.5 and 1.4). Fractures of the medial malleolus may also be observed in association with fractures of the tibial shaft. There they tend to represent the distal extension of a torsional force (Fig. 32); but, they are also seen frequently in fractures of the distal tibial segment. In the latter case, they are of minor significance, since the lateral ligamentous complex of the ankle joint usually remains intact. It is for this reason that a fracture line in the medial malleolus should not be taken as evidence that the corresponding tibial fracture is metaphyseal or even articular. This question is determined only by the location of the main tibial fracture or by the course the fracture line takes in the weightbearing articular surface.

On the other hand, a concomitant fracture of the medial malleolus may indicate the degree of displacement and, thereby, reflect the severity of the injury, even though it is not used as a categorizing criterion. We thus follow earlier rating systems, which either fail to mention [46] or disregard the medial malleolus [84, 173] when assessing the severity of the fracture.

If fractures of the medial malleolus were to be included in the classification, this would cause confusion and misunderstanding in terms of the main injury. For example:

> Our case data contain 397 extraarticular fractures; 48 of these show a concomitant fracture of the medial malleolus. To base the classification on this criterion would mean that all of these fractures would have to be considered as articular, namely, complete, circular fractures of the C type. Examples of this are given in Figures 39, 60, 69, and 74.
>
> Articular B- and C-type fractures, in which a concomitant fracture of the medial malleolus is more common, would turn from simple splits into complex injuries (B1 and B2 would become B3, and C1 and C2 would become C3). Examples are given in Figures 113, 115, 176, and 177.
>
> The only solution to the following classification problems thus requires that medial malleolar fractures be disregarded in the rating system.

This approach is also supported by the fact that this type of concomitant injury has no effect on the outcome of the main tibial fracture. Moreover, the operative technique in fractures of the medial malleolus is standardized and unlikely to cause major problems. The vertical and the oblique fractures are treated by screw fixation, and the small avulsion fracture is usually treated by tension band wiring. Nevertheless, we thought it reasonable to analyze the fracture of the medial malleolus in connection with the complete injury.

Of the 1077 fractures of the distal tibia in our study, a concomitant fracture of the medial malleolus was found in 266, or 25%. Their percentage is limited in extraarticular fractures (48 of 397, or 12%), but the number increases in articular fractures, in particular when more complex forms are present: 22% (64 cases) in B-type and 39% (154 cases) in C-type fractures. Comparatively, they are most common in the groups B3 and C3, i.e., in complex articular fractures. Their exact distribution is depicted in the box on p. 275, and explained in the detailed analysis of the patient data in the Appendix, section 3.2.

When a fracture of the medial malleolus coexists with a fracture of the distal tibia, it runs in the sagittal plane and is visualized on the AP radiograph. Three classic types are encountered (Fig. 37).

1.1.1. Vertical Fracture

The vertical fracture is seen with any form of tibial fracture. In simple extraarticular fractures, it is the dominating feature, and in these instances it represents mainly the terminal extension of a torsional component (Fig. 39). In complex fractures of the tibial metaphysis and articular tibia, a varus force appears to play a role in addition to the rotatory component (Fig. 133). Simple varus pressure often leads to an adjacent, anteromedial depression of the joint surface (Fig. 115). In varus angulation, we also find the combination with a fibular bending fracture, which in most cases is localized above the malleoli (Figs. 127, 133) (see also section 1.3.6). However, a vertical fracture of the medial malleolus may also occur together with an intact fibula. Then it is only slightly displaced (Fig. 177).

1.1.2. Oblique Fracture

This form is the most common pattern found among our case data (Fig. 37). The flatter the angular distance, the more pronounced the displacement. In the severe articular fractures of the C2.3 and C3 types, we often find an irregular or partition fracture of the medial malleolus.

1.1.3. Small Transverse Fractures (Figs. 37 and 40)

Small transverse fractures are found at the level of the articular line or distal to it. No more than 17 cases are found in our documentation. Thus, this fracture pattern is rare. Marked displacement is always present, reflecting that the injury is produced partly by shearing but sometimes also by avulsion forces. The fractures are evenly distributed among the fracture types A, B, and C. In contrast to malleolar fractures, they are unrelated to the level of the fibular fracture. In the former, the small fracture of the medial malleolus is usually associated with a fibular shaft fracture. This association was found only four times in our patients.

1.1.4. Fissures of the Medial Malleolus in the Frontal Plane

The frontal and the oblique view sometimes reveals fissures in the medial malleolus. We found nine such cases, six of them in extraarticular epiphyseal fractures (see section 4). It should be noted, however, that the corresponding fracture line is poorly depicted on standard radiographs. Systematic investigation of the implants in the medial malleolus suggests that such fracture lines are far from rare, particularly in partial articular fractures of the B type (Fig. 119).

1.1.5. Deltoid Ligament

Disruption of the deltoid ligament is a common injury in malleolar fractures, in particular in the C-type fracture involving the fibular diaphysis. Rupture of the ligament is equivalent to a fracture of the medial malleolus. On radiographic studies it is recognized by a widening of the medial joint space. This type of injury is not found in association with the distal tibial fracture, a phenomenon pointed out by Weber [207]. Even in the comprehensive illustrative material of Jahna et al. [84], only one questionable case was found. The situation is suspected only once in our case data (Fig. 52). The only explanation for the absence of this injury would be that shearing forces at the articular level are of minor significance in distal tibial fractures (see p. 53). Disruption of the deltoid ligament may serve as a discriminating feature for the differentiation between distal tibial fractures and malleolar fractures (see section 1.4).

1.1.6. Sagittal Articular Split

A fracture extending into the weightbearing articular surface must be considered a sagittal articular split and not a fracture of the medial malleolus. It tends to be oblique and may be clearly distinguished from the pure fracture of the malleolus. The medial malleolus is then part of a large, usually anteromedial, articular fragment that extends far posteriorly (Fig. 38).

> Fractures of the medial malleolus must be ignored for the classification.

Examples

Illustrative radiographs of fractures of the medial malleolus are given in Figures 39 and 40. The morphology of medial malleolar fractures is further illustrated in:

- Figures 60, 74, 115, and 133: vertical fractures
- Figures 69, 99, 113, 125, and 177: oblique fractures
- Figures 114, 175, and 176: transverse fractures

Figure 37. Schematic of fractures of the medial malleolus. **A.** Vertical and oblique fracture. **B.** Transverse fracture at the level of the interarticular space and distal to it.

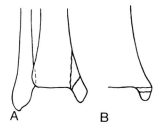

A   B

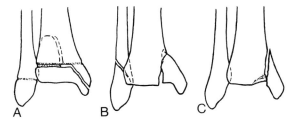

Figure 38. Schematics of fracture patterns not considered fractures of the medial malleolus. **A.** Triplane fracture with an unfused epiphyseal plate: vertical fracture line in the posterior tibial wall (frontal plane); partial epiphysiolysis (transverse plane), sagittal or oblique fracture of the medial malleolus, often extraarticular; classified as an extraarticular oblique fracture (A1.2). **B.** Sagittal fracture of the weight-bearing articular surface, classified as a partial articular fracture (B1.2). **C.** Depression of the articular surface close to the medial malleolus, classfied as a medial depression fracture (B2.2).

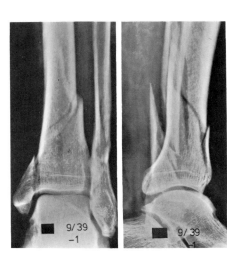

Figure 39. A vertical fracture of the medial malleolus, here the distal end of a spiral wedge fracture of the metaphysis. Laterally, some contact exists between the main fragments. The posteromedial wedge extends far into the diaphysis. The injury presents no pilon fracture and is classified as A2.3. The fibular shaft shows a long spiral wedge fracture distally.

Figure 40. A small transverse fracture of the medial malleolus distal to the joint line (probably an avulsion). *Left:* Partial articular fracture of the tibia (posterior wall intact), anterior split (frontal plane); the injury presents a pilon split fracture classified as B1.1. The valgus position *(right)* shows an impacted fracture of the fibula above the syndesmosis. (The same case is shown in Figure 175 to illustrate the operative technique.)

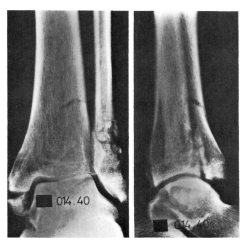

1.2. Fractures of the Articular Margin

Once proximal and medial lesions have been identified, the damage to the articular margin is examined.

1.2.1. Fractures in the Sagittal Plane (evident on the AP film)

Splits on the medial side, which may closely approach the medial malleolus, involve the weightbearing articular surface. Thus they characterize a pilon fracture (see also Fig. 38B). Lateral splits are often located at the margin. If they run obliquely, they may be hard to detect on the standard x-ray film. We interpret them as follows:

Small avulsion fragments of the anterior tibiofibular ligament at the ventral tubercle (of Tillaux-Chaput) are extraarticular. We consider them part of a malleolar fracture and have excluded them from this study.
Larger fragments are found in children with an unfused epiphyseal growth plate, but they are also found in the adult. When they involve the joint, they are categorized as pilon fracture (see also Figs. 58G and 98B).

1.2.2. Fractures in the Frontal Plane (evident on the lateral film)

Isolated fractures of the anterior margin may extend to the medial malleolus; then the fibula is usually intact. The main challenge, however, is given by fragments of the posterior tibial margin. Here, a split is present in the mechanically most delicate part of the weightbearing articular surface.

If there is a typical fracture of the external malleolus, the posterolateral fragment, which is produced by shearing forces in external rotation and not by axial forces, will be subgrouped under this main injury. It will then be classified as a malleolar fracture (segment 44) (Fig. 41). In the AO classification of 1987 [132, 134], it is allocated either to subgroup .3 or to the main group B3. This type of injury is often referred to as a *trimalleolar fracture,* a term denoting the presence of lateral, medial, and, in addition, posterior bony components. Typical malleolar fractures showing a posterolateral fragment have thus been excluded from this study. In French-speaking countries, the authors continue to assign the posterolateral fragments to the pilon fracture and not to the malleolar fractures [32].

The differentiation between trimalleolar fracture and pilon fracture may occasionally be difficult (see also section 1.4). Attention should be paid to:

■ Posteromedial fragments: they do not involve the posterior tubercle, run obliquely, and may extend into the medial malleolus. Illustrations of these fragments have been provided by Gay and Evrard [46] (Fig. 83). In the systematic analysis, they are allocated to group B1.

- Posterolateral fragments: these may present the articular component of a tibial fracture of which the center is located at the diaphysis. A striking finding is that the fibula is often preserved (Fig. 42). In this situation, two separate fractures occur at the same bone. The articular component presents a simple partial split requiring separate coding and classification (segment 43). Another argument supporting this division is the fact that frequently there is no anatomic connection between the diaphyseal and the articular fracture (see also Appendix).
- The rare occurrence of isolated posterolateral fragments as the only lesion visible on the radiograph is very likely to be associated with additional tears of the ligamentous complex (syndesmosis and interosseous membrane). Gay and Evrard [46] have reported five cases and Decoulx et al. [36] have reported one case. Our case data contain only one instance of an isolated posterolateral fragment. To allocate posterolateral fragments not to malleolar fractures but to pilon fractures would be justified in those cases in which there is an additional depression of the articular surface (Fig. 111). This important concomitant injury involves the center and not the periphery of the tibial articular surface and is far from rare [57]. With some exceptions, it is not recognized on standard films, which explains why the injury is usually interpreted and classified as a malleolar fracture. We did not find such a case among the case data compiled at the AO documentation center. Two examples taken from our personal patient population are given in Figure 114.

> When a posterolateral fragment is associated with both a distal oblique fracture of the fibula and a torn deltoid ligament, it is certainly part of a malleolar fracture (trimalleolar) (see Figure 41A).

Examples

Radiographs of fractures of the articular margin are shown in Figures 53 and 101.

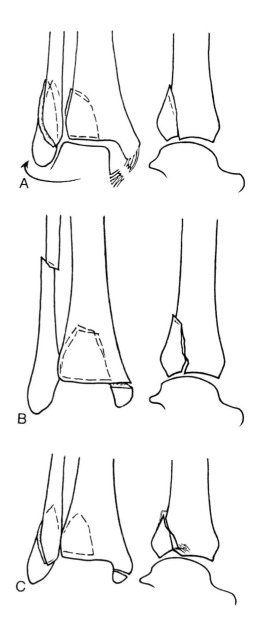

Figure 41. Typical posterolateral articular fragments (Volkmann's triangle) in malleolar fractures. **A.** Type B malleolar fracture: a long oblique fracture of the lateral malleolus at the level of the syndesmosis. **B.** Type C malleolar fracture: fracture of the fibular diaphysis and horizontal fracture of the medial malleolus. **C.** Depression of the tibial joint surface by the talar trochlea. This pattern ought to be classified as a partial articular fracture of the distal tibia, but initial recognition of these depressions is rare.

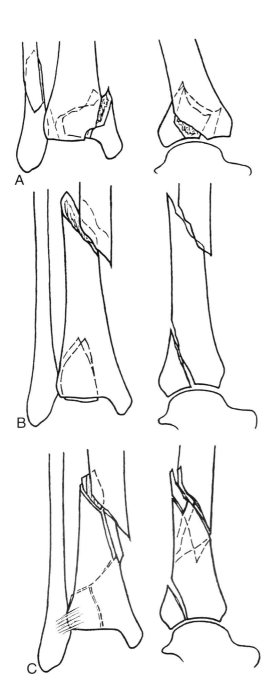

Figure 42. Posterior articular fragments classified as partial tibial fractures (B1). **A.** Anterior and lateral views of a posteromedial oblique fracture including the medial malleolus into the large block. **B.** Combination of a posterolateral isolated articular fragment with an anatomically unrelated oblique fracture of the tibial diaphysis in segment 42. As a fracture of segment 42, it requires a separate classification. The fibula is intact. **C.** Combination of a posterolateral articular fragment with a spiral fracture of the diaphysis. The lesion is anatomically related to the fracture of the tibial diaphysis in segment 42. The fibula is intact.

1.3. Fibular Fracture and the Syndesmotic Complex in Fractures of the Distal Tibia

1.3.1. General Remarks

The comparison of malleolar fractures with fractures of the distal tibia reveals a basic difference with regard to the significance and the involvement of the fibula. In fractures of the ankle, the dominating feature determining classification, diagnosis, and therapy is given by the fibular fracture [57]. Rotation is the principal mechanism of injury. It causes disruption of the tibiofibular ligaments and sometimes of the interosseous membrane, which stabilizes more proximally. It is often combined with an injury to the medial side of the joint (fracture of the medial malleolus or rupture of the deltoid ligament) [207]. Fibular fractures distal to the articular line (type-A malleolar fracture) are thought to result from other mechanisms.

At the level of the syndesmosis or above the ligaments, the fibular fracture (type-B malleolar fracture) shows a very characteristic, almost specific morphology: a long oblique or spiral fracture with the tip of its main distal fragment extending dorsally (Fig. 41A).

The forces prevailing in the distal tibial fracture, on the other hand, appear to be those of axial compression and bending. Involvement of the fibula is of minor importance. It is displaced along with the tibia since it remains attached to it through the intact ligaments of the syndesmosis.

In contrast to the malleolar fracture, the appropriate formula here is: The higher the fibular fracture, the more stable the mortise. Exceptions to this rule certainly exist: disruption of the syndesmosis with fracture of the fibula was found by Börner [14] in 7 of 102 cases.

Our data contain four cases of fibular fracture with a normal mortise where a positioning screw was inserted. Rupture of the syndesmosis is mentioned in only two surgical reports. Failure to report explicitly the presence of a torn ligament cannot be determined in retrospect. This question was specifically searched for in group C1 (see Appendix). Manifest displacement of the mortise is, however, a rare event. If the fibula is fractured, the syndesmosis may generally be assumed to be intact.

Rieunau and Gay [165], in 1956, were the first to recognize that realignment and sometimes even reduction of the tibial fracture could be achieved by internal fixation of the fibula alone. The intact distal tibiofibular connection is the reason why after reduction and proper stabilization the fibular fracture becomes an indispensable indicator and stabilizer for the length and the axis of the tibia. This constitutes the basic principle underlying the operative technique of the AO [173], recommended in 1968 and confirmed repeatedly since then: internal fixation of the fibula must be the first therapeutic step. Subsequently, the tibial fracture is dealt with (see pp. 158 to 160). The same approach has also been recommended recently in fractures of the distal tibial shaft [79].

1.3.2. Multifragmentary Fractures of the Fibula

Whereas internal fixation of the simple fibular fracture is hardly complicated, reduction and stabilization of the multiple fracture (wedge, comminution, bone loss, segmental fracture) are highly challenging. Investigation of our patient data [57] revealed a rapid increase in surgical and technical errors with the latter fracture pattern. This observation led to categorization of the multifragmentary diaphyseal fracture of the fibula as main group C2 in the classification of malleolar fractures [132, 134]. In line with this division, we initially intended to assign to its own subgroup all distal tibial fractures associated with a concomitant multifragmentary fracture of the fibula. This classification was introduced within the AO in 1980 but was not pursued further (see also [128] and Fig. 155).

After detailed analysis of the case data, it became obvious that this procedure would have led to the subordination of the most varying tibial fracture patterns to an accessory finding, namely the concomitant fibular injury. The main fracture would have been subject to illogical grading systems and ambiguous, clinically untenable classifications. Another reason why the idea of taking the fibular lesion as a classifying criterion was abandoned is the fact that the fibula may remain intact in almost any form of distal tibial fracture.

1.3.3. Intact Fibula

The fibula may remain intact in the most varied forms of distal tibial fracture. First of all, this occurs in cases without gross displacement of the tibial fragments, a situation observed even with more complex fracture patterns. If the fracture is extraarticular, the varus position of the articular surface indicates preservation of the syndesmotic ligaments (Fig. 44A).

If the fibula has remained intact in a grossly displaced articular fracture, tibial fragments remain attached to the fibula through one or both syndesmotic ligaments (Fig. 44B–D). These fragments serve as an indicator for the reduction of fragments that constitute the articular surface of the tibia. An illustrative case is depicted in Figure 49.

When the entire articular surface of the tibia is impacted upward into cancellous bone, signaling complete disruption of the syndesmotic ligaments, this is considered a distinct group by Weber. In our patients, this morphologic pattern has been evident only once and suspected in three other cases (Fig. 47). The literature provides little information. The most reliable series is Börner's [14], who reported on 102 cases: tears of the tibiofibular ligaments (possibly not more than one) were found in 7 cases, even though the fibula was fractured. When the fibula remained intact, he found rupture of the syndesmosis in 19 cases.

1.3.4. High Fibular Fracture (Figs. 43 and 44E)

When the main fracture is located at the distal tibia, it is—in contrast to malleolar fractures—only rarely associated with a high fibular fracture. Among our patients, we find only five cases involving slight dislocation. They all show the morphology characteristic of torsional forces: in the three patients operated on, no tears of the syndesmotic ligaments have been reported. The other two patients were treated conservatively. Again, the morphology is different from the Maisonneuve-type fracture seen in malleolar fractures (Fig. 60).

If the fibula is fractured, the syndesmotic ligaments are usually intact. If the fibula is preserved, some tibial fragments are usually attached to the fibula through the syndesmotic ligaments. Upward impaction of the entire tibial joint surface into cancellous bone with disruption of the syndesmotic ligaments is rare.

1.3.5. Fibular Fracture with the Tibia in Valgus Position

Axial malalignment is usually associated with fracture of the fibula, since the latter remains tied to the tibia through the intact ligamentous complex. This causes characteristic fracture patterns that may be clearly differentiated from the typical appearance of malleolar fractures. They are most obvious with valgus and varus angulation, less so in antecurvature and recurvation.

The most common finding is fracture of the fibula with the tibia in the valgus position. Although four such cases are mentioned by Gay and Evrard [46], a detailed description is lacking since the authors' analysis of tibial fractures focuses on the frontal plane (lateral x-ray view).

Fracture of the fibular shaft is generally associated with shortening and lateral displacement. But the characteristic pattern consists in the wedge fracture (Fig. 45A), as was pointed out by Böhler [13]. Through the intact syndesmosis, compression and bending forces are applied to the diaphysis, which leads to expulsion of a wedge.

The morphology of the suprasyndesmotic valgus fracture of the fibula is clearly different from that of the typical oblique malleolar fracture of type B, in which the distal main fragment extends posteriorly and proximally (Fig. 41A). Proximal to the tibiofibular ligaments, where cortical bone merges into cancellous bone, it is the structure of the bony tissue around the fracture site that determines whether cortical fragmentation or impaction into cancellous bone will occur (Fig. 45B, C). Illustrations of such cases are provided by Schatzker [177], who places special emphasis on the valgus position. Small cortical fragments maintaining their relationship with the periosteum are not subject to devitalization. If the main fragments are gently reduced without stripping, callus will form without delay while the fragments are being secured with a buttress plate (Fig. 155). Decoulx et al. [36] provide us with an illustration of such a fracture, on which they do not comment. But when cancellous bone is impacted into cancellous bone, reduction is followed by a defect (Fig. 45C). Failure to recognize this gap, to fill it in with a graft, and to provide it with additional mechanical support will result in secondary bony collapse with shortening of the fibula. Pseudarthrosis may follow (Fig. 175). Distal to the syndesmotic ligaments, valgus angulation may be associated with cancellous impaction of the fibula, if the fibula, unable to escape because of its bonds to the capsuloligamentous complex, is compressed the moment the tibia is driven into the valgus position (Figs. 112, 176).

1.3.6. Fibular Fracture with the Tibia in Varus Position

The main forces involved here are tension and bending. The characteristic appearance is the short and oblique fracture similar to the form observed at the fibular diaphysis immediately above the malleoli or to the less common, typical avulsion fracture below the malleoli (Fig. 46). Illustrative radiographs are found in the works of Decoulx et al. [36] and Gay and Evrard [46].

The valgus or varus deformity of a fibular fracture may sometimes be so characteristic as to allow inference of the position of the main tibial fracture at the time of injury. The postinjury radiograph does not always reflect the circumstances of the accident. If a foot is grossly displaced, reduction at the site of the accident is a first-aid measure that is performed long before the postinjury radiograph is taken. The first radiographs may be of poor quality, and sometimes the documented radiograph is obtained with the foot already in traction.

Valgus or varus position with the typical concomitant fracture of the fibula is common in extraarticular fractures of main groups A2 and A3, and in schematic drawings they were preferred for visualization (Figs. 54 and 64). They occur just as often with complete articular fractures of type C. In partial fractures of type B, axial malalignment is far less frequent, which also holds true for the typical fibular fracture (see Appendix for details).

The damage to the fibula is disregarded in the categorization of groups and subgroups. It should be recorded, of course, for therapeutic and prognostic reasons. A so-called complementary code number has therefore been reserved for documentation (see Appendix).

The typical diaphyseal fracture of the fibula with the tibia in valgus position shows a wedge or complex pattern. In the metaphysis, it may be complex or impacted. With the varus position, the fibular fracture is oblique.

Examples

Illustrative radiographs of an intact fibula and typical fibular fractures are given in Figures 47 to 51. Further illustrations are provided in Figures 56, 62, 99, 101, 107, 116, 119, 120, 132, and 183. For further case reports of typical, concomitant fibular fractures with axial malalignment:

Fractures in valgus position: Figures 40, 61, 67, 68, 74, 121, 122, 125, 126, 176, and 181.

Fractures in varus position: Figures 63, 66, 102, 115, 123, 124, 127, 133, 178, and 182.

Figure 43. Schematic of two different patterns of injury with fracture below the head of the fibula. *Left:* High fibular fracture as an element of malleolar fracture (Maisonneuve's fracture). It is associated with complete disruption of the syndesmotic ligaments and the interosseous membrane. Medially, there is either disruption of the deltoid ligament or fracture of the medial malleolus. *Right:* In the distal tibial fracture, the distal ligaments remain, with rare exceptions, intact (see Figure 60).

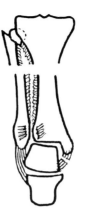
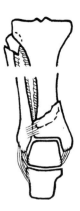

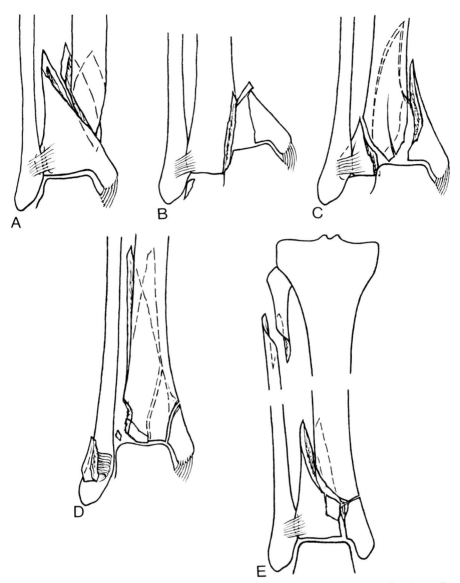

Figure 44. The tibiofibular syndesmosis and fracture of the distal tibia (the contours of typical radiographs are outlined). **A.** Extraarticular spiral wedge fracture. The fibula is intact; the articular surface is in varus angulation; there are no signs indicating displacement of the mortise; the syndesmosis is assumed to have remained intact. **B.** Partial articular split fracture of the tibia with small flake fragment of the talus; the fibula and syndesmosis are intact (see also Figure 56). **C.** Complete split fracture of the tibia. The lateral articular fragment includes the fibular notch, and through the syndesmotic ligaments, it is connected to the intact fibula (see also Figure 48). **D.** An extreme example showing an intact fibula: the articular surface of the tibia is impacted upward with multiple articular splits extending into the diaphysis. An anterolateral tibial fragment (Tillaux-Chaput) remains attached to the fibula through the intact anterior syndesmotic ligament. **E.** Subcapital spiral fracture of the fibula with shortening. There is apparent upward impaction of the tibial articular surface with an intact syndesmosis (see Figure 60).

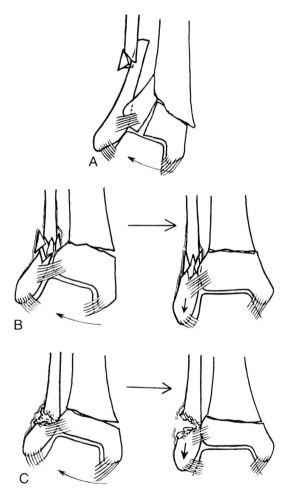

Figure 45. Typical fractures of the fibula in the valgus position. **A.** Wedge fracture of the diaphysis. **B.** Complex fracture above the syndesmotic ligaments with multiple cortical fragments. They maintain their periosteal attachments and are not subject to devitalization. Following realignment, fracture union will occur under buttress protection. **C.** Impaction of the fibula (cancellocancellous) immediately above or at the level of the syndesmosis. Realignment will produce a defect requiring a cancellous bone graft.

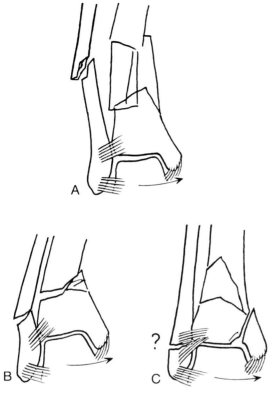

Figure 46. Schematic showing typical fractures of the fibula in varus angulation. **A.** Oblique fracture of the diaphysis. **B.** Oblique fracture above the syndesmosis. **C.** Transverse fracture with anteromedial depression. The status of the syndesmosis unclear.

Figure 47. Impaction of the entire articular surface with rupture of the syndesmosis. This rare case of upward impaction involves the complete tibial joint surface. An essentially sagittal split of the tibial articular joint surface takes an oblique course and is not displaced. A small, posterior articular fragment is seen (connected to the fibula through the posterior syndesmotic ligament?). The fibula is intact; whether its tip is displaced distally cannot be determined. Classified as C1.1.

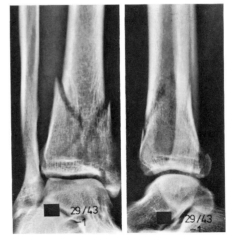

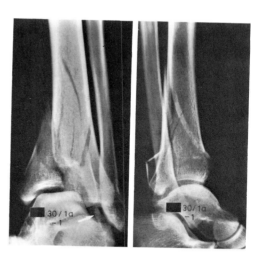

Figure 48. Complete sagittal articular fracture of the tibia (completing its circle in the metaphysis) with extension into the diaphysis. Classified as C1.3. The fibular and syndesmotic ligaments are preserved. *Arrow* indicates talofibular diastasis with a small avulsion fragment.

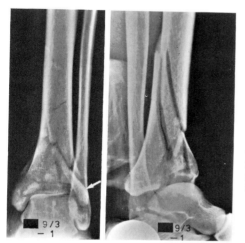

Figure 49. Intact fibula with complete, complex articular fracture of the tibia with multiple splits and depression. Only one articular fragment may be identified posterolaterally. Anterior dislocation of the talus; extension into the diaphysis. Classified as C3.3. The fibula is connected to the large, posterolateral tibial fragment (posterior syndesmotic ligament). Anteriorly, a small fragment of the tibial syndesmosis (Tillaux-Chaput) establishes the connection to the fibula *(arrow)*.

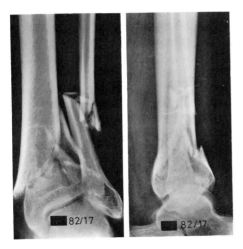

Figure 50. Wedge fracture of the fibular dia-physis in the valgus position. The tibial joint surface shows a lateral articular split in the sag-ittal plane (due to the projection, it is translu-cent). Metaphyseal impaction with lateral wedge. Classfied as C2.1.

Figure 51. Cancellocancellous impaction of the fibula in the valgus position in a 33-year-old patient. The tibia shows a complete frac-ture with an anterolateral split and depression as well as impaction in the distal metaphysis. Classified as C2.1 (subdivision with depres-sion).

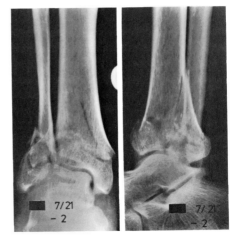

1.4. Differentiation from Malleolar Fractures

Malleolar fractures are defined as injuries to the bones and ligaments that surround the weightbearing articular surface of the tibia and stabilize the joint. The clinical picture is dominated by the combination of fracture of the fibula and disruption of the syndesmotic ligaments (or by equivalent avulsion fractures at the ligamentous attachments). Fractures of the medial malleolus or disruption of the deltoid ligament are common.

If the posterior lip of the tibia is sheared off as a posterolateral fragment (the so-called Volkmann triangle), this is assigned to malleolar fractures in the English, Scandinavian, and German literature. In French-speaking countries, it is considered the main injury. Because of the involvement of the weightbearing articular surface, it is interpreted as a pilon fracture. The French categorization distinguishes only bimalleolar fractures and pilon fractures [32, 36, 46, 47].

Distal articular fractures of the tibia are characterized by damage to the weight-bearing articular surface (split, depression) (Fig. 52). Additional injuries to the surrounding structures are subgrouped under this finding. Lesions of the tibiofibular syndesmotic ligaments are uncommon (see section 1.3). If these definitions are taken as guides, only three situations are encountered in which differentiation of the two injuries is ambiguous: (1) fractures involving the anterolateral tubercle of Tillaux-Chaput; (2) the presence of posterolateral shear fragments; and (3) the rare incidence of a fracture of the posteromedial tibial edge, including the medial malleolus, and introduced in the classification as malleolar fracture of the main group A3 [132, 134] (Figs. 42 and 83). It is recommended that the last-named be assigned to the malleolar fracture if it occurs in combination with rupture of the fibulotalar ligamentous complex or with an infraligamentous avulsion fracture of the lateral malleolus.

As already outlined in section 1.2.1, the minor avulsion fracture at the tubercle of Tillaux-Chaput is thought to form part of the malleolar fracture. It was excluded from this study because in analogy to the simple, extraarticular avulsion fracture of the posterior syndesmotic ligament, there is, in the adult, no involvement of the articular surface. On the other hand, large anterolateral fractures, which are clearly articular, have been included (Fig. 105; see also section 6.3).

A more difficult situation arises with the assessment of certain posterolateral fragments: if a typical fibular fracture (obliquely intraligamentous or diaphyseal in combination with a small fracture of the medial malleolus) and simultaneous disruption of the syndesmotic ligaments are present, the classification as malleolar fracture is justified (Fig. 41A). But if areas of depression are found at the articular surface of the tibia, this would qualify as a pilon fracture (Fig. 111). Because it is difficult to appreciate on the x-ray film, the injury is generally classified as malleolar fracture. As the AO case data do not describe such a case, an example has been taken from our own patient data (Fig. 114).

Vertical and dorsal fragments extending far proximal toward the diaphysis are assigned to the articular tibial fracture, particularly if they are located more to the posteromedial side. In these cases they show a morphology similar to that of fragments of the anterior margin (Fig. 100). The allocation is also unambiguous in those cases where a posterior fragment coexists with an intact fibula. This pattern is not included in the spectrum of malleolar fractures. Consideration of these criteria will largely prevent borderline assessments (see also Fig. 53).

In summary, we may say that fragments of the posterior margin should be classified as malleolar fracture if the following criteria are met: a short, dorsolateral, oblique marginal fragment; a typical, intraligamentous, oblique fibular fracture of the malleolar B type; disruption of the mortise; and tear of the deltoid ligament.

The classification as partial articular tibial fracture (B1) is more likely to be valid in the presence of a vertical fragment extending far proximally or located at the posteromedial side; additional fissures in the weightbearing articular surface in another plane; depression at any site (B2); an intact fibula; and a horizontal fracture of the medial malleolus with a nondiaphyseal fracture of the fibula.

Malleolar fracture: Torsional forces. The higher the fibular fracture, the more extensive the damage to the tibiofibular ligaments.

Distal tibial fracture: Compression and bending forces. The higher the fibular fracture, the more stable the mortise.

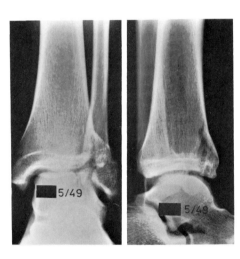

Figure 52. A borderline case between malleolar fracture and articular fracture of the tibia. A short, oblique fracture of the fibula below the syndesmosis; widening of the medial joint space (rupture of the deltoid ligament—the single case in our series). Split depression of the anterolateral articular surface; fracture of the lateral talar margin. The decisive feature for classification is the articular split depression. Classified as B2.2.

Figure 53. Another borderline case between malleolar fracture and articular fracture of the tibia. A long oblique fracture of the tibia starts at the level of the syndesmosis and runs sharply upward; morphologically, it resembles a B-type malleolar fracture. A slightly more posteromedial articular fragment tapers off proximally. In addition, there is a sagittal split of the medial articular surface outside the medial malleolus *(arrow)*. The decisive features for classification are the two splits of the articular surface and the slightly more posteromedial articular fragment. Classified as B1.3.

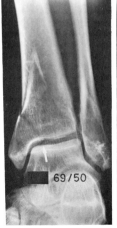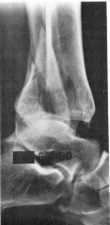

2. CONCOMITANT INJURIES

A fracture of the distal tibia is frequently combined with other injuries. While the victim's pain is centered on one area, concomitant injuries may easily escape the examining physician's attention. Lesions frequently occurring in the neighborhood of and at a greater distance from the site of pain are described in the literature. Because our case data concentrate on the tibia and its distal segment, we only offer an incomplete description of concomitant injuries. Figure 54 indicates the sites of adjacent lesions on the same extremity.

2.1. Proximal Tibial Fractures

The most common additional fracture in this region is probably the fracture of the tibial shaft. It affects the same bone but another segment, and therefore requires separate coding. It coexists most frequently with the partial articular split (B1), but may occasionally also be observed with other articular fracture patterns. Even though simultaneous fracture of the tibial plateau is less frequent, it is particularly grave because both articular surfaces have been injured. If several fractures occur at the same bone, the indication for surgery is of course mandatory. Depending on the type of fracture, intramedullary nailing, in the case of an isolated articular split of type B, or plate fixation is performed on the tibial shaft. Recently, external fixation has also been performed (see Appendix).

2.2. Concomitant Injuries to the Talus

Concomitant injuries to the talus do not involve the tibia. Recording and classification in the same context are therefore precluded. They must, however, be observed because of their intimate relationship with the distal tibial fracture and the considerable influence they have on its management and prognosis. Such injuries were rated as being of greater severity and assigned to their own group by Weber in 1967 [207].

Concomitant fractures of the talus require surgical intervention. Because of the danger of necrosis and rapid deterioration, the surgeon may be tempted to perform primary or very early secondary arthrodesis rather than reconstructive surgery. Flake fragments are highly arthrogenic and require restoration of anatomic congruence and stable fixation for proper healing.

A concomitant talar fracture is, however, uncommon. Songis-Mortreux [184] reported 6 cases out of 106 pilon fractures, Börner [14] reported 4 cases out of 102, and Hourlier [80] reported 1 case out of 84. Our data include no more than three cases. Two of the talar flake fragments were observed in pilon B-type fractures; only one occurred in combination with a severe pilon fracture of type C3 (see also Figs. 52, 56, and 135).

2.3. Disruption of the Distal Ligamentous Connections

Partial or complete disruption of the fibulotalar ligamentous complex is rare. Börner [14] is the only author to mention two cases. The injury is evident in the series of Trojan and Jahna [196], but was not commented on. The same applies to the material of Jahna et al. [84]. Our data contain some cases. Two morphologic patterns may be distinguished: (1) diastasis between the fibular joint surface and the trochlea of the talus with the talus being medially subluxated (Fig. 55A); (2) distal displacement of the fibula as a result of a relative lengthening while the articular surface of the tibia is displaced proximally. In such cases there is no visible fibulotalar diastasis (Fig. 55B). In both forms the fibula is either intact or shows an undisplaced diaphyseal transverse fracture (slight varus drift) that is unable to prevent axial displacement (Fig. 178).

There is no association with disruption of the syndesmotic ligaments. The lateral fragments of the tibia maintain the ligamentous conjunction with the fibula (see section 1.3 and Figs. 48, 56, 119, and 126). Tears of the distal fibular ligaments apparently go easily unnoticed at operation; sutures are not mentioned in the surgical reports. Our data contain one case in which screw fixation of a small avulsion fracture was performed. This concomitant injury heals under the protection of the main proximal lesion. In our follow-up, there were no findings pointing to such an initial injury. In the case of conservative treatment (traction), an additional factor of instability would arise making reduction more difficult and jeopardizing ligamentotaxis.

2.4. Calcaneal Fractures

The association of pilon fractures with calcaneal fractures appears to be quite frequent, in contrast to the combination with talus fractures. The coexistence with calcaneal fractures was mentioned by Böhler [13]. The calcaneal fracture may be present on the same extremity in addition to the pilon fracture, but may also occur on the contralateral leg. Börner [14] reports one case; Macek [110], three; and Hourlier [80], two cases. Songis-Mortreux [184] reported on six cases on the same leg, and seven on the opposite leg. Although such cases are included in our data, their exact number cannot be determined (x-rays out of focus or incomplete).

2.5. Remote Injuries

Depending on the type of accident (fall from a height, traffic accident, etc.), remote injuries are reported in combination with the pilon fracture. After a fall, fractures of the spine prevail. They are particularly noteworthy, since they may not display any external signs or symptoms and require a systematic clinical examination to be detected. In traffic accidents, a preponderance of femoral and pelvic fractures is seen. Cerebrocranial injuries should also be mentioned here.

The most common additional fractures affect the tibial shaft and calcaneus. Talus fractures are rare. The most common remote injuries are fractures of the spine, the cranium, the pelvis, and finally the femur.

Examples

A radiograph illustrating several combination injuries is given in Figure 56. For examples of additional fractures of the talus, see Figures 52 and 135.

Radiographs showing the tear or avulsion fracture of the fibulotalar ligamentous complex are provided in Figures 47, 48, 56, 119, 126, and 178.

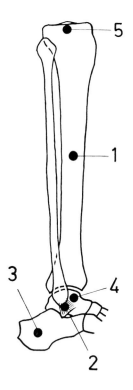

Figure 54. Injuries in the vicinity of the distal tibial segment. The injuries are numbered according to the frequency of the concomitant injury. *1*, Fractures of the tibial shaft. *2*, Tears of the distal talofibular ligaments. *3*, Fractures of the calcaneus. *4*, Fractures of the talus. *5*, Fractures of the tibial plateau.

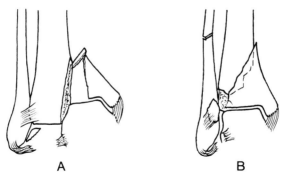

A   B

Figure 55. Tears of the ligaments between the tip of the fibula and the bones of the foot. **A.** Talofibular diastasis with rupture of the distal ligamentous complex (anterior talofibular ligament, posterior talofibular ligament, and calcaneofibular ligament). The ligaments of the syndesmosis remain intact. Partial fracture of group B1 (see also Figure 56). **B.** Avulsion fracture of the talofibular and calcaneofibular ligamentous attachments after distal displacement of the fibular tip or upward impaction of the tibial articular surface; no talofibular diastasis. Anterolateral tibial fragment connected to the fibula through the anterior syndesmotic ligament. Intact fibula or slightly dislocated transverse fracture of the diaphysis. This pattern occurs predominantly in complete tibial fractures of type C.

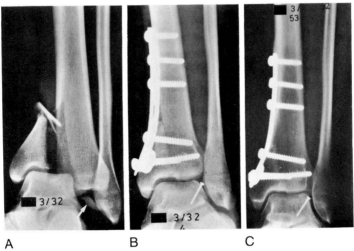

A   B   C

Figure 56. A. Partial sagittal split of the articular surface; laterally sheared-off fragment of the articular margin of the talus *(arrow)*, talofibular diastasis (torn distal ligament) with intact fibula resulting from a fall in a suicide attempt of a 26-year-old psychiatric patient. Closed fracture. Further injuries: distal fracture of the radius and fracture of the opposite calcaneus. **B.** Four weeks after emergency internal fixation with T-plate and screw fixation of the talar fragment. **C.** At 1 year, the joint is free of arthrosis; a very fine irregularity has resulted from the osteochondral defect with density medially. Healing of the talar fragment; no irritation at the implant interface.

3. AXIAL MALALIGNMENT

When analyzing our case data, our attention was drawn to the frequency and the significance of axial malalignment, a finding pointed out as early as 1951 by Böhler [13]. But since then, axial malalignment has attracted little interest, even in recent publications [32].

3.1. Axial Malalignment in a Recent Fracture

Axial malalignment is most frequent with impacted fractures and complex metaphyseal fractures (A2.1, A2.2; also C2.1 and C2.2). Interestingly enough, it is also often found in simple oblique or wedge fractures, but rarely in partial fractures (group B). It is noteworthy that trap-door depressions (see section 6.3.2) always prove axial malalignment at the time of the accident. If the talus subsequently glides back into its original position, axial realignment of the foot will occur (Fig. 120). Angulation is a frequent finding in impacted metaphyseal and complete articular fractures. Because the leg is more or less fixed in its faulty position, the injury is easily recognized. Variations, however, occur (cf. also Appendix, subgroups A2.1 and C2.1).

As we have already emphasized, the postinjury radiograph does not always reflect conditions immediately after the accident. In order to preserve the soft tissues, gross displacements are reduced at the site of accident. Thus the quality of the first radiographs is not always acceptable (see section 2.2 and Fig. 30), and the film available is often the second or third radiograph.

After a simple depression, the talus often glides back spontaneously into its original position (Fig. 120). The incidence of initial axial malalignment is certainly much higher than what is suggested by the radiographs in the documentation. Another indicator besides depressions may be the characteristic pattern of the fibular fracture (see section 1.3.5).

Abbreviations used in the systematic analysis (see Appendix, section 3) are the following: *VL*, valgus; *VR*, varus; *RC*, recurvation; *AC*, antecurvature (see section 1.2.2). Combinations are common, but recurvation and antecurvature are found only in complete fractures (group C).

Long fractures extending into the diaphysis are generally associated with a lesser degree of axial malalignment. The combination of axial deviation with spiral fractures or highly complex articular fractures (C3) is extremely rare. The most common is dislocation into valgus deformity (almost 200 cases, or about one fifth of our patient population), followed by dislocation into varus angulation (almost 90 cases, or about one twelfth of our patients). We confine ourselves here to an analysis of these two types of dislocation. Although the combination with antecurvature or recurvation is frequent, the drift into varus or valgus angulation dominates the injury, not least in terms of late follow-up results. Isolated recurvation or antecurvature is uncommon and, with few exceptions, shows no relevant long-term effects.

It is striking that we often find the combination of dislocation into valgus angulation with an open fracture, i.e., with damage to soft tissues. Mere coincidence is unlikely, as some subgroups are rarely associated with open fractures (e.g., the impaction subgroups A2.1 and C2.1), but when they are, they always present in the valgus position (see Appendix, section 3.2, groups A2 and C2). The combination of displacement into valgus angulation and open fracture is also frequent in extraarticular wedge fractures (group A2.2) and articular split fractures with metaphyseal multifragmentation (group C.2.2). The damage to the soft tissues then is located predominantly on the medial side. Open fractures in the varus position, on the other hand, are less frequent and, on the whole, less likely to give rise to major problems (cf. examples in section 3.2.2).

The dominating axial deviation is the valgus position (often combined with soft tissue damage), followed by the varus deviation. Recurvation and antecurvature are less relevant.

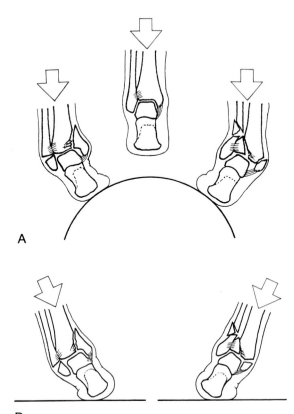

Figure 57. Schematic representation of the mechanism of injuries in valgus or varus fractures by the foot and body striking an oblique surface vertically (**A**) or a horizontal surface obliquely (**B**), respectively. See also the schematics of Böhler (Figure 80) and Gay and Evrard (Figure 84).

3.2. Secondary Deformity

On a late follow-up, secondary deformity was found in 29 of 601 patients (about 5%). It was never observed to occur after simple fractures but only following wedge and complex fractures, in particular of the metaphysis. The findings in secondary deformities are now described.

3.2.1 Dominance of Position at the Moment of Impact

There is a constant correlation between the deformity and the displacement at the time of the accident; the direction of a secondary deformity is always in the direction of the original deviation: a drift into the valgus position at the moment of impact will always turn into a valgus deformity; a drift into the varus position will turn into a varus deformity. The deformity is caused by asymmetric and delayed fracture healing of the metaphysis. Another factor is the traction effect of the soft tissues (deep scarring, possibly muscular contracture?). An exception is depicted in Figure 211 (not included in our case data).

3.2.2. The Fibula as Lateral Pillar (cf. section 3.4)

A well-buttressed fibular fracture functioning as a ''lateral pillar'' [63, 79, 185] will almost always help to prevent a secondary valgus deformity (Fig. 150). This is shown in some cases where an early secondary internal fixation of the fibula was performed. Our data contain only two exceptions to this rule. If the syndesmosis is intact in the varus position, the lateral implant will exert a tension band effect. Initially the AO group feared a possible collapse of the tibial bone into the varus position [173]. Accordingly, the medial implant was first thought to act as a buttress only, but this interpretation needs to be revised in terms of the significance of a valgus deformity. Frequently, the medial implant comprises only the epimetaphysis and acts as a neutralizing connection to the diaphysis (cf. Fig. 142). Of 29 secondary deformities, 22 were present in the valgus position. In 10 cases, they resulted from failure to perform internal fixation of the fibula, and once from a technically insufficient fibular fixation. In 11 cases, the reasons for the deformity remained unclear. In two, deformity occurred even though a technically correct fibular fixation had been performed. Secondary deformity could not be prevented by the application of a second tibial plate (laterally, 2 cases; anteriorly, 1 case). Six cases of secondary varus deformity were observed despite a medial plate (as a result of devitalization beneath the implant?) (Fig. 205).

Secondary recurvation was seen only once. Following a technically faultless internal fixation, the original position was regained (Fig. 182).

Our patient data so far do not allow assessment of the clinical relevance of these deformities, particularly the problem of subsequent late osteoarthrosis. This requires that more time elapse between the time of surgery and the follow-up (about 1 year in the majority of our patients).

Examples

Illustrative radiographs showing typical axial malalignment:

TYPE A FRACTURES: valgus position in Figures 67 and 68; varus position in Figures 63 and 66.

TYPE B FRACTURES: valgus position in Figure 40; varus position in Figures 102, 113, 115, and 133.

TYPE C FRACTURES: valgus position in Figures 50, 51, 121, 122, 126, and 181; varus position in Figures 123, 124, 127, and 137.

4. FRACTURES WITH AN UNFUSED EPIPHYSEAL GROWTH PLATE

We shall discuss epiphyseal fractures, as the ABC classification is based on the location of the injury, and the AO documentation also includes fractures of some children and young adults that were operated on. The classification corresponds to that outlined in the *Manual of Internal Fixation* (third edition) [133]. When the fracture affects the joint, priority must be given to meticulous restoration of anatomic congruence. As the indications for surgery are identical to those in the adult patient, we may safely assume that our data give a realistic impression of the natural relations between adolescents and adults. The majority of extraarticular fractures in adolescents are treated nonoperatively. In our data, only a small minority of such injuries are included, and in these cases surgery was necessary because the fractures were irreducible or open. Even though fractures passing within the medial malleolus and not involving the weightbearing articular surface are far from rare, they had to be excluded from the study for systematic reasons (see section 1.1.1). (Fig. 58A, B).

Supramalleolar epiphyseal fractures passing almost vertically through the metaphysis (exceptionally extending to the diaphysis) are equivalent to the extraarticular oblique fractures and, accordingly, are classified as A1.2 (Fig. 58C). The purely traumatic separation of the epiphysis is the biomechanical equivalent of an extraarticular transverse fracture and is classified as A1.3 (Fig. 58D).

Simple articular fractures involving the weightbearing articular surface are common. They correspond to partial splits and are assigned to group B1.2. The dislocation is oriented either medially (Fig. 58F) or laterally (Fig. 58G). Its interpretation as an articular fracture becomes ambiguous in the case of a small lateral fragment resembling morphologically a tibial avulsion fracture of the anterior syndesmotic ligament at the tubercle of Tillaux-Chaput. A clear differentiation may prove to be difficult in some cases. At their proximal and distal terminations, these injuries may run in different planes so that with inclusion of the physeal separation a total of three planes is affected by the lesion (the so-called triplane fracture) (cf. also section 1.1.4) (Fig. 58E).

True rarities are the complete articular fractures combined with a traumatic, circular separation of the epiphysis or a smaller dorsal metaphyseal fragment. Our data contain only one case (Fig. 212). The corresponding morphology in the adult is the C-type fracture.

In adolescents, metaphyseal and partial articular fractures involving several planes are dominant.

Examples

Radiographic examples of fractures with an unfused epiphyseal plate are provided in Figures 33, 62, 105, 106, 124, and 212.

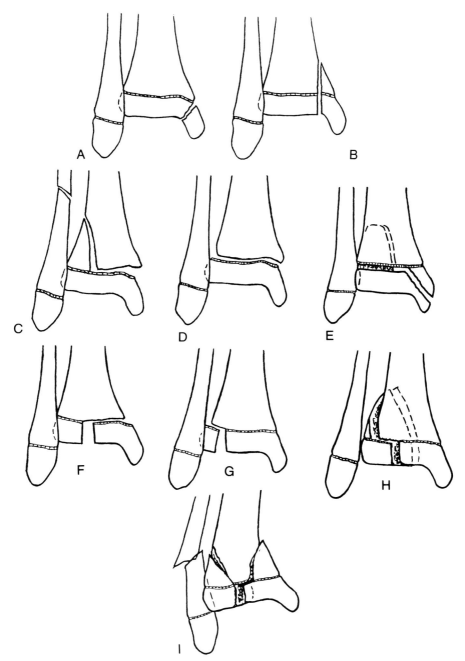

Figure 58. Fractures involving the growth zone. **A, B.** Isolated oblique and vertical fractures of the medial malleolus, neither involving a fracture of the distal tibia (see pp. 44 to 48.) **C.** Extraarticular epiphyseal fracture. **D.** Traumatic epiphysiolysis. **E.** Triplane fracture. **F.** Partial articular fracture with epiphysiolysis medially. **G.** Partial articular fracture with epiphysiolysis laterally. **H.** Partial articular fracture with metaphyseal components. **I.** Complete articular fracture (extremely rare; see Figure 212).

5. FRACTURES OF THE DISTAL TIBIAL METAPHYSIS

Any assessment of distal metaphyseal fractures must consider the clinically relevant features that are detectable on the standard x-ray film. To this end, we use the grading system laid down and explained in the *Comprehensive Classification of Fractures of Long Bones* [134] for all locations on long bones:

- Simple fractures are separated into spiral, oblique, and transverse fractures.
- In multifragmentary fractures, the question to be asked is whether after reduction there is contact between the main fragments.

5.1. Simple Fractures

Spiral fractures are always closed. Thus they cause little damage to the soft tissues (Fig. 59A). Oblique fractures are the most common. They are encountered as either an epiphyseal fracture in the adolescent (Fig. 58C) or as an oblique fracture in the adult (Fig. 59B). Transverse fractures, in which the angle between the fracture line and a vertical line on the tibial axis is below 30 degrees on every plane, are thus less frequent. This group also includes the purely traumatic physeal separation seen in the adolescent.

5.2. Multifragmentary Fractures

Here we are confronted with a fracture pattern which, if it occurs in the distal tibia, is associated with certain peculiarities applicable only by analogy, if at all, to other fracture sites on long bones. Distally, the metaphyseal cone of the tibia widens symmetrically. Unlike the distal femur or the distal humerus, it does not end in two clearly distinguishable pillar-supported condylar compartments. The sectional view passes from the diaphyseal triangular shape over to the oval shape of the metaphysis and then to the rectangular articular surface (Figs. 2 and 6). Any laterality of the fracture patterns is therefore nonexistent or nonspecific. Splits, axial malalignments, and impactions are distributed all over the bony circumference. Classification systems characteristically employed with the distal femur and the proximal tibia are based on a division according to the sagittal and the frontal planes. These cannot be adopted for the distal tibia. The typical morphologic forms are the wedge fracture, the metaphyseal impaction, and multiple fragmentation.

5.2.1. Wedge Fractures

In wedge fractures some direct contact between the main fragments is preserved after reduction. The wedge may be simple or composed of multiple fragments. Extension into the diaphysis is comparatively frequent and must be taken into account. One wedge fragment lies with its major portion in the diaphysis. The mechanism of injury may sometimes be inferred from the morphology. (A classification based on the mechanism of the injury was favored by Böhler [13].) In extraarticular fractures the mechanism of torsion is most clearly revealed by long curved fracture lines extending into the diaphysis. The shorter the fragments, the more problematic the interpretation.

5.2.2. Metaphyseal Impaction

This morphology appears to be nearly specific for the distal tibial segment, not only for the purely extraarticular forms (type A) but also for fractures with additional splits in the joint (type C). M. E. Müller et al. [132, 134] define *metaphyseal impaction* as "interpenetration of thin, cortical shells into cancellous bone." In addition to this corticocancellous impaction, there exists also a cancellocancellous impaction in the area of the medial and distal metaphysis (Fig. 65). As a result of the impaction, such fractures are stable, tend to be displaced toward the axis but only slightly to the side, and, subsequently, are almost always closed. On the radiograph, the impaction is often revealed by typical densities of the cancellous bone structure. Such impactions of the proximal metaphysis are known from the knee and elbow, where they are adjacent to the ball-shaped head of the femur or humerus. This limits the functional consequences of any axial malalignment.

At the distal segments of radius and tibia the impactions occur in the immediate neighborhood of the joint cavity. There, they lead to disturbing deformities and functional impairment. Similar injuries are also found at the metacarpal metaphyses. Because the distal metaphyses of femur and humerus show a compartmental structure in the frontal plane, pillar fractures of different forms, but not impaction, will occur if asymmetric forces are applied.

Although the distal radius and the tibial metaphysis show many similarities, three differences have to be pointed out:

1. The distal tibia resembles a cone. The shape on cross section proceeds from the rectangular articular surface, to the oval shape of the metaphysis, to the triangular form of the diaphysis, but the reduction in sectional diameter from distal to proximal is insignificant (with the exception of the nonweightbearing medial malleolus) (Figs. 6 and 15). The distal radius has the shape of a trumpet. There is a sudden reduction in diameter from the broad joint surface to the diaphysis; the differences in cross section are significant (Figs. 6 and 15).

2. The morphology corresponds to the zone of uniform cancellous bone, which in the tibial metaphysis is broad and in the radius is narrow. Impactions in the tibia are therefore often of the cancellocancellous type; those in the radius are more likely to be corticocancellous (Fig. 15).

3. The ankle has a hingelike, tight ligamentous stabilization corresponding to the cylindrical shape of the joint cavity (Fig. 16). This leads to poor tolerance of axial malalignment, in particular of a drift into varus or valgus angulation. The radius is stabilized by ligaments by adaptation to the function and shape of the joint

cavity (dome, goblet) and allows motion in every plane. Consequently, malalignment will lead to far less impairment.

Another difference between the distal radius and the distal tibia appears to be the relation between impaction and osteoporotic disease: at the radius, extraarticular impaction is characteristic of menopausal women. In pilon fractures, impactions occur soon after fusion of the epiphyseal plate. The mean age of the patients was 42 years with a male preponderance (cf. Appendix).

When an impaction is removed by reduction, a cancellous defect arises and the fracture becomes unstable. If this gap is not filled in with a graft and buttressed, secondary bony collapse will occur. Again the situation is different from the distal radius, where, in contrast to metaphyseal bone subject to loadbearing, after reduction and conservative treatment a cancellous bone defect may heal spontaneously with newly formed bone. If the distal tibia is impacted, this may affect the entire cross section or only part of it. Combinations with splits are common (Fig. 65).

Analysis of our patient data has shown that in metaphyseal impaction a contact between the main fragments is always preserved after reduction. As this constitutes a key criterion in the classification, the fractures are considered as being noncomplex. Accordingly, they are allocated to group A2 together with the wedge fractures.

> Impaction is a typical pattern in metaphyseal fractures. It may be corticocancellous or cancellocancellous.

5.2.3. Complex Fractures

In this fracture type there is no contact between the main fragments. Therefore at least four fragments are present. Two morphologic forms are distinguished: (1) fractures with few fragments, clearly identifiable and reducible; and (2) fractures with multiple, smaller fragments hardly discernible and, sometimes, irreducible. Their vitality is questionable. Internal fixation requires cancellous grafting. With both forms, a significant number of open fractures is seen.

5.2.4. Extension to the Diaphysis

The extension of complex and wedge fractures into the diaphysis is used as an accessory criterion in classification. It certainly implies increased instability and biologic deterioration since two areas with separate blood supplies are involved. The surgical management is therefore complicated by additional technical difficulties.

> Extension of a fracture of the distal segment into the diaphysis should always be looked for.

5.3. Summary of Criteria and Classification

In summary, the following criteria are used to classify fractures of the distal tibial metaphysis:

  1. Simple fracture—spiral, oblique, transverse (A1, Fig. 59)
  2. Multiple fracture, in which the contact between the main fragments is preserved (A2, Fig. 64)—impaction, simple or multiple wedge formation
  3. Complex fracture (no contact between the main fragments) (A3, Fig. 70)—large distinct fragments, multiple smaller fragments (devitalization)

The course of the fracture line into the diaphysis is used to distinguish the third subgroup (A3.3) in A2- and A3-type fractures. The injury is allocated to this group if one wedge fragment extends with its major portion into the diaphysis. Concomitant injuries, e.g., axial malalignment, fibular fractures, fractures of the medial malleolus, serve as additional indicators when the degree of severity is assessed, but they are disregarded for purposes of classification. For details and numeric distributions, see also the Appendix, section 3.

Examples

Radiographic examples of extraarticular fractures:

Simple fractures: Figures 60–63.

Wedge and impacted fractures: Figures 71–74.

Further examples of extraarticular fractures are illustrated in Figures 33, 34, 39, and 187.

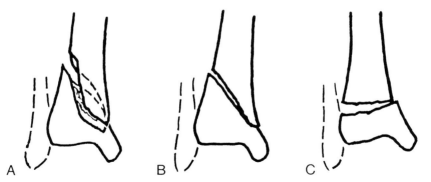

Figure 59. Typical simple fractures of the metaphysis. **A.** Spiral fracture *(A1.1).* **B.** Oblique fracture *(A1.2).* **C.** Transverse fracture *(A1.3)* (for definitions, see p. 75).

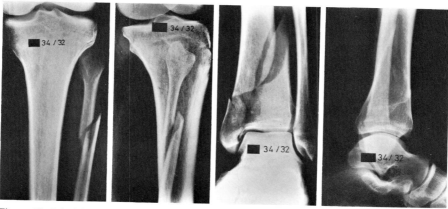

Figure 60. Spiral fracture of the tibial metaphysis. The articular surface has not been injured. Spiral fracture of the proximal fibula with shortening (similar to a Maisonneuve malleolar fracture). No signs indicate displacement of the mortise (surgical report unrevealing). Vertical fracture of the medial malleolus. Classified as A1.1.

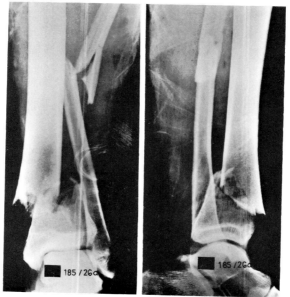

Figure 61. Simple oblique fracture of the metaphysis, evident on the lateral radiograph. Classified as A1.2. Slight drift into valgus with typical wedge fracture of the fibular diaphysis.

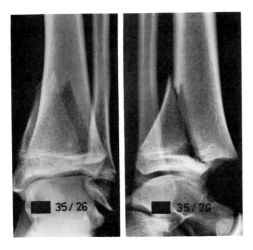

Figure 62. Extraarticular epiphyseal fracture. The oblique fracture line takes a posteromedial course starting at the partial anterior epiphyseal detachment. Classified as A1.2.

Figure 63. Transverse fracture of the metaphysis. The angle formed with a line perpendicular to the tibial axis does not exceed 30 degrees in any of the planes. Classified as A1.3. Varus position; fracture of the fibular diaphysis with a small bending wedge.

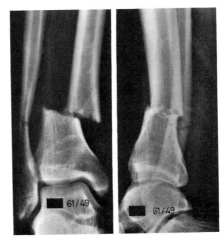

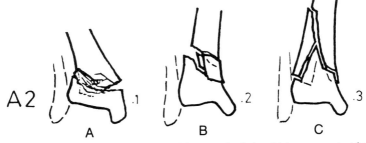

Figure 64. Typical multifragmentary fractures of the metaphysis in which some contact between the main fragments has been preserved *(A2)*. **A.** Impaction fracture *(A2.1)*. **B.** Simple or multifragmented wedge fracture *(A2.2)*. **C.** Extension into the diaphysis *(A2.3)*.

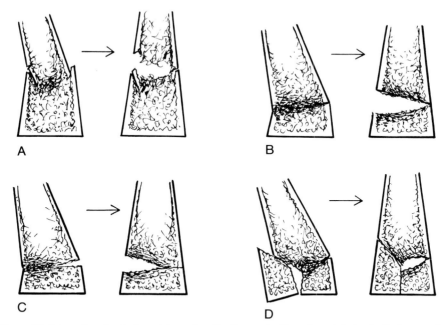

Figure 65. Schematic of metaphyseal impaction. Realignment will produce defects. **A.** Corticocancellous impaction of the proximal metaphysis. **B.** Cancellocancellous impaction involving the entire width. **C.** Partial cancellocancellous impaction. **D.** Partial impaction with expulsion of a wedge.

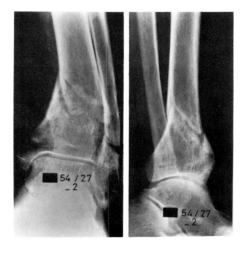

Figure 66. Extraarticular impaction fracture. Posteromedially, the contact between the main fragments is preserved. Varus position with typical bending fracture of the fibula (see also Figure 46) above the syndesmotic ligaments. Classified as A2.1.

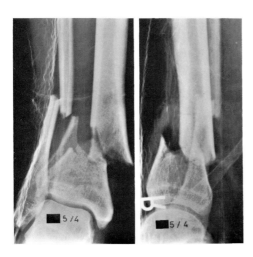

Figure 67. Oblique fracture of the metaphysis with significant lateral displacement; a large, lateral wedge fragment; valgus position; and oblique fracture of the fibular diaphysis.

Figure 68. Extreme example of group A2: multifragmented metaphyseal wedge with bone loss. Posterolaterally, contact is preserved between the main fragments (clearly evident on the lateral radiograph *[arrow]*). The fissure probably reaches up into the joint. Transverse fracture of the fibular diaphysis. Slight drift into valgus angulation and recurvation; closed fracture. Classified as A2.2.

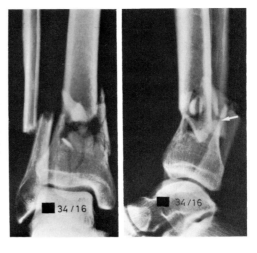

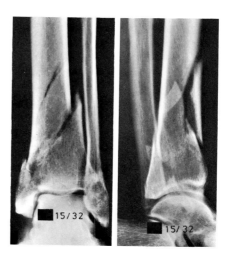

Figure 69. Spiral fracture of the metaphysis. The proximal wedge lies mostly in the diaphysis. Oblique fracture of the distal fibula at the level of the syndesmosis. No ligamentous lesion was mentioned in the surgical report: Slight upward impaction of the entire articular surface, steep oblique fracture of the medial malleolus. Closed injury. Classified as A2.3.

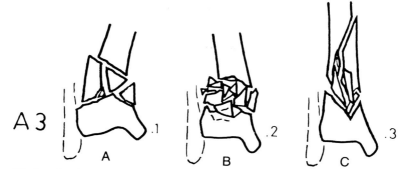

Figure 70. Complex fractures of the metaphysis. Any contact between the main fragments has been lost. **A.** Several, clearly identifiable wedge fragments *(A3.1)*. **B.** Multiple smaller fragments *(A3.2)*. **C.** Extension into the diaphysis *(A3.3)*.

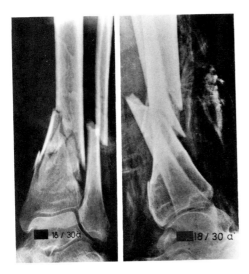

Figure 71. Fracture of the metaphysis; multi-fragmented wedge composed of large fragments; no contact between the main fragments. The anteromedial fragment lies mostly in the metaphysis (borderline case). A first-degree open oblique fracture of the fibular diaphysis without concomitant injuries, sustained in a traffic accident. Classified as A3.1.

Figure 72. Complex extraarticular fracture, multifragmented wedge, no contact between the main fragments, and valgus position. A typical example of a diaphyseal fibular wedge fracture. Classified as A3.2.

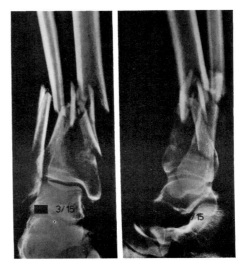

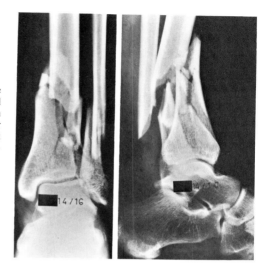

Figure 73. Extraarticular complex fracture of the spiral type. Complex metaphyseal fracture in which contact between the main fragments has been lost. The large, anterior wedge fragment extends with its greater part into the diaphysis. First-degree open fracture. Classified as A3.3.

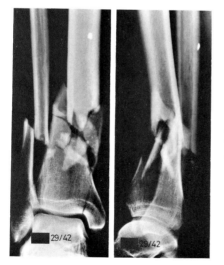

Figure 74. Complex fracture of the metaphysis without contact between the main fragments. Two small fragments of the wedge extend predominantly into the diaphysis; oblique fracture of the fibular diaphysis; vertical fracture of the medial malleolus. Classified as A3.3.

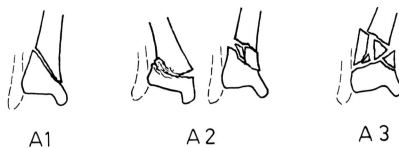

A1   **A 2**   **A 3**

Figure 75. Summary of the typical morphologies of extraarticular fractures: *A1*, simple fracture; *A2* impaction or wedge fracture (some contact between the main fragments preserved after reduction); *A3*, complex fracture without contact between the articular and the diaphyseal main fragment.

6. THE PILON FRACTURE

Whereas the proximal articular surface of the tibia is referred to as a plateau, the distal surface articulating with the trochlea of the talus has a quadrangular shape with its arch in the sagittal plane. Occasionally it is called a *plafond* (Fr. ''ceiling''). The area of the weightbearing portion has been given as about 17 cm² [164]. There is no compartmental structure, neither at the articular surface nor at the cylindrical metaphysis.

6.1. The Concept and Definitions

In French-speaking countries, the distal end of the tibia is called the *pilon*. The word *pilon* means ''pestle'' or ''rammer,'' and the verb *pilonner* means ''to ram,'' ''to stamp.'' Fracture of the pilon always implies damage to the weightbearing articular surface. The latter does not include the medial malleolus (see section 1.1).

The French radiologist Destot was the first to use the term *pilon tibial* in his seminal book *Traumatismes du pied et rayons X* published in 1911 [37]. He distinguished malleolar fractures not involving the articular surface of the tibia from lesions affecting the weightbearing joint surface. In German-speaking countries, these fractures were initially described as *Stauchung* (compression), a term reflecting the mechanism of the accident [13, 83, 196]. The word *éclatement* (''explosion'') is also used by the French [33, 93], while in the early Anglo-American literature, the descriptive expression ''fractures of the lower end of the tibia involving the ankle joint'' is common [168]. Later ''explosion'' [20, 116] and ''fractures of the tibial plafond'' [146] are found. The foregoing illustrates clearly why the French term *pilon tibial* is much more applicable and precise when we attempt to characterize both the lesion and the mechanism of injury. It is for this reason that the term has lately become widely adopted. Special attention should be paid to the spelling since faultless rendering of French orthography is rare. Occasionally, a misspelling is commented on [113]. The word *pylône* (pylon) is rendered as "bridge" or "stone archway."

Credit for the first description of the pilon fracture and also for the first two internal fixations goes to Albin Lambotte [93]. He operated in 1905 and 1906 on two such fractures: one with a cerclage only, the other with an additional screw for the articular split. He called the injury *fracture de l'épiphyse* (Fig. 79). Pilon fractures are uncommon. They used to be observed as the result of a work accident (fall from a height) [13]. Reimers [159] estimated their percentage to be about 1.7% of all tibial fractures. With the popularization of alpine skiing in the late 1950s, their numbers started to increase. The problem then engaged local traumatologists, especially the young Association for the Study of Internal Fixation (ASIF). The proportion of pilon fractures was estimated to reach 5% according to Rüedi et al. in 1968 [173], 15% according to Heim and Näser in 1976 [67], and about 10% according to Rüter in 1978 [175]. In skiing accidents, the figure has been decreasing since about 1975 as a result of improved equipment. Currently these fractures are again increasingly observed after a fall from a height (including suicide attempts) and even more so following traffic accidents. Recently the percentage of tibial fractures is reported at 2.6% by Möller and Krebs [123], 7% by Bourne et al. [20], and to 5% by Bone [16].

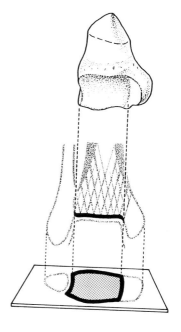

Figure 76. Schematic of the weightbearing articular surface of the tibia. Viewed from below, the horizontal line is in the sagittal section. Viewed from above, the articular surface projects onto a flat surface.

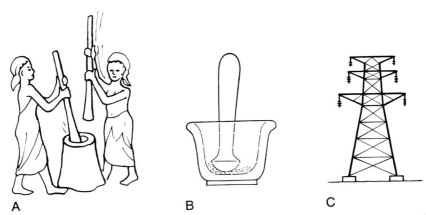

Figure 77. A–C. Illustrations regarding the word *pilon:* **A.** Women in Southeast Asia pounding *(pilonner)* rice with wooden clubs. **B.** A pestle in a mortar. **C.** A pylon *(pylône)*, used to buttress high-tension wires, is a completely different structure.

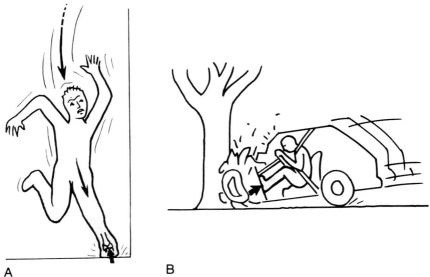

Figure 78. Frequent mechanisms creating pilon fractures. **A.** A fall from a height. **B.** An automobile accident with the driver's foot on the brake.

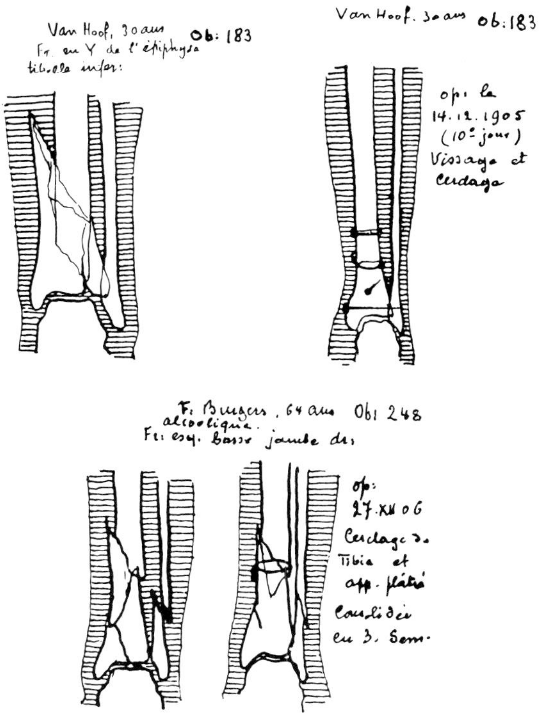

Figure 79. Illustrations of articular fractures and internal fixations drawn by Albin Lambotte in 1905 and 1906 [93]. Lambotte refers to the injury shown as "epiphyseal Y-fracture." In our classification, it would be assigned to group C1.3. Stabilization was performed by screw fixation of the articular component and cerclage wiring of the diaphysis.

6.2. Classifications and Therapeutic Concepts

In his book on fracture treatment, Lorenz Böhler [13] devoted two detailed chapters to fractures of the distal end of the lower leg: the analyses of extraarticular (pp. 1896–1903) and intraarticular fractures (pp. 1910–1934) were carried out separately. Böhler's description is largely based on the mechanism of the accident. Since conservative treatment prevailed at the time, the categorization was oriented more on causative factors (rotation, shearing, compression, bending) rather than on morphologic features. If axial malalignment was observed, valgus and recurvation deformities were dealt with in the context of extraarticular fracture patterns, and varus deformity with the articular forms. Therapeutic management consisted mainly of reduction with a splint and later plaster fixation. In severe forms, permanent traction or pins in plaster were applied.

Screw fixation was recommended in the case of major wedge fragments, particularly when these were located on the posterior or lateral side. Cerclage was advised for irreducible diaphyseal components. The radiologic examples concentrate on split fractures, the most common fracture pattern seen at the time. Partial fractures occurred frequently, whereas complex injuries of the articular surface itself were only occasionally seen. Later (1955), Böhler himself made radiologic contour drawings and schematic illustrations which were included in subsequent editions of his book.

We have reproduced these drawings without modification to honor the extraordinary perception of this past master (Figs. 80 and 81). Although Böhler recognized and illustrated the phenomenon of depression, neither he nor his pupil Jahna seemed to pay particular notice to it.

Worth mentioning in this connection is Figure 80A, which anticipates the Gay and Evrard scheme [46] that was subsequently adopted by Weber [207] and by Rüedi et al. [173]. It is, however, unlikely that the capsules and ligaments are torn the way that is indicated in the figure. This would have produced fragment necrosis, a complication discussed only with surgical treatment. (see Chapter 4, section 5.4.5).

Since 1956, several working groups have started to analyze the morphology of pilon fractures in an attempt to improve the prognosis by implementing new therapeutic concepts. Internal fixation as an alternative treatment was mentioned in 1956 by Trojan and Jahna [196]. They recognized the deep fibular position and the anterolateral tibial fragment and fixed it with a screw from the lateral side (cf. also section 2.3 and Fig. 55B).

In 1956, Rieunau and Gay [165] recommended stable fixation of the fibular fracture alone by medullary wiring to stabilize and reduce the tibia fracture. This procedure was combined with plaster fixation.

In 1961, Decoulx et al. [36] made a detailed study of 48 pilon fractures, but this figure included 15 cases of a posterolateral wedge in a malleolar fracture. The term *éclatement* (''explosion'') was used for severely comminuted and torsional fractures. Surgical management was suggested for those cases where anatomic conditions allowed it (major fragments, steps in the joint line).

In 1963, Gay and Evrard [46] summarized the current literature and published a classification now widely used in French-speaking countries. It concentrates on the morphologic aspects for fracture differentiation. The authors' data are based on 241 cases, but 159 cases of articular posterolateral wedge fragments are included. With the exception of six oblique splits, these must be assigned to malleolar fractures. This leaves 88 cases, to which 5 cases of an ''isolated'' posterior wedge fragment have to be added. We may, then, discuss 82 fractures in which the lesion is not confined to the posterior margin. Four groups are distinguished according to the main criteria: (1) anterior marginal fractures (''*fractures marginales antérieures*''), 33 cases (Fig. 82); (2) a combination of anterior and posterior wedge fragments (''*fractures bi-marginales*''), 24 cases (Fig. 85); (3) supramalleolar fractures extending to the articular surface (''*fractures supra-malléolaires à propagation articulaire*''), 22 cases; and (4) pure sagittal fractures that are depicted on the AP radiograph, 3 cases. Multiple and severely comminuted fractures are assigned to these main categories and are found in all four groups. A more detailed analysis was not attempted.

The illustrative drawings and radiographs focus on the lateral view showing the weightbearing concavity *(plafond)*. This presentation is restrictive, stylized, and unrealistic (Fig. 85). A detailed analysis is given in terms of the morphologic aspects and concomitant injuries, particularly the fracture of the fibula. Experiments on cadaver bones are dealt with in an addendum. These studies suggest that the morphologic variety of the fractures results from the position of the foot at the moment of impact (Fig. 84). The same interpretation had been made by Böhler [13]. The therapeutic and prognostic conclusions to be drawn from the survey of Gay and Evrard are limited: surgical treatment is recommended for major displaced articular fragments, but not for complex fractures.

In 1963, *Technik der operativen Frakturenbehandlung* was published by the AO-ASIF group. In this book, Allgöwer [1] describes the individual steps of the tactical approach and the operative technique and is the first to point out the metaphyseal defect which requires filling with autologous cancellous bone chips [1, 129].

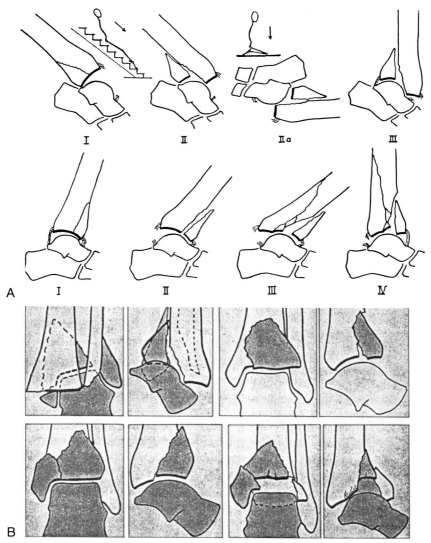

Figure 80. Drawings from Lorenz Böhler [13] showing the genesis and morphology of compression and shearing fractures of the lower end of the distal tibia. Emphasis is placed on partial fractures in both planes. Descriptions and illustrations of depressions are provided. Dislocation into varus angulation is dominating. An intact fibula is always shown together with a tibial fragment (intact syndesmosis). **A.** Shearing fractures in the frontal plane. The drawings are almost identical with subsequent schemas by Gay and Evrard [46], Weber [207] and Rüedi [172]. The capsuloligamentous tears are unlikely to have been demonstrated by biopsy. **B.** Fractures produced by compression and shearing in the frontal plane. Böhler, however, always drew both planes. [From Böhler L (1951). *Die Technik der Knochenbruchbehandlung,* eds 12, 13. Vienna, Maudrich.]

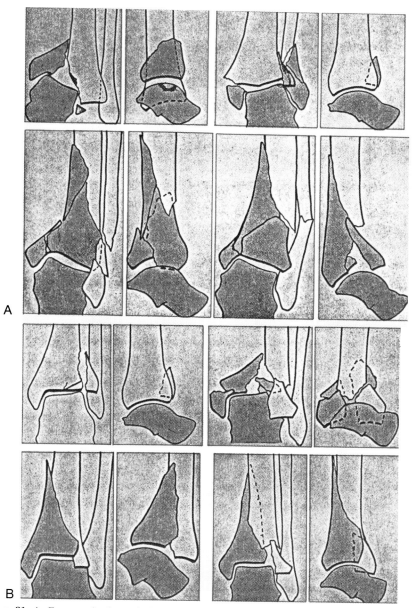

Figure 81. A. Fractures in the sagittal plane caused by compression and shearing. **B.** Compression fractures with expulsion of an anterolateral tibial wedge (cf. legend to Figure 80). [From Böhler L (1951). *Die Technik der Knochenbruchbehandlung,* eds 12, 13. Vienna, Maudrich.]

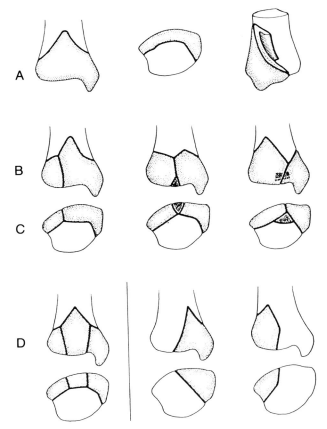

Figure 82. Anterior, marginal fragments of various morphologic patterns; depressions are implied. Where the fracture line takes an oblique or crescent-shaped course, it includes the medial malleolus. [From Gay R, Evrard J (1963). Les fractures récentes du pilon tibial chez l'adulte. *Rev Chir Orthop* 49:397–512.]

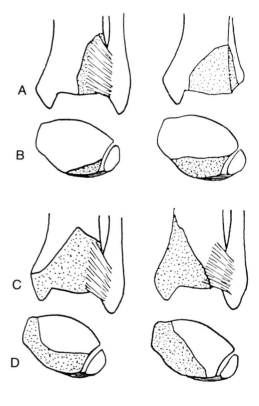

Figure 83. Marginal, posterior fractures of various morphologies. Also, in this type of fracture the fracture line may include the medial malleolus. [From Gay R, Evrard J (1963). Les fractures récentes du pilon tibial chez l'adulte. *Rev Chir Orthop* 49:397–512.]

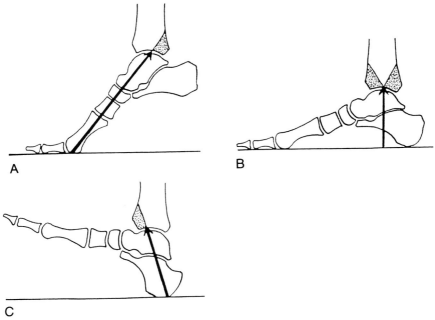

A

B

C

Figure 84. Diagram explaining the mode of origin of the various fracture patterns by the position of the foot at the moment of impact. This scheme, markedly influenced by Böhler (see Figure 80), was later adopted by Weber [207] without modification. **A.** Complete, so-called bimarginal fractures. **B.** Posterior marginal fragments. **C.** Anterior marginal fragments. [From Gay R, Evrard J (1963). Les fractures récentes du pilon tibial chez l'adulte. *Rev Chir Orthop* 49:397–512.]

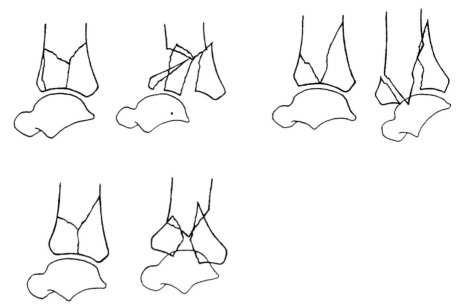

Figure 85. Complete pilon fractures. *Left,* fracture lines; *right,* dislocations. The drawings reproduce the radiologic contours of lateral projections. Because the Gay and Evrard classification of complete fractures is based entirely on this aspect, it is not realistic. [From Gay R, Evrard J (1963). Les fractures récentes du pilon tibial chez l'adulte. *Rev Chir Orthop* 49:397–512.]

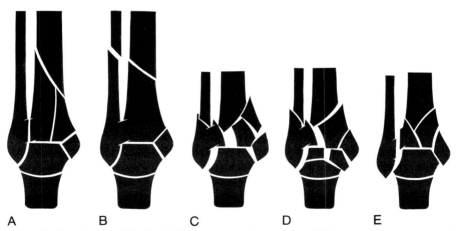

A   B   C   D   E

Figure 86. Classification of distal tibial fractures according to Weber [207] based on the pathology of the syndesmosis. **A, B.** Fracture of the lower leg with involvement of the ankle joint and intact fibula corresponding to our subgroup C1.3. **C–E.** The three forms of impaction fractures: **C,** fibular fracture with intact syndesmosis; **D,** fracture of the talus as the main characteristic; **E,** intact fibula and rupture of the syndesmotic ligaments. It is noteworthy that in all schematic drawings, a similar fracture of the medial malleolus is shown. [From Weber BG (1967). *Die Verletzungen des oberen Sprunggelehkes.* Bern, Huber, pp. 145, 165.]

In 1967, Weber recognized and illustrated three patterns of intraarticular compression fracture at the distal tibia (Fig. 86). Weber recognized the combined fracture of both tibia and fibula in which the syndesmosis and the talus remain intact. An additional fracture of the talus is considered a special form. A fracture in which the fibula is intact and the syndesmotic ligaments are torn as a result of metaphyseal impaction is assigned to a third category. Rupture of the syndesmosis is the central issue in Figure 86, reflecting the problems of malleolar fractures, the main topic of his monograph.

In 1968, the AO operative technique, published in 1963, was codified by Rüedi, Matter, and Allgöwer [173]. Their assessment was based on severity and took into account the following criteria: fragment gap and displacement, simple articular incongruence, severe articular incongruence with multiple steps in the joint line, shortening and defect of the tibia, and complex fibular fracture. A scoring system was introduced describing three degrees of severity. Later, the authors ceased to recommend this classification since it allows insufficient consideration of the complexity of the injury.

The study analyzes the late results of 82 fractures operated on. It was the first publication on the systematic internal fixation of complex fractures at this location that was widely accepted internationally. The first edition of the *Manual of Internal Fixation,* published in 1969 [130], reviews the AO operative technique for complex fractures with a supramalleolar defect.

In 1970, Bandi [4, 5] analyzed the pilon fracture of the skier on the basis of biomechanical aspects. In his opinion, the mode of origin of the supramalleolar impaction at the moment of brisk deceleration is the result of the combined forces of compression, bending, and torsion under the influence of the tension band effect of the gastrocnemius and soleus muscles (Fig. 87).

Heim [55], in 1972, described the morphologic features of the severe pilon fracture with regard to its surgical management (Fig. 88): a large fragment of the medial malleolus, depression of the anterior tibial margin with impaction of cancellous bone into the distal metaphysis, and an anterolateral fragment of the tibia, which, in the case of fibular fracture, remains fixed to the fibula through the anterior syndesmotic ligament. If a fracture line involves the posterior wall of the tibia, recurvation results. In the analysis presented, we find that numerous fractures of the C2 and C3 types display these elements (see Appendix, section 3.4, group C2). Coonrad [31], in 1970, was the first to describe an anterolateral depression.

In 1972, Heim and Pfeiffer [69] also described the anteromedially depressed fracture of the articular surface combined with a vertical split of the medial malleolus (Fig. 90). Illustrations show the technique of reduction, the packing of the cancellous bone defect with cancellous bone chips locally harvested, and the stabilization by means of horizontal screws. A clinicoradiologic example is included.

In 1973, Vichard and Watelet [202] stressed the prognostic significance of an isolated, partial depression fracture of the articular surface requiring surgical treatment. The lesion was mainly observed on the anteromedial side and was referred to as a *fracture de transition.* In 1977, Stampfel and Mähring [185] introduced the term *Übergangsfraktur* ("transitional fracture") to describe the fluid boundaries between malleolar fractures and complex pilon fractures. They pointed out, however, that such depressions could be observed anywhere on the periphery of the articular surface (Fig. 91). These forms correspond to what we classify as B2 partial depression fracture.

In 1978, a new classification of pilon fractures was introduced by Rüedi and Allgöwer [171], one that is still widely used in many countries. Only complete fractures are included and three types are recognized: the simple split without significant displacement (type I), the split with significant articular incongruence (type II), and the complex fracture of the articular surface itself and metaphyseal multifragmentation (type III) (Fig. 92). This classification also figures in the second edition of the *Manual of Internal Fixation* [131].

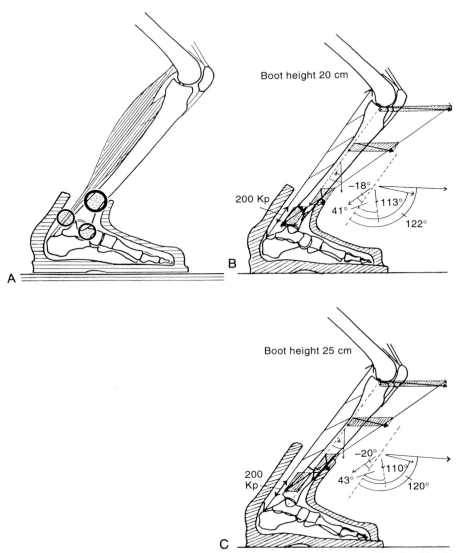

Figure 87. Calculation of the critical overload sites in the distal lower leg and ankle of a skier the moment he or she comes to a sudden halt when running into an obstacle. Influenced by the tension band effect of the calf muscles, the vectors of the acting forces turn downward at the moment of deceleration and produce compression and shearing in the fracture area. **A.** Critical overload sites. **B.** Calculation with boot height of 20 cm. **C.** Calculation with boot height of 25 cm: the forces acting on the distal tibia remain more or less unchanged. The area likely to fracture moves upward a few centimeters. [From Bandi W (1974). Die distalen intraartikulären Schienbeinbrüche des Skifahrers. *Aktuel Traumatol* 4:1–6.]

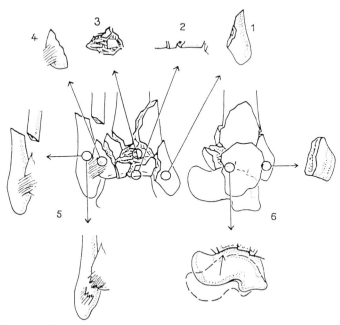

Figure 88. Elements typical of the severe pilon fracture in the skier. *1,* Fracture of the medial malleolus. *2,* Complex depression of the anterior tibial margin. *3,* Area of multifragmentation in the metaphysis. *4,* Anterolateral tibial fragment. *5,* Fracture of the fibula. *6,* Fracture of the posterior tibial wall. [From Heim U (1972). Le traitement chirurgical des fractures du pilon tibial. *J Chir* 104–309.]

Figure 89. Screw fixation of a simple complete pilon fracture. [From Heim U, Pfeiffer KM (1973). *Small Fragment Set Manual.* Heidelberg, Springer, p. 181.]

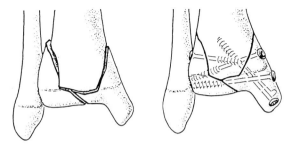

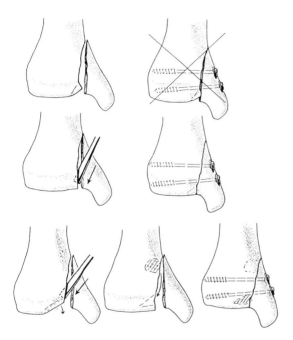

Figure 90. Medial depression of the tibial articular surface and its operative reduction (with a local cancellous bone grafting, if necessary). [From Heim U, Pfeiffer KM (1973). *Small Fragment Set Manual.* Heidelberg, Springer, p. 221.]

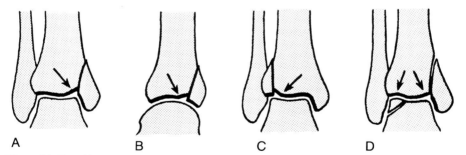

A   B   C   D

Figure 91. Transition to pilon fracture. The various sites of depressions of the articular surface are shown: **A.** A-type dislocation fracture; **B.** Posterior wedge. **C.** C-type dislocation fracture. **D.** Atypical pattern. [From Stampfel O, Mähring M (1977). *Komplikationen und Ergebnisse 40 operierter Pilon-tibial-Stauchungsfrakturen.* In Proceedings of the Austrian Surgical Society, Graz, pp. 639–642.]

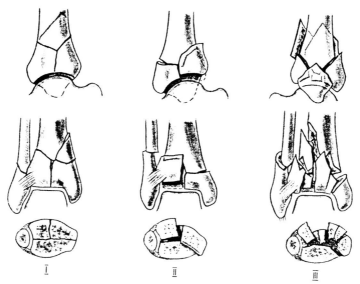

Figure 92. Complete pilon fractures. *Type I*, Circular, undisplaced T-shaped fracture. *Type II*, Same fracture pattern, but with steplike dislocation of articular elements. *Type III*, Complex fracture of the articular surface with multifragmentation of the metaphysis. [From Müller ME, Allgöwer M, Schneider R, et al (1977). *Manual der Osteosynthese*. Heidelberg, Springer.]

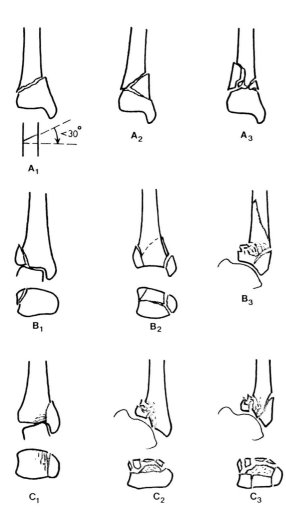

Figure 93. Heim and Rüedi's classification of fractures of the distal segment of the tibia. *A,* Extraarticular fractures; *B,* articular splits; *C,* articular depression fractures. Partial articular fractures are classified as B_1 and C_1, complete articular split fractures as B_2 and B_3, partial complex fractures as C_2, and complete complex fractures as C_3. This scheme served as groundwork for the AO documentation in the years 1980–1987. [From Müller ME, Engelhardt P (1982). Verletzungen des Halte- und Bewegungsapparates. In Berchtold R, Hamelman H, Peiper H-J (eds). *Arbeitsbuch Chirurgie.* Munich, Urban & Schwarzenberg, pp. 489–561.]

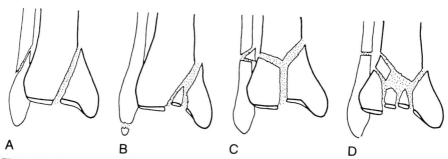

A   B   C   D

Figure 94. Classification of pilon fractures according to Vivès et al. [203]. Anterior view. **A.** Partial simple fracture. **B.** Partial complex fracture. **C.** Complete simple articular fracture. **D.** Complex articular fracture. [From Vivès P, Hourlier H, De Lestang M, et al (1984). Etude de 84 fractures du pilon tibial de l'adulte. *Rev Chir Orthop* 70:132.]

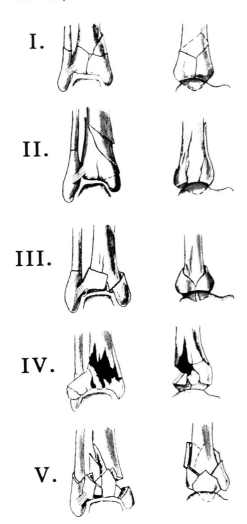

I.

II.

III.

IV.

V.

Figure 95. Classification of complete pilon fractures according to Ovadia and Beals [146]. *I,* Undisplaced fracture. *II,* Minimally displaced fracture. *III,* Displaced fracture composed of several large fragments. *IV,* Displaced fracture with several large fragments and additional bone loss in the metaphysis. *V,* Displaced and disintegrated articular fracture. [From Ovadia DV, Beals RK (1986). Fractures of the tibial plafond. *J Bone Joint Surg [Am]* 68:544.]

On the basis of comparatively few patients (23 cases), Kellam and Waddell [88], in 1979, differentiated between an A (rotational) type and a B (compression) type.

Also in 1979, Jahna, Wittich, and Hartenstein [84] published their monograph *Der distale Stauchungsbruch der Tibia* (''Distal Compression Fracture of the Tibia''). In this study, 583 cases were treated in line with the multiyear experience of the Böhler school. Posterolateral wedge fragments were assigned to malleolar fractures and excluded from the investigation. Surgery was mainly performed in displaced split fractures and for certain elements in complex fractures (to reduce depressions). The authors emphasized the adverse prognostic significance of primary lateral displacement (instability of the mortise) in their series. Their classification is based on morphologic aspects and comprises the following criteria: intra-articular fissures, anterior tibial wedge fragments, anterolateral wedge fragments with ventral subluxation, fracture of both the anterior and the posterior half of the tibia, varus or supination fractures, and irregular complex fractures. The classification comprises three degrees of severity:

Type I: no articular incongruence
Type II: articular incongruence without subluxation
Type III: articular incongruence with "subluxation and marked displacement or dissociation

Small areas of depression are thought to be of minor importance and not further considered. Management consists of a well-positioned transcalcaneal drill wire, prolonged traction, and subsequent plaster fixation followed by a period of immobilization. The indications for surgery correspond to those listed by Böhler [13]. If large and dislocated wedge fragments are present, these are fixed with screws.

We believe that Jahna et al. have overemphasized the significance of a subluxated trochlea. Once traction is applied, numerous cases previously classified as type III in terms of severity turn out to be simple splits with a comparatively large displacement.

An uninjured ligamentous apparatus is, of course, a prerequisite for ligamentotaxis to be carried out. Instability is increased by torn ligaments and is an obstacle to reduction when traction is applied (possibly diastasis of the joint space). For internal fixation, however, the finding is irrelevant in terms of the technical and prognostic aspects (see section 2.3).

Although the therapeutic concept of Jahna et al. differs from today's strong reliance on surgical methods, their conservative treatment has produced impressive and unique results. Theirs is also the only monograph published so far on pilon fractures. Meticulous analysis of the case data was performed. It provides us with precious information and suggestions that we will repeatedly refer to in this book.

Because long follow-ups were carried out in almost all cases, the discussion and analysis of the problem of arthrosis are particularly useful. It is noteworthy that these largely correspond to the comprehensive postoperative series carried out by Rüedi and Allgöwer [171].

In M. E. Müller and Engelhardt's chapter on fractures in the surgical workbook *(Arbeitsbuch Chirurgie)* [128] a classification of distal tibial fractures is recommended, which was elaborated on in 1979 by Heim and Rüedi. The classification was primarily designed for the internal documentation of the AO-ASIF but was not published at the time. The classification is based on the ABC principle, which has been used within the AO-ASIF for several years now. The classification system was published in 1984 by Rüedi [169]. In this classification, the extraarticular metaphyseal fracture is also allocated to type A. All forms of articular split fractures, including those with metaphyseal impaction, are assigned to B-type fractures. All depression fractures of the articular surface are assigned to type C (Fig. 93). Fractures with a complex fibular fracture are combined in a separate subgroup. For the first time, partial and complete articular fractures are differentiated. Our study has evolved from this classification. With regard to fractures of the fibula, the reader is referred to section 1.3.

With surgical management in mind, a simplified classification was proposed by Vivès et al. [203] in 1984. The anterior view of the fracture is considered, and, again, partial and complete fractures are differentiated, each into a simple and a complex form (Fig. 94).

In 1986, Ovadia and Beals [146] summarized the data on 169 fractures gathered from different clinics. The authors used the term *tibial plafond*. Although the classification is largely based on the Rüedi and Allgöwer system of 1977 [171], the authors recognize five fracture types. Displaced articular fractures are separated into a group showing a large metaphyseal defect (type IV), and a group dominated by complex morphology of the articular surface (type V) (Fig. 95). In 1987, M. E. Müller et al. [132] published *Classification AO des fractures* (published in English in 1990 as *The Comprehensive Classification of Fractures of the Long Bones*) [134]. All long bones are considered. The classification is based on morphology and structured according to the ABC principle of the AO, arranged in three groups and three subgroups, each further subdivided into three categories. In addition to defining the segments, Heim contributed an analysis and classification of the distal tibial segment and malleolar fractures. The main groups of Heim's study correspond to those presented in this book. In the meantime, the classification has become widely established on an international level (with the exception of the French-speaking countries).

All these grading systems and classifications reflect the difficulties inherent in an attempt to differentiate the complex pilon fracture in detail. Whereas the mechanism of the injury (compression, explosion, *éclatement*) was featured in earlier works, today the morphologic aspect is coming to the fore. One objective of this study is to categorize such terms as "irregular multifragmentary fracture" [84, 196] and "comminuted fracture with bone defect" [54, 121].

In the early 1980s, soft tissue problems started to attract increasing attention, a development observed while the number of postoperative infections appeared to increase [121, 127, 149]. Infections were the result of accident-related primary lesions (contusions, open fractures) seen in traffic accidents (multiple trauma) and falls and skin necroses resulting from inadequate surgical approaches or operative wound trauma. Somewhat later it was observed that fragment vascularity was often impaired by the trauma of surgery. One should therefore abstain from direct reduction and fixation of areas of severe comminution. Instead, these should be reduced indirectly and fixed at some distance. Important research in this area has been performed primarily by Tscherne and colleagues [198–201] and by Mast and co-workers [116–118]. An excellent review of these problems and some solutions are given by Schatzker and Tile [177], whose decision-making algorithm for pilon fractures is depicted in Figure 140. The scheme may be helpful in unclear situations. Thus an all-embracing approach to pilon fractures has developed over the past years, which includes bony lesions and the damage to soft tissues, and these have been incorporated in the major setting of complete body trauma.

Since the publication of the German edition of this book in 1991, several clinical papers have appeared, which should be considered here. They are based in part on earlier case reports, which means that they are of special value with regard to late follow-up results [43, 115]. In part, they document techniques that have ceased to be generally accepted.

The most comprehensive series published by one author is that of Beck [7], who in 1993 reported on 380 cases during the years 1972–1985, including 256 patients followed for a mean observation period of 7.5 years. Other publications have examined recent trends with regard to indications and techniques. Special emphasis is placed on the evaluation and the management of soft tissue damage and on the prevention of infection by reducing the number of implants (minimal internal fixation, general rejection of the plate). The external fixator is being increasingly used [103, 141, 142], either alone or in combination with percutaneous reduction maneuvers. Few tibial implants are being used [10, 11]. These publications are referred to in later chapters.

In 1991, M. E. Müller et al. published the third edition of *Manual of Internal Fixation* [133]. It depicts the division of segment 43 as we previously worked it out. The curved end of the lower tibial incision is no longer shown. The operative reduction and fixation should first consider whether the fibula is intact and whether the fracture is simple or complex. The external fixator and the distractor are recommended in certain situations, especially when the skin conditions are precarious. The cloverleaf plate, the distractor as an aid to reduction, and the external fixator as frame construction are illustrated.

In 1991, congresses were held in Vienna and in Paris at which pilon fractures were one of the main topics. The proceedings of these two meetings are now available. At the congress of the Société Française de Chirurgie Orthopédique et Traumatologique (SOFCOT) in Paris in November 1991, Copin and Nérot [32] presented their study of 706 pilon fractures from nine French university hospitals. This material also contains 48 cases with a posterolateral fragment that the German-speaking and to a great extent the English-speaking countries assign to malleolar fractures. The dominant feature determining classification consists in the differentiation between partial (306) and complete (400) fractures.

Dislocation of the trochlea in relation to the tibial axis *(translation)* receives special attention as a further criterion for differentiation. A particularly unfavorable prognosis is attached to an anteriorly shifting talus.

The terms employed by Copin and Nérot are strongly related to French usage. Definitions are not provided, and their use within the text is inconsistent, which makes any comparison difficult. The terms we consider important, such as depression, impaction, and cancellous defect (adequate filling), are hardly mentioned. Although the concomitant injuries involving the fibula, medial malleolus, or ligaments are mentioned, they are not analyzed.

The sections dealing with therapeutic management also include 189 conservatively treated fractures and reflect the current, manifold diversity of concepts and techniques in France. This permits only a limited outlook and few conclusions can be drawn. Nevertheless, in the chapters dealing with operative techniques and complications, we shall refer to individual case reports from this comprehensive study.

H. Tscherne and J. Schatzker organized and presided over the joint meeting of the German, Austrian, and Swiss Societies for Traumatology together with the North American Trauma Association in Vienna in May 1991. In their monograph *Major Fractures of the Pilon, the Talus and the Calcaneus* [201], all aspects of pilon fractures are examined by independent authors. In the following chapters, we repeatedly refer to this work. One series [7] has already been mentioned.

> The French term *pilon tibial* coined by Destot in 1911 has proved to be most fitting for morphologic and pathogenetic reasons. It is now accepted by scientists of all languages.

6.3. Fractures of the Weightbearing Articular Surface

The ankle joint has a small articular surface without discernible compartments or pillars that would allow a classification on an anatomic basis. The fact that axial malalignment or possible damage to the surrounding structures (fibular fracture, medial malleolus) must be ignored in the classification but taken into account as accessory findings makes the situation even worse.

The mechanisms of injury are complex, and to assess them reliably from radiologic studies is rarely feasible. In analogy to the approach adopted for other bones we therefore decided to base our classification exclusively on morphologic criteria.

If the weightbearing articular surface of the tibia is injured, two basic patterns are found: split and depression. Initially, we intended to categorize articular fractures according to these basic patterns. Split fractures (B) would then have been opposed to depression fractures (C). The preliminary study, performed in 1979 and first published in 1982 [128] has already been mentioned. We subsequently abandoned this classification because it was inconsistent with the general and well-organized system that had been chosen in the AO classification [132]. In this classification, articular fractures are divided into two major groups: partial (B) and complete or circumferential (C) fractures. The basic elements split and depression must then be assigned to the appropriate group. If the typical morphologic patterns of the metaphyseal fracture—impaction and multifragmentation—are then combined with these basic injuries (see section 5.3), a clinically relevant, uniform, and well-organized arrangement is obtained for the entire distal tibial segment, which at the same time serves as a guide to management and prognosis. A prerequisite for classification is that such injuries of the articular surface undergo a detailed, morphologic analysis.

Only two basic patterns exist in fractures of the articular surface: split and depression.

6.3.1. Split

A split fracture may be produced by various mechanisms. The pattern of displacement consists in steplike incongruences of the joint surface, possibly dehiscence and, less frequently, axial rotation. These three basic types of dislocation are illustrated schematically in Figure 96. If there is no interposition, such dislocations may be removed by the following external reduction maneuvers: by the application of traction on the ligamentous apparatus, the integrity of which is maintained—the so-called ligamentotaxis—or the application of compressive and shearing forces. If the anatomy of the articular surface is completely restored, a split fracture will not lead to posttraumatic osteoarthrosis, since it produces only insignificant damage to the cartilaginous tissues. If the articular edge is fragmented but not grossly dislocated, the periosteal and capsuloligamentous connections are preserved, and devitalization will not occur. We therefore do not necessarily agree with the interpretation of Gay and Evrard [46], the first classification of Rüedi et al. [173], and the system of Jahna et al. [84], all of whom consider steplike incongruence to be a direct indication of increased severity or poor prognosis.

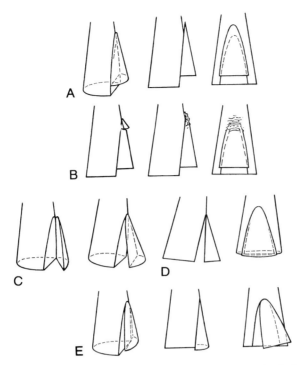

Figure 96. Diagrams showing the patterns of how the split of a conus may be displaced. **A.** Displacement of the whole split fragment. **B.** Proximal impaction or split. **C.** Unilateral dehiscence (gaping). **D.** Diastasis with bilateral dehiscence. **E.** Axial rotation.

Splits may occur in the frontal plane (visualized on the lateral radiograph) as well as in the sagittal plane (visualized on the AP film). They may be oblique or bent, and in these cases may appear unclear or blurred because of overshadowing or because the splits are visualized simultaneously on different x-ray projections.

The question whether a simple split or multiple splits are present may be hard to answer using standard radiographs only, particularly when the split is oblique or bent.

We have tried to illustrate these problems by means of a simple scheme (Fig. 97). Even the use of a tomogram or computed tomography (CT) scan will not always allow a clear differentiation, but this question is of academic interest only since practical reasons require the use of simple documents for classification. The relevant question to ask is not whether there is a double or a T-shaped split in the articular surface, but whether it is not more than an undisplaced fissure. The latter must be clearly distinguished from a depression or a dislocated complex fracture. In practice, the differentiation is not too demanding. The criterion determining group allocation is the split as opposed to the depression. Isolated splits are common.

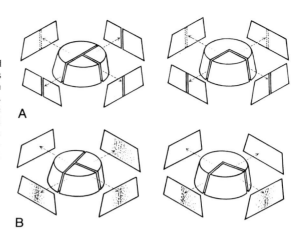

Figure 97. Diagram of a truncated conus demonstrating the various forms in which a split may appear on the conventional radiograph. **A.** When the x-rays run parallel to the split, a sharp picture will be obtained on the film close to the split, and a blurred picture on the film on the opposite side. **B.** When the beam and the split are not parallel, the film will be unclear or negative, and its interpretation questionable.

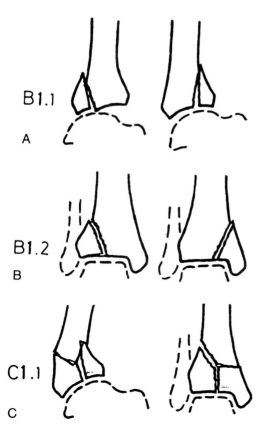

Figure 98. The classification of simple splits. **A.** Splits in the frontal plane, posterior or anterior *(B1.1)*. **B.** Splits in the sagittal plane, lateral or medial *(B1.2)*. **C.** Splits in complete fractures *(C1.1)* (Y- and T-forms). The split may be located in the frontal as well as the sagittal plane. Because *the fracture is circular in nature,* it would be unrealistic to divide it according to planes.

To consider the planes of the split is only feasible in partial fractures (type B). In these fractures, part of the articular surface has remained intact and the continuity with the diaphysis is preserved. The plane of the split may then be inferred from the position of the intact part of the joint. The procedure is particularly useful in partial complex fractures or situations difficult to interpret for other reasons. Again, an oblique fracture line may be challenging, but only when the definite allocation of the fracture to individual subgroups has to be made.

Partial splits classified as B1 are therefore divided into two types: splits in the frontal plane (easier to recognize on the lateral view), where the intact part of the joint is situated posteriorly or anteriorly (Fig. 98A), and splits in the sagittal plane (easier to recognize on the AP view) with a preserved lateral or medial articular portion (Fig. 98B).

Partial fractures occasionally coexist (predominantly in the frontal plane) with fractures of the diaphysis. The latter present a second anatomic location in another segment of the same bone, and require separate recording and codification (see also Appendix, section 3.3). Such cases were described in 1960 by Witt [216] as "double fracture."

Pure splits are also frequently found in complete circumferential fractures (type C). A differentiation according to planes, however, cannot be made since there is no anatomic connection between the joint and the diaphysis. Simple splits are allocated to group C1. If, in addition, there is a complex metaphyseal component (impaction or multifragmentation), these fractures, in analogy to extraarticular fractures, are classified as C2.

Examples

Radiographic examples of simple articular splits: Figures 99–107

Further radiographic examples:

Partial fractures (B): Figures 40, 53, and 56,

Complete fractures (C): Figures 47 and 178.

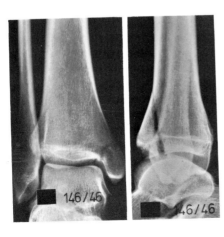

Figure 99. Radiograph of a partial articular fracture, anterior split (frontal plane, evident on the lateral radiograph). Diastasis, no step, intact fibula. Oblique fracture of the medial malleolus. Classified as B1.1.

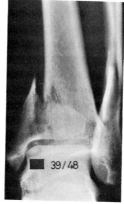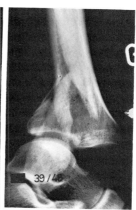

Figure 100. A partial articular fracture. Posteromedial, obliquely running split, predominantly in the frontal plane including the medial malleolus. Oblique fracture of the distal fibular diaphysis. The lateral radiograph suggests a trough-shaped depression, but this was excluded by the postoperative findings (see Figure 174). Classified as B1.1.

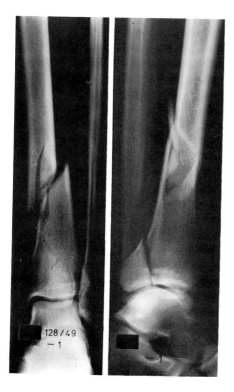

Figure 101. Combination of a partial, articular split fracture with fracture of the tibial diaphysis (of segment 42, to be classified separately). The posterior split in the frontal plane corresponds morphologically to a posterolateral wedge fragment (Volkmann's triangle). There is no malleolar fracture; the fibula is intact. Classified as B1.1.

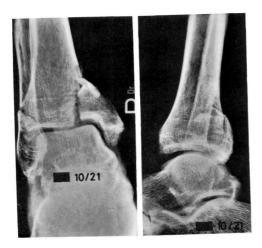

Figure 102. Partial articular fracture, sagittal split, and steplike incongruity (evident on the anteroposterior (AP) film of the medial articular surface; varus position; typical oblique fracture of the fibula above the syndesmosis. Classified as B1.2.

Figure 103. Partial articular fracture; anterolateral split in the sagittal plane. Fissure of the fibula at the level of the tibial fracture. Classified as B1.2.

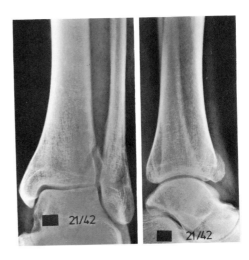

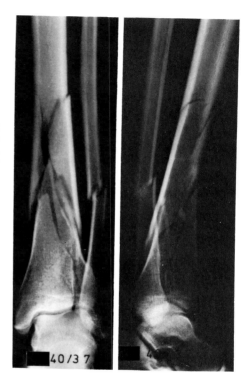

Figure 104. Combination of an articular split with fracture of the tibial diaphysis (segment 42). Separate codification. Partial, lateral split in the sagittal plane; oblique fracture of the fibular diaphysis. Classified as B1.2. This is an unusual borderline case for classification. It is analogous to the posterior split (B1.1) combined with a diaphyseal fracture of the tibia (see Figure 101). In spite of the morphologic and functional relationship with the fracture of the diaphysis, the case has not been allocated to group C1.3, since an individual and complex fracture center exists in the tibial diaphysis (see also Figure 118).

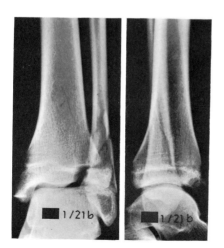

Figure 105. Partial articular fracture in an adolescent. Despite the angular shape of the anterolateral fracture of the epiphysis, it is clearly evident on the AP film; spiral fracture of the fibula above the syndesmosis. Classified as B1.2.

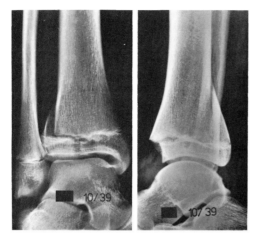

Figure 106. Epiphyseal fracture in an adolescent. Sagittal, oblique (therefore blurred on the radiograph) split with partial, lateral epiphysiolysis continued as a posterior split in the frontal plane (triplane fracture); intact fibula; articular split evident on the AP radiograph. Classified as B1.2.

Figure 107. Complete articular split (taking a circular Y shape in the metaphysis). Articular fracture line on the AP radiograph; in addition, a second, lateral split is suggested. On the lateral radiograph, the interpretation is unclear; no axial malalignment; fibula intact. Classified as C1.1.

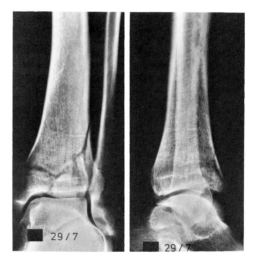

6.3.2. Depression of the Articular Surface

General Remarks

Depression of an articular surface is caused by the sharper and stronger end of one bone ramming into another. The bone end that is driven into the other tends to be convex. The bone that is depressed usually shows a concave shape resembling a pan or plate. The depressed area consists of a section broken off the articular surface; continuity with the surroundings is partially or completely destroyed. The overlying cancellous bone will be crushed, or the surrounding fragments will be driven apart and the depressed articular portion will be trapped in between. This leads to an apparent widening of the contours on the radiograph (Fig. 109). This is a well-known morphologic feature in fractures of the proximal tibial plateau. There, depressions are predominantly found at the lateral condyle, and in most cases they are associated with a split. Medial or isolated, or hollow-shaped and central depressions are less common. They are also observed in certain basal fractures of the short bones of the hand and foot where they often occur in partial fractures [71]. Whether the depressed area has preserved its vitality is always questionable, since depression always implies damage to the cartilaginous tissues.

The depressed bone remains trapped, preventing reduction by traction (ligamentotaxis) or external compression. Depression is therefore a clear and unambiguous indication for surgery. The operative approach depends on the location of the depression (see Chapter 4, section 3.4.3).

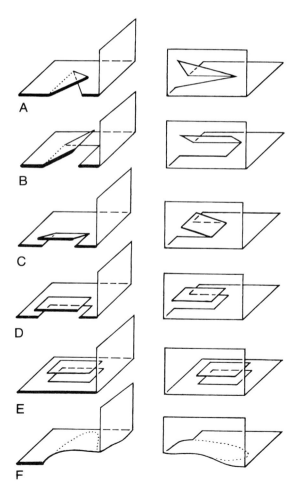

Figure 108. Geometric drawings showing—in analogy to simple depressions of a joint—gapings in or detachments out of a surface area containing a side wall. The figures on the *right* correspond to those on the *left* but are turned at 90 degrees, producing completely different appearances. Marginal lines are in the foreground and therefore drawn as *thick lines.* Central and more distant or superimposed lines are drawn as *thin lines.* **A.** Triangle; may be confused with a trap-door depression. **B.** Trap-door depression. **C.** Trap-door depression in the second plane; may be confused with a pestle-formed depression. **D.** Marginal, pestle-formed depression. **E.** Central, pestle-formed depression. **F.** Trough-like depression. The diagrams are supposed to illustrate why marginal depressions are often only evident on one radiologic projection. Another objective is to aid in the interpretation of poor focusing or superimposition effects. True pestle-formed depressions must be evident in two planes.

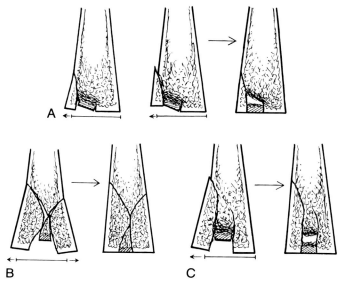

Figure 109. Schematic of split depressions. The depression displaces the split, and widening of the epiphysis ensues. **A.** There is only a slight displacement in the trap-door depression; a defect remains after restoration of the articular surface. **B.** Pestle-formed depression with a strongly built depressed fragment; marked displacement and widening of the epiphysis. No defect remains after reduction. **C.** Pestle-formed depression with compression of cancellous bone; only minor displacement and widening of the epiphysis. After reduction, a defect remains which must be packed.

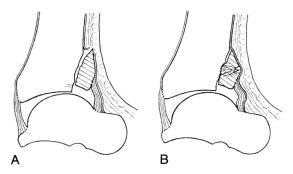

Figure 110. Vascularity of marginal fragments. Even when displaced with the periosteum stripped off, they remain vital because of their attachments to the articular capsule (see also Figure 27). **A.** Split. **B.** Depression.

Basic Patterns of Depression

Depressions of the distal tibial joint surface give rise to diagnostic, surgical, and prognostic problems. To facilitate their understanding, depressions may be depicted as geometric figures viewed from two different planes or angles (Fig. 108), the objective being to explain the optical illusions that may be encountered on the standard radiograph.

Basically, we have to distinguish between the more common triangular or trap-door depressions and the less frequent pestle-form and trough-shaped depressions (Fig. 112). The triangular depression consists in an angular, upward impaction. It has a broad base tapering toward the apex. The base of the triangle remains attached to the surrounding articular surface. The trap-door or winglike depression corresponds to a flap two sides of which have been driven upward. On one projection, a horizontal line appears which may be taken for the pestle form. But at the base of the square, one side has maintained its contact with the surrounding structures so that in a trap-door depression, there is no complete devitalization.

The pestle-form depression consists of a circular area that has been punched out. The depressed fragment is separated and has been driven upward. Connection to the bony surroundings is interrupted. A trap-door depression is often mistaken for a pestle-form depression, since on one projection, the former is visualized as a horizontal line (see Fig. 108C). To prove the diagnosis of a pestle-form depression, visualization on two projections or tomographic evidence is necessary.

If, in front of the depressed area, another fragment is split off, the latter remains attached to the joint capsule and will not be subject to devitalization. The depression is concealed and therefore more difficult to expose or reduce (Fig. 110).

The trough-shaped depressions known from the tibial plateau and the femoral head present a rare finding hard to identify. On radiographs of the distal tibia, these patterns are often simulated by overshadowing or superimposition.

Frequency and Mode of Origin at the Distal Tibia

At the tibial plafond, depressions are produced by the effects of impaction caused by the opposing talus with its trochlea or edges. Böhler [13] was the first to point out this injury. Although he provided illustrations (Fig. 80), he did not attempt any further analysis. Depressions were reported by Gay and Evrard [46] and roughly outlined by two schematic drawings (Fig. 82). To our knowledge, the first description of a depression on the lateral side of the articular surface was made by Coonrad [31] in 1970. Heim and Pfeiffer [69] described it in connection with fractures of the medial malleolus. Vichard and Watelet [202] and, later, Stampfel and Mähring [185] discussed its special features (Fig. 91). Recently, Tile [192], Mast [118], and Caffinière et al. [24] have studied the problem. Depressions are less common than pure splits and may occur in any part of the tibial joint surface. They are almost always associated with a split in front. The most common location is at the anteromedial or anterolateral side. Our case data contain a total of 117 cases, or slightly more than 10% of the total fractures of the articular surface.

The split may be considered as the first phase of the injury since it affects the stronger, peripheral zone of the joint, which is buttressed by a cortical wall and less vulnerable to impaction and compression. Once the split has occurred, the weaker, purely cancellous bone lying behind is more likely to be compressed. The inverse sequence, i.e., depression followed by a split, is conceivable for other locations, in particular for the area adjacent to the medial malleolus. Without weightbearing function, the medial malleolus barely supports the adjacent cancellous bone. At this site, where depressions are particularly frequent, they would constitute the early phase of the injury. With varus pressure increasing, the medial malleolus would then split off (vertical form). But other depressions may also result from such a two-phase process. A precise analysis of the mechanism of injury is impossible. A noteworthy finding is that the majority of depressions are observed in those areas where the subchondral mineralization and the cartilaginous covering are particularly pronounced (see Figs. 8 to 14). The reason why in some cases only a split is produced while in others it is combined with depression is not clear. There is no evidence suggesting that depression would occur only in subjects with impaired cancellous bone structure, e.g., in the elderly. In the adolescent before epiphyseal maturity, impaction and depression are extreme rarities. One case was reported by Vichard and Watelet [202]. But soon after growth is completed, both morphologic patterns are frequently observed in our patients. Analysis of partial depression fractures (B2) and also of complete fractures (C1.2) reveals that several patients in the age group 17 to 23 years are affected. Moreover, the average age of the patients in these groups is low. For details, see Appendix, section 3.3, Group B2.

Trap-door and pestle-form depressions require a different management (see Fig. 161).

X-Ray Diagnosis

On the radiograph, depressed areas may be clearly appreciated as dense lines if they lie more or less parallel to the beam. Usually, this is the case in one projection only. Clear visualization on the second projection is possible only if the depression is of the pestle form. But the image of central depressions remains blurred because of surrounding radiopaque structures.

Trap-door depressions are usually visualized on the radiograph as a sharply bent angle. If the talus glides back into its original position, an asymmetric, angular opening of the joint line will ensue. Paradoxically, major depressions, in which the trochlea of the talus remains subluxated, are more readily missed. The use of the tomogram and the CT scan may improve the recognition and interpretation of depressions.

The identification of a depressed fracture is only possible if the surrounding structures are intact or consist of major fragments. In case of a complex injury of the articular surface, i.e., if dissociation is present, it is therefore not possible to distinguish an individual depression fracture, even though it is certainly part of the injury as a result of the compression forces.

Significance and Prognosis of Depression Fractures

If reduction is not at all or only partially achieved, the persisting incongruence of the articular surface will lead to lax and insufficient joint stabilization and thus inevitably to secondary arthrosis.

We know that the various parts of the tibial joint surface are subject to different amounts of functional load [207]. The outcome of a depression therefore largely depends on the site and the extent of the lesion. Posterolaterally, it is more severe than posteromedially, and an anterolateral injury appears to be less serious than an anteromedial lesion [211]. The analysis of our patients, however, has shown that the prognosis of depression is always worse than that of the pure split (see Appendix, group B). For operative treatment this means that both high precision and, for biological reasons, very delicate handling are crucial.

Damage to the Cartilage in Depression

The damage to the cartilaginous tissues cannot be assessed from the radiograph. Although the morphology may provide some information, it is the surgeon's observation at operation that is important. A detailed description by the surgeon is essential in complex fractures. Another factor of prognostic significance is the condition of the cartilage of the trochlea of the talus (see section 2.2).

Classification of Partial Depression Fractures (B2)

In these fractures one part of the joint has remained intact. Depressions combined with a split may therefore be classified according to planes, as the injury is usually better visualized on one of the two radiographic views. In case of doubt, guidance is provided by the intact part of the joint.

To start with, fractures in the frontal plane are easier to recognize on the lateral radiograph; they are summarized in subgroup B2.1. The intact part of the joint is then located posteriorly (more common) or anteriorly.

Posterior depressions, in which the anterior part of the joint has remained intact, are not included in this group of patients. They are occasionally found in malleolar fractures (Volkmann's triangle with an additional area of depression), and should theoretically be assigned to this group (cf. section 1.4, Figs. 41 and 111A). If the fracture is located in the sagittal plane (better evident on the AP view), the intact part of the joint is either lateral (more often) or medial (Fig. 111B). These fractures belong to subgroup B2.2.

Classification of Complete Fractures with Depression

Depressions are also far from rare in this type of fracture. Here, it would be impractical to base the classification on fracture planes, as no part of the joint has remained intact.

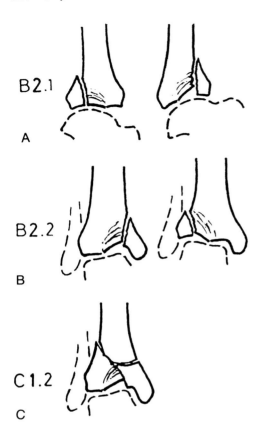

Figure 111. Classification of simple depressions. **A.** Depressions and splits in partial fractures occurring in the frontal plane (evident on the lateral radiograph) are classified as *B2.1*. They may be located on the posterior or anterior side. **B.** Split depressions in the sagittal plane of partial fractures (evident on the AP radiograph) are allocated to *B2.2*. They may be located either laterally or medially. **C.** Simple split depressions in simple complete (circular) fractures are assigned to the distinct subgroup *C1.2* irrespective of the plane of the depression.

Figure 112. The classification of various, typical patterns of depression fractures drawn from radiographs. **A–I.** Partial fractures. **J–M.** Complete fractures. **A.** Anterior depression (B2.1) (see Figure 113). **B.** Posterior depression (B2) (see Figure 114). **C.** Central, pestle-formed depression (B2.1) (see Figure 177). **D.** Anterior, trough-like depression (B2.1). **E.** Medial depression (B2.2) (see Figure 115). **F.** Lateral depression (B2.2) (see Figures 51 and 52). **G.** Marginal, lateral depression (B2) (see Figure 176). **H.** Central, sagittal depression (probably trap-door) (B2.3) (see Figure 183). **I.** Trough-shaped depression, medially (B2.2). **J.** Central pestle-formed depression (C1.2) (see Figure 179). **K.** Combined pestle- and trough-shaped depression. There is impaction of the unfractured, posterior articular surface. **L.** In cases in which the impacted posterior wall is not associated with an additional depression, the ''folding-roof'' type is formed [185]. **M.** Disintegration of the articular surface; no impaction but fracture of the posterior wall. The determination whether a pestle-formed or trap-door depression is present cannot be made. Classified as C3.1 (see Figure 134).

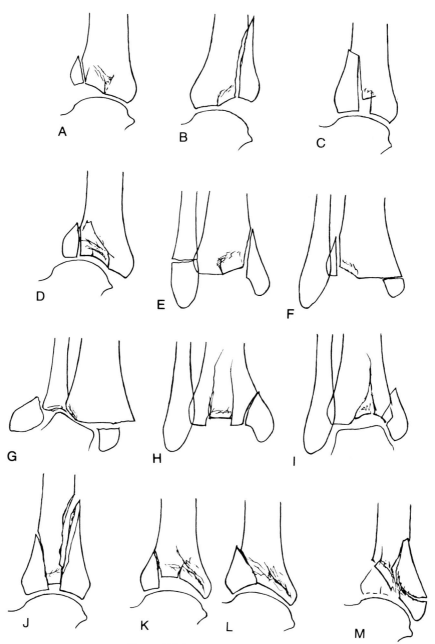

Figure 112 *See legend on opposite page*

Simple fractures are often associated with depression, and are then classified in subgroup C1.2 (Fig. 111C) as opposed to the purely articular split fractures (C1.1) (see Fig. 98C). We may also observe small articular depressions, in which the main feature consists of metaphyseal impaction or multifragmentation (C2.1 or C2.2). Separate analysis is carried out in connection with the corresponding subgroups (see Appendix, section 3.4, Group C2).

Depressions are less common in fractures that extend far into the diaphysis. They are dealt with in the discussion of subgroups C1.3 and C2.3 (see Appendix, section 3.4).

> Depressions of the tibial plafond are frequent. They are easier to detect in partial fractures, but also exist in complete fractures.

Examples

Illustrative radiographs of split depressions: Figures 113–116. Further examples are given in Figures 52, 176, and 199.

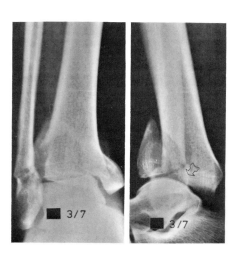

Figure 113. Partial fracture with depression in the frontal plane (evident on the lateral radiograph) and a split in front. Anterior subluxation of the talus; varus position with typical, oblique fracture of the fibula at the level of the syndesmosis; oblique fracture of the medial malleolus. Classified as B2.1.

Figure 114. Posterior depression of the tibial articular surface in the frontal plane (evident on the lateral radiograph). In the foreground is a small, triangular posterolateral fragment of the articular margin. Oblique fracture of the fibula above the ligaments, transverse fracture of the medial malleolus distally. This case must be classified as B2.1. The example was not taken from the base data analyzed but from the author's personal series where it was recorded under malleolar fracture.

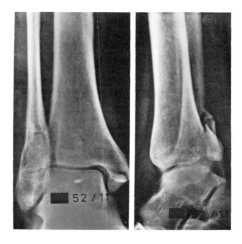

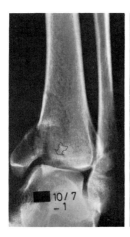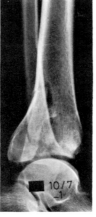

Figure 115. Partial articular fracture (lateral part of the joint intact). Anteromedial depression in the sagittal plane, better seen on the AP radiograph. Posteromedial split; varus position; typical fracture of the fibula at the level of the ligaments; vertical fracture of the medial malleolus. Classified as B2.2.

Figure 116. Complete (circular) articular fracture taking a Y-shape in the metaphysis. Anteromedial depression in the frontal plane, better seen on the AP radiograph. The lateral split is located in the sagittal plane; the fragment including the medial malleolus is articular. Slight recurvation, intact fibula. Classified as C1.2 (borderline C3.1). This clearly illustrates why a classification according to fracture planes is not feasible in complete fractures.

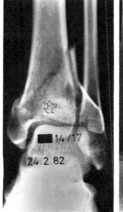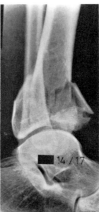

6.3.3. Metaphyseal and Diaphyseal Morphology of Articular Fractures

Articular fractures always extend to the metaphysis and sometimes even to the diaphysis. Analysis of the morphology further proximal has revealed the same characteristic features found in extraarticular fractures. These allow grading the injury according to severity and in agreement with clinical signs and symptoms (see section 5.3).

The assessment of extraarticular fractures is based on the following four criteria: (1) metaphyseal wedge, (2) metaphyseal impaction, (3) complex metaphyseal fracture with multifragmentation, and (4) extension into the diaphysis. Articular fractures have no distal main fragment. By definition, this precludes the finding of a wedge with contact preserved between the main fragments. Multiple metaphyseal components are therefore only present in multiple splits, impactions, or comminution.

Multiple Fracture Lines in the Metaphysis

Multiple fracture lines occur also in partial articular fractures. They present an obstacle to reduction and stabilization. The thin, cortical shell of the metaphysis allows good recognition on the x-ray film. In B-type fractures, individual subgroups (B1.3 and B2.3) may be established on the basis of this property (Fig. 117A, B).

Because in partial fractures one part of the articular surface has preserved its integrity, these lesions are usually confined to the distal end. In contrast to other groups, we deal here with a fracture in which the property ''extension into the diaphysis'' is neither suited nor practicable for subgroup designation.

Partial articular fractures of the distal humerus, the distal radius, and the distal femur display similar morphologies [132, 134]. The classification of these fractures, including subgroup designation, is likewise based on the multiple metaphyseal split but not on the rare finding of extension to the diaphysis.

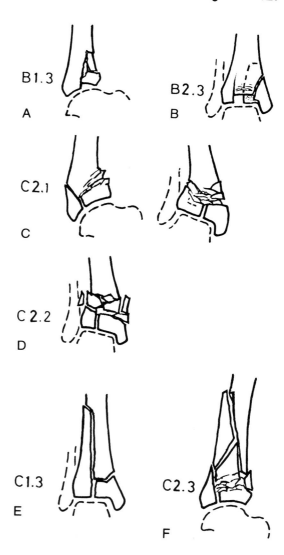

Figure 117. Simple articular fractures presenting with multiple or complex morphologic patterns in the metaphysis and diaphysis. **A.** Partial fracture, simple articular split, multifragmentary in the metaphysis *(B1.3)*, depicted in the frontal plane (lateral radiograph). **B.** Partial fracture with depression, multifragmentary in the metaphysis *(B2.3)*, depicted in the sagittal plane (AP radiograph). **C.** Complete fracture, simple articular, with impaction of the metaphysis *(C2.1)*, depicted in the frontal and sagittal planes. **D.** Complete fracture, simple articular, with a zone of multifragmentation in the metaphysis *(C2.2)*. **E.** Complete articular fracture, simple articular, extending into the diaphysis *(C1.3)*. **F.** Complete fracture, simple articular, with metaphyseal impaction or multifragmentation, extending into the diaphysis *(C2.3)*.

Metaphyseal Impaction

Metaphyseal impaction is characteristic of the distal tibial fracture. In the extraarticular forms, preservation of contact between the main fragments is observed after reduction. Articular fractures, in which there is no main fragment distally, cannot show this sign.

In complete circular articular fractures, the variability of both the site and the plane of the split precludes their use for differentiation into subgroups. Complete articular fractures in the adult are characterized by the frequent combination of split with impaction (the largest group in our series) (Fig. 117C). The form corresponds to the classic pilon fracture of the skier, and presents the basic model for the standardization of the AO operative technique. Somewhat stylized drawings of the impacted fracture combined with an articular split were made by Heim [55]. Its mode of origin was analyzed by Bandi [4] in 1970 (Fig. 87).

Metaphyseal impaction and articular split may coexist with depression of the articular surface, but in this case the depression is limited and not deep (a mitigating effect due to the metaphyseal impaction?). Such depressions are therefore not assigned to an individual subgroup, but subordinated to the main group criteria split and impaction. We refer the reader to the details given in the systematic analysis of group C2 in the Appendix, under section 3.4, and to Fig. 125).

We noted that the average age of patients who showed an articular split in combination with metaphyseal impaction was lower (mean age, 43 years) than that of patients with pure extraarticular impaction (mean age, 57 years). With involvement of the articulation, a significant preponderance of males was found (see Appendix, section 3.2, Group A2, and section 3.4, Group C2).

Metaphyseal Multifragmentation

In extraarticular fractures, this was recognized as an individual fracture pattern and classified as such. It is far from rare in articular fractures. In such cases, we find the combination of an articular split with a multifragmentary fracture of the metaphysis (Fig. 117D). Its differentiation from the multiple split described in partial articular fractures (B type) is simple. Like the impacted fractures, the injury is completely circular, which is why fragmentation and displacement of the metaphyseal elements have taken on completely new dimensions.

These fractures are also far more severe than impacted fractures. In most cases, they result from traffic accidents or a fall from a height. Open fractures are common (more than one third of all cases). The technical problems encountered with internal fixation and the prognosis are very different from the situation in impacted fractures. The average age of patients is 45 years with a marked preponderance of males (see also Appendix, section 3.4, subgroup C2.2). This fracture type may also be associated with small depressions of the articular surface adjacent to the split. The finding is considered accessory and assigned to the main group of split with complex metaphyseal fracture. Close analysis of our series, however, reveals a more unfavorable prognosis for these injuries when compared to simple splits. Admittedly, the numbers are small. The arthrosis may result from the surgeon's failure to detect the accessory finding at operation while he or she was concentrating on the predominant metaphyseal injury.

Combinations of articular split with metaphyseal features are impaction and complex pattern.

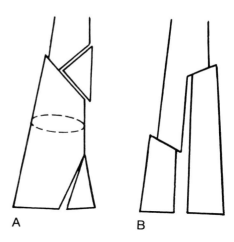

Figure 118. Schematic of a partial articular fracture with an unrelated fracture of the diaphysis (subgroup B1.1; see Figure 101) and a complete simple articular fracture which completes its circle in the diaphysis (subgroup C1.3, Figures 127 and 128). **A.** In a partial fracture, there is a distinct fracture center in the diaphysis. The tibial cylinder shows an intact section in the upper metaphysis (in some cases a fissure may be present). **B.** In a complete fracture, the displaced articular split passes continuously through the center of the cylinder into the diaphysis.

A   B

Extension of the Fracture to the Diaphysis

Extension of the fracture to the diaphysis is the fourth morphologic criterion taken from metaphyseal fracture patterns and is combined here with articular fractures. The finding is seen in many end fractures of other long bones where it is occasionally used for the classification of subgroups (distal humerus, C3.3; distal femur, C3.3; distal radius, C2.3 and C3.3). In other locations, extension into the diaphysis is expressed by a so-called additional code number (proximal tibia, proximal radius) [132, 134]. Extension into the diaphysis is common in complete articular fractures of the tibia. This serves for subgroup designation; in the simple articular split, the fracture line divides and becomes circumferential only in the diaphysis (Figs. 117E and 118). This characterizes subgroup C1.3. In fractures with complex morphology of the metaphysis (impaction, severe comminution), the diaphyseal component consists of one or several fragments located predominantly further proximal. Thus the subgroup C2.3 is made up (Fig. 117F). If the articular surface shows a complex fracture pattern (C3), extension into the diaphysis is used to form subgroup C3.3 (see Fig. 131C). In fractures of subgroups C1.3 and C2.3 with extension into the diaphysis, individual cases of a small additional depression of the articular surface have been found (Fig. 128) (cf. Appendix, section 3.4).

Examples

Radiographs illustrating the metaphyseal and diaphyseal morphology of simple articular fractures: Figures 119–129
Further radiographs:
Multiple metaphyseal splits in partial fractures (B1.3 and B2.3): Figures 53, 177, 183
Metaphyseal impaction (C2.2): Figures 50, 51, 185
Multifragmentation of the metaphysis (C2.2): Figure 181
Extension into the diaphysis (C1.3 and C2.3): Figures 48 and 178

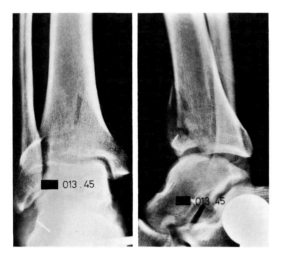

Figure 119. Radiograph of a partial articular fracture (intact posterior wall) taken with the foot in traction. Antero-medial split including the medial malleolus (lateral radiograph, frontal plane); a second, anterolateral split (sagittal plane, AP radiograph). The fibula is intact; downward displacement of the tip with a small talar avulsion fracture of the distal ligamentous attachments *(arrow)*. Classified as B1.3.

Figure 120. Partial articular fracture (posterolateral wall intact). Large, pestle-shaped depression of the anterior margin (evident on both radiographs). Lateral and medial splits in the sagittal plane (better seen on the AP radiograph); a large, posteromedial fragment including the medial malleolus, the tip of which shows a small avulsion fracture *(arrow)*; intact fibula. Classified as B2.3. This case illustrates clearly the increased severity of the injury when compared to the depression depicted in Figure 115. In this case, classification according to fracture planes poses problems. Orientation is provided by the narrow, intact posterolateral wall.

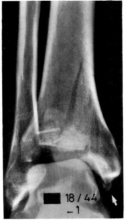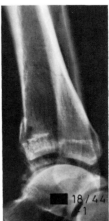

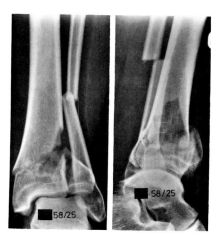

Figure 121. Lateral articular split with partial impaction of the metaphysis medially; valgus position; transverse fracture of the fibular diaphysis. Classified as C2.1.

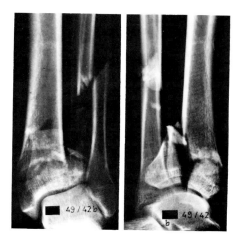

Figure 122. Lateral radiographs showing wide dehiscence of the articular split; anterolateral impaction; valgus position; antecurvature and oblique fracture of the fibular diaphysis. Classified as C2.1. In Figure 185, the same case also serves to illustrate the operative technique, course, and result.

Figure 123. Articular split (sagittal) and impaction of the metaphysis; recurvation, oblique fibular fracture of the distal diaphysis. The articular split and fibular fracture may be taken as initial evidence of varus angulation. Classified as C2.1. In Figure 182 the same case serves to illustrate the operative technique, course, and result.

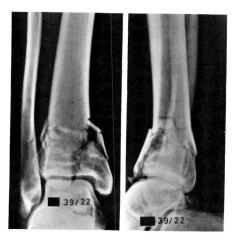

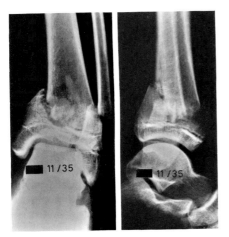

Figure 124. A single case of a complete articular fracture with an unfused epiphyseal plate in a 14-year-old boy who sustained a closed injury in an accident. Oblique (blurred picture) sagittal articular split taking a Y shape in the metaphysis; partial impaction medially with cancellous bone loss (to be inferred from its course; see also Figure 212). Varus position; typical oblique fracture of the fibula above the syndesmosis. Classified as C2.1.

Figure 125. Combined articular split, impaction of the metaphysis, and small depression. The postinjury radiographs were taken with the foot in traction. The articular split takes an oblique course (widening of the epiphysis on the lateral radiograph). The depression is located anteriorly and centrally, the partial impaction is predominantly anteromedial. Laterally is an area of multifragmentation; oblique fracture of the fibular diaphysis; undisplaced fissure of the medial malleolus. Presumably, the status after primary drift into valgus angulation. Classified as C2.1; subdivision with depression (see p. 310).

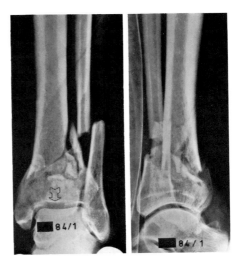

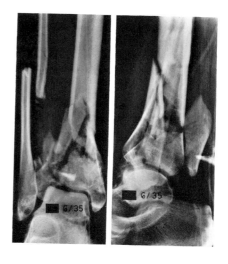

Figure 126. Articular depression with multifragmentation in the metaphysis in a 36-year-old woman. Articular split with depression laterally *(AP film)* and anteriorly *(lateral film)*. Metaphyseal multifragmentation with a large posterolateral expelled wedge, clearly distinguishable from impaction. Valgus position; diaphyseal fracture of the fibula with multiple, small fragments; oblique fissure in the medial malleolus. Classified as C2.2. Borderline to C3.2; second-degree open fracture.

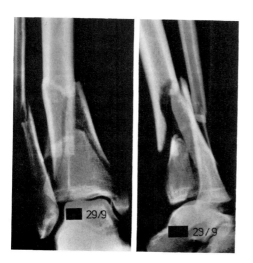

Figure 127. A simple articular split extending into the diaphysis (see Figure 118). Dehiscence of the articular split in the frontal plane *(lateral radiograph)*. The fracture completes its circle at the metaphyseal-diaphyseal border; two wedge formations. Varus position; typical, oblique fracture of the fibular diaphysis. Classified as C1.3.

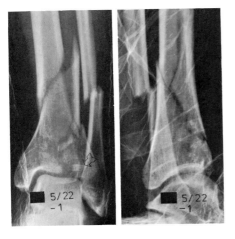

Figure 128. Complete articular fracture. Split with an additional, pestle-formed depression anterolaterally. The fracture extends into the diaphysis; spiral element with apparent varus angulation in the transportation cast. Classified as C1.3.; subdivision with depression. In Figure 179, the same case illustrates the operative technique, course, and result.

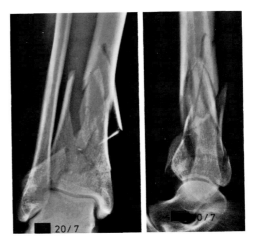

Figure 129. Articular split laterally *(AP radiograph)*, posterior split frontally *(lateral film)*. Circular area of multifragmentation in the metaphysis; extension into the diaphysis. Slightly displaced transverse fracture of the fibula distally. The second fibular fracture in the upper metaphysis is not shown on the radiograph (accident at work). Classified as C2.3.

6.3.4. Disintegration of the Articular Surface

This term denotes a complex injury of the weightbearing articular surface; it is descriptive of, and restricted to, the lesion. The designations found in the literature are not precise and do not indicate whether the severe pilon fracture is to be understood only as a complex injury of the metaphysis (impaction, multipart fracture). If so, the damage to the joint could be limited to the split. A comparison of the various designations used illustrates the problem:

Multifragmentation, multifragmentary with bone defect [13, 54, 145, 160, 173, 175, 211]

Comminution [22, 123, 149, 172]

Complexe [46, 203]

A better expression was coined by K. H. Müller, "Zermörselung der Gelenkpfanne," or "crushing of the articular surface" [127]. Although it is less ambiguous, its true meaning can only be revealed by the simultaneous viewing of illustrations, e.g., type III of Rüedi and Allgöwer [171], which is also depicted in the *Manual of Internal Fixation* [131]. The same holds true for the term *complexe* used by Vivès et al. [203]. In the AO classification [132, 134], *complexe* is confined to diaphyseal and metaphyseal lesions. A severe injury of the articular surface is referred to as *plurifragmentaire* (multifragmentary). In our opinion, this term fails to describe all aspects of the comprehensive morphology of the severe pilon fracture. When we use the word *disintegration,* we mean that the articular surface consists of multiple, unconnected, and displaced elements. We observe the combination of multiple splits and depressions. The identification of the latter is impossible, because they cannot be related to any intact part of the joint.

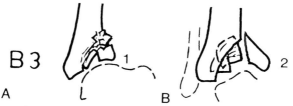

Figure 130. Disintegration of the articular surface in a partial fracture; there is a complex injury to most of the articular surface (disintegration) in partial fractures. **A.** Posterior wall is intact. Fracture is predominantly in the frontal plane (B3.1). **B.** Lateral wall is intact. Fracture is predominantly in the sagittal plane (B3.2).

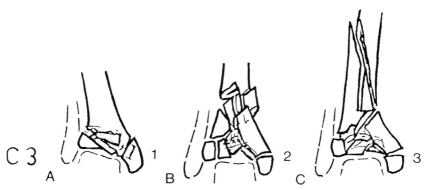

Figure 131. Disintegration in a complete articular fracture. **A.** The lesion is confined to the epiphysis and distal metaphysis (C3.1). **B.** The injury includes the proximal metaphysis (C3.2). **C.** The injury extends into the diaphysis (C3.3).

It is obvious from the morphology that a significant devitalization must have occurred. To achieve anatomic restoration of the surface is either extraordinarily difficult or impossible, in which case the fracture must be considered as inoperable. The unfavorable prognosis of this fracture pattern is also demonstrated by the results of our late follow-ups (see Appendix). To distinguish a disintegrated articular surface from the simpler articular split-depression is not always easy. Radiographs taken in various projections are required if confusion of superimpositions with depressed segments or severe comminution is to be avoided. Most cases present with axial malalignment or impaction. But if a preoperative tomogram or CT scan was precluded, some cases remain in which the definitive diagnosis can only be made at operation. When classifying such cases in our series, we always took into account the postoperative radiograph and—where possible—the short- and long-term follow-up. Disintegration of the articular surface is no common injury, but with its spectacular morphology it is extraordinarily impressive.

In partial fractures (type B), disintegrations are, by definition, rare. Group B3 represents 1.3% of our patients and comprises 16 cases. We then have a very complex, fractured part of the articular surface. The division into subgroups is based on the intact portion of the joint. It is noteworthy that the anterior wall of the tibia is always fractured (cf. also Appendix, section 3.3, Group B3, and Fig. 130).

Complete articular fractures (C3) with disintegration of the articular surface are more common (45 cases, or 4%). The division into subgroups is based on the extent of the disintegration: if the injury is confined to the epiphysis and distal metaphysis, it is distinguished from lesions that also involve the proximal metaphysis. A further subgroup is recognized in fractures with some fragments extending into the diaphysis (see also Appendix, section 3.4, and Fig. 131).

Disintegration of the articular surface produces destruction comparable to a jigsaw puzzle. This dramatic pattern is seen in B- and C-type fractures, but is not common.

Examples

Radiographs illustrating a disintegrated articular surface: Figures 132–137
Further examples:

Partial fracture of the B3 type: Figure 186
Complete fractures of the C type: Figures 49 and 190

Figure 132. Partial complex articular fracture. The anterior parts of the joint are broken off and too disintegrated to allow identification of details. Intact posterior tibial wall and intact fibula; vertical fracture of the medial malleolus. Classified as B3.1.

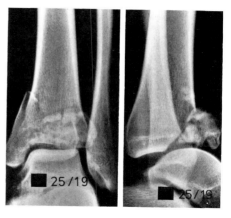

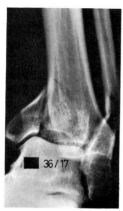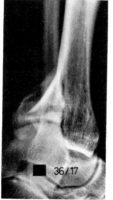

Figure 133. Partial fracture with disintegration of the articular surface. Fracture predominantly in the sagittal plane; multiple posteromedial fragments; the anterolateral portion of the joint is intact. Varus position; typical, oblique fibular fracture above the syndesmosis; vertical fracture of the medial malleolus. Classified as B3.2.

Figure 134. Complete complex articular fracture confined to the distal metaphysis; combination of extensive multifragmentation with depression of the articular surface. The details are unidentifiable. Varus recurvation; transverse fracture of the fibula through the syndesmosis. The defect suggests an initial drift into valgus angulation. Classified as C3.1.

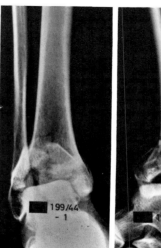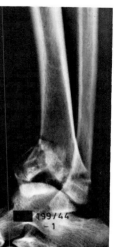

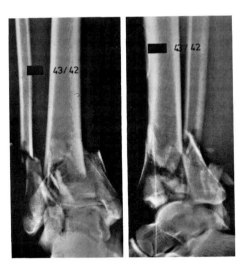

Figure 135. Disintegration of the articular surface. Major posteromedial fragment; split medial malleolus; small anterolateral fragment. Central, pestle-formed depression; area of multifragmentaton in the metaphysis extending into the middle of the upper metaphysis; oblique fracture of the fibula at the junction between diaphysis and metaphysis; sagittal gaping split of the trochlea of the talus. Classified as C3.1.

Figure 136. Complex articular fracture in which three major elements may be recognized; (1) a large posteromedial fragment including the medial malleolus, (2) a smaller anterolateral fragment, and (3), in between, an area of multifragmentation with a major, marginal anterior fragment. The area of multifragmentation is located in the metaphysis. Slight valgus position, oblique fracture of the fibular metaphysis. Radiograph taken in traction: striking dehiscence of the joint line (ruptured ligaments?). Although the tibial joint surface is less severely destroyed than is the case in Figure 135, the lesion is more complex than a split depression. It is possible that the impaction was removed by the application of traction. Classified as C3.2. Closed injury. Following internal fixation, the course was favorable with only slight arthrosis.

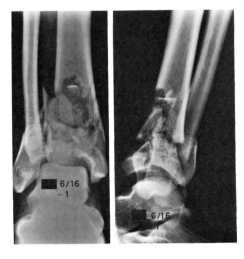

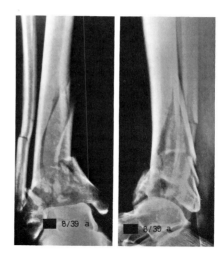

Figure 137. Complex articular fracture extending into the diaphysis. Articular combination of crushing and depression. The only major element consists of a posteromedial fragment including the medial malleolus. Wedge extends into the diaphysis. Varus position, segmental fracture of the fibula. Closed injury; 55-year-old patient; accident at home. Classified as C3.3.

6.4. Features of the Pilon Fracture Relevant for Classification

The explanations given in the preceding chapters allow a logical and clinically relevant classification of pilon fractures.

B-type fractures are partial articular fractures in which one part of the articular surface is preserved and has maintained its anatomic continuity with the shaft.

Group B1 comprises split fractures. These are subdivided according to planes:

B1.1: partial articular split in the frontal plane (anteriorly or posteriorly), better visualized on the lateral view (Fig. 98A).

B1.2: splits in the sagittal plane (laterally or medially), better visualized on the AP view (Fig. 98B).

If splits are depicted on both projections (bent or double fracture line), the classification is determined by the intact articular portion. Fractures difficult to classify are rarely encountered.

If a pure articular split coexists with multiple fracture lines in the metaphysis, this is classified as B1.3 (Fig. 117A).

Extension of the fracture lines to the diaphysis is rare.

Group B2 comprises all simple depressions combined with a split.

B2.1: depressions combined with a split in the frontal plane (anteriorly or posteriorly), better visualized on the lateral view (Fig. 111A).

B2.2: depressions combined with a split in the sagittal plane (medially or laterally), better visualized on the AP view (Fig. 111B).

If a depression coexists with multiple fracture lines in the metaphysis (rarely extending to the diaphysis), it is classified as B2.3. (Fig. 117B).

Group B3 comprises all partial fractures in which there is local disintegration of the articular surface (complex articular morphology). The intact portion of the articular surface tends to be small; its position determines the further division into subgroups:

B3.1: partial disintegration of the articular surface preserving the posterior wall of the tibia, better visualized on the lateral view (Fig. 130A).

B3.2: local disintegration of the articular surface preserving the lateral or medial tibial wall, better visualized on the AP view (Fig. 130B).

The subgroup B3.3 denotes the rare morphology of multiple metaphyseal-diaphyseal fragments.

In C-type fractures, there is complete anatomic separation between the joint and the diaphysis. At the metaphysis (or diaphysis), the entire circumference is involved.

Group C1 comprises all complete fractures with a simple articular and metaphyseal morphology (articular split and depression):

C1.1: articular splits with a simple metaphyseal component (Y- or T-shaped type). A differentiation based on fracture planes is impracticable (Fig. 98C).

C1.2: articular split and depression; there is simple but circumferential involvement of the metaphysis (Fig. 111C).

C1.3: this group includes the basic patterns of C1.1 and C1.2, but the fracture lines extend far into the diaphysis; in some cases the articular split becomes circumferential only in the diaphysis (T- and Y-shaped type) (Fig. 117E).

Group C2 comprises all circumferential fractures in which the articular fracture pattern is simple but the extension into the metaphysis or diaphysis shows a complex morphology.

C2.1: fractures with articular split and metaphyseal bone impaction (in some cases the split is associated with a small depression) (Fig. 117C).

C2.2: fractures with articular split and complex metaphyseal fracture (Fig. 117D); occasionally, a minor depression is observed in addition to the split.

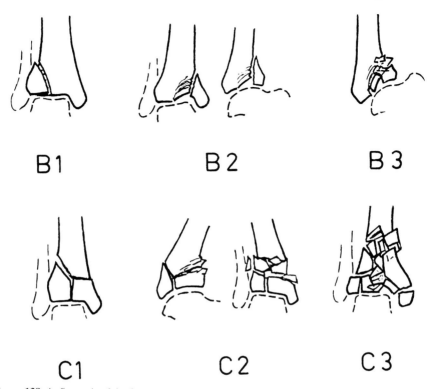

Figure 138. A. Synopsis of the features of B-type, partial pilon fractures: *B1,* split; *B2,* depression plus split; *B3,* partial disintegration of the articular surface. **B.** Synopsis of the features of complete C-type pilon fractures; *C1,* simple articular, simple metaphyseal fractures (V- or T-shaped); *C2,* simple articular, metaphyseal impaction, or complex; *C3,* articular and metaphyseal disintegration.

C2.3: articular and metaphyseal fracture, corresponding to subgroups. C2.1 and C2.2; at least one fragment extends with its major portion into the diaphysis (Fig. 117F).

Group C3 comprises all complete fractures with a complex articular component: disintegration of the articular surface (Fig. 131):

C3.1: disintegration confined to the joint and the distal metaphysis.

C3.2: disintegration also involves the proximal metaphysis.

C3.3: disintegration of the articular surface and involvement of the metaphysis plus fracture elements extending far into the diaphysis.

The categorization of the individual fracture may prove to be challenging. To provide some help, a systematic approach is offered in Chapter 3 by means of questions and answers. Case reports are provided as examples.

■ *Chapter 3*

Classification and Documentation

1. THE CONCEPT, MEANING, AND PRACTICAL EXPERIENCE

The classification of fractures is an essential precondition of scientific terminology. Precise definitions are indispensable if we want to establish a mutual understanding between basic scientists and clinicians.

Classification is based on current knowledge. The history of medicine has seen succeeding classifications. Those of the nineteenth century, achieved by clinical experience and experiments and reinforced by the authority of the teachers, were long accepted. With the introduction of x-ray photography, a decisive change came about, so that subsequent classifications of fractures have been based on the morphologic aspects and their mode of origin. At the time, the prevailing mechanism was the work accident (involvement of the tibia as the result of a fall from a height). These genetic classifications (Böhler [13], Lauge-Hansen [99]) were predominantly guided by the mechanism of the injury and laid the groundwork for conservative treatment, i.e., reduction and immobilization. The same tradition holds true when we consider the modern-day deceleration injury, i.e., the high-velocity trauma [16, 19, 100].

We can in some cases deduce the mechanism of the accident from the morphology (e.g., if the fracture shows a torsional component). Small expulsions and comminution may also indicate high-velocity trauma. Classifying fractures on the basis of origin requires taking the patient's history. Anyone who has taken patient histories is well aware of their unreliability, particularly with respect to situations surrounding an accident. Even in isolated injuries, the history may be of little help. In a patient with multiple trauma, the history is generally futile.

The more ample and variable the patient data, the more difficult the assessment of the mechanism of injury. But if we want to obtain generally applicable conclusions, it is essential to have highly diversified and comprehensive patient data.

Furthermore, recent decades have seen an increasing reliance on the operative treatment of complex and, in particular, metaphyseal and articular fractures. This requires an understanding of the biomechanical conditions and the technical difficulties of the operative intervention and its complications. Increasing attention must be paid to prognostic aspects. Modern classifications and rating systems are thus highly differentiated.

When skeletal lesions are to be evaluated, the morphologic classification is now generally used. Soft tissue damage, however, must be evaluated separately, and we often see a divergence between these two injury components.

For the morphologic classification, the AO-ASIF group adopted the ABC system [132, 134]. It was introduced by Weber [207] for the classification of malleolar fractures, and for which it has been internationally accepted. This tripartite system, which is further divided and subdivided by groups of three, has a solid biological foundation. It has been revised and modified for other sites.

Whereas the A groups contain the comparatively simple fractures with a favorable prognosis, there is an increase in the degree of severity in B and C. The classification of diaphyseal fractures is based on their complexity. A-type fractures are simple. The B type comprises wedge fractures in which there is contact between the main fragments. The C type comprises so-called complex fractures in which there is no contact between the main fragments.

The same arrangement cannot be used for terminal segments. There, the A type designates an extraarticular, metaphyseal fracture, and the B and C types designate articular fractures. The B type denotes partial fractures in which part of the articular surface has remained intact and maintained its anatomic continuity with the shaft, whereas C-type fractures are complete fractures with total disruption of the anatomic connection between articular surface and diaphysis.

In the *Manual of Internal Fixation* [131], the ABC principle is roughly outlined for the following locations: distal humerus, distal femur, pelvis, and malleolar fractures including epiphyseal lesions. In 1979, it was extended by the AO-ASIF to include all fractures of the extremities, and since then it has been the basis for the AO-ASIF documentation.

M. E. Müller and Engelhardt, in 1982 [128], were the first to apply the ABC principle to all bones of the human skeleton. It was systematically revised by Müller and colleagues in 1987. Their monograph [132] laid the groundwork for the discussion of the distal segment of the lower leg. But the full scope of the classification, not least in terms of its practical significance, will be revealed only when documented and comprehensive case material of injured patients is compiled. This will enable us to compare, measure, and evaluate the individual case in the setting of a large group.

Lorenz Böhler, more than anyone, deserves credit for appreciating clearly and for the first time the necessity of thorough documentation. His standard work [13] is based on regular follow-up and documentation of patient data.

Influenced by M. E. Müller, the young AO-ASIF group realized that documentation was one of its most essential tasks. Documentation is of special value in comparatively rare injuries where the experience of the individual traumatologist would be too limited to appreciate large-scale relationships, for obtaining valid data for the implementation of a therapeutic concept, and for the prognostic evaluation. An adequate documentation should comprise all cases treated, recording not only the initial phase of treatment but the entire healing process. This provides guidelines for therapeutic management, and also provides useful prognostic information. We thus find a close and mutual relationship between documentation and classification: both the reliability and the practicability of a classification depend on the size of the documentation of coherently recorded case reports. Only then may fundamental rules and principles be worked out and distinguished from incidental findings. But for a reasonable documentation, we need a coherently structured and uniformly applied classification.

This explains why earlier classifications, being based as they were on a restricted or selected patient population, may appear biased today. It also explains why a valid documentation requires the constant and arduous work of all those involved, and why its utility to the clinician depends on continuous revision. The individual physician, at risk of losing some of his original enthusiasm over the years, may not always be fully aware of these relationships. Today, access to the data should be open to anybody interested in their evaluation. Classification and documentation therefore must be modified to meet the requirements of electronic data processing. The 1987 AO-ASIF classification has been designed with this in mind, and the establishment of decentralized documentation is now under way.

The AO documentation center in Bern (since 1993, in Davos, Switzerland) where more than 40 clinics have regularly filed their data over the years, fulfils the task of recording all cases treated and of documenting the initial treatment. But follow-up studies are incomplete, which is limiting in terms of the prognostic aspects. The percentage of follow-up studies in the distal tibial segment, which appears to be of wider interest, is fortunately higher than for any other site (see Appendix, section 1).

One of the objectives of this book is therefore to demonstrate the value of a comprehensive documentation to aid in the analysis of an extraordinarily challenging fracture.

Documentation and classification show a constant interaction. While a systematic and large-scale documentation forms the basis for a comprehensive classification, the classification is important for prognosis and is the basis for management concepts.

---

2. SUMMARY OF THE CRITERIA FOR THE CLASSIFICATION OF DISTAL TIBIAL FRACTURES

Extraarticular fracture with its center at the metaphysis = A
    Simple fracture = A1
        Spiral = A1.1
        Oblique = A1.2
        Transverse = A1.3
    Multifragmentary fracture in which some contact between the main fragments
        is preserved = A2
        Impaction of the metaphysis = A2.1
        Simple or fragmented wedge = A2.2
        One fragment with its major portion in the diaphysis = A2.3
    Complex fracture (no contact between main fragments) = A3
        Large fragments = A3.1
        Multifragmentary = A3.2
        Extending into the diaphysis = A3.3

Partial articular fracture (one part of the articular surface intact) = B
    Pure articular split = B1
        Frontal split (anteriorly or posteriorly) = B1.1 (lateral view)
        Sagittal split (medially or laterally) = B1.2 (AP view)
        Multifragmentary in the metaphysis = B1.3
    Split-depression = B2
        Frontal (anteriorly or posteriorly) = B2.1 (lateral view)
        Sagittal (medially or laterally) = B2.2 (AP view)
        Multifragmentary in the metaphysis = B2.3
    Disintegration of the articular surface (complex) = B3
        Posterior wall intact = B3.1 (lateral view)
        Lateral or medial wall intact = B3.2 (AP view)
        Extending into the diaphysis = B3.3
Complete (circular) fracture = C
    Simple articular fracture = C1
        Articular split = C1.1
        Depression plus articular split = C1.2
        Extending into the diaphysis = C1.3
    Simple articular fracture, multifragmentary metaphyseal fracture = C2
        Articular split (plus depression) plus metaphyseal impaction = C2.1
        Articular split (plus depression) plus metaphyseal multifragmentation = C2.2
        Articular split plus metaphyseal impaction or multifragmentation plus extension into the diaphysis = C2.3
    Disintegration of the articular surface (complex) = C3
        Confined to the distal metaphysis = C3.1
        Extending into the proximal metaphysis = C3.2
        Extending into the diaphysis = C3.3

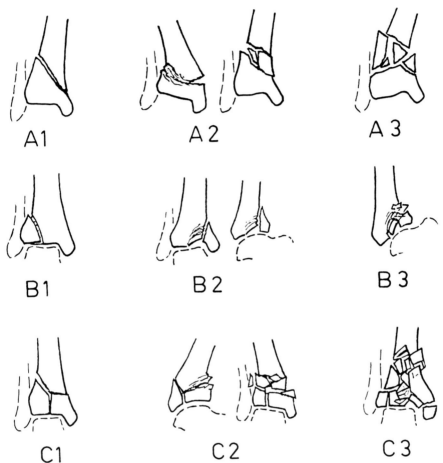

Figure 139. Synopsis of the features of extraarticular and pilon fractures for classification. *A1,* simple fracture; *A2,* impaction and wedge fracture in which, after reduction, some contact between the main fragments remains; *A3,* complex fracture without contact between the articular and the diaphyseal main fragment; *B1,* split; *B2,* split plus depression; *B3,* partial disintegration of the articular surface; *C1,* simple articular, simple metaphyseal (V- or T-shaped); *C2,* simple articular, metaphyseal impaction, or complex; *C3,* articular and metaphyseal disintegration.

3. PRACTICAL APPROACH TO THE CLASSIFICATION OF DISTAL TIBIAL FRACTURES (SEGMENT 43) ACCORDING TO THE ABC PRINCIPLE OF THE AO-ASIF

Systematized questions and answers. (Fractures of the medial malleolus are not considered.)

Extraarticular fractures = A
   Is the center of the fracture at the metaphysis? (See Fig. 31) If yes = A

Questions in A-type fractures:

Is the fracture simple? If yes = A1
   Subgroups:
      Spiral = A1.1
      Oblique = A1.2
      Transverse = A1.3 (for definition, see section 5)
Is there after reduction some contact between the main fragments? If yes = A2
   Subgroups:
      Metaphyseal impaction = A2.1 (for definition, see section 5.2.2)
      Simple or fragmented wedge = A2.2
      One fragment with its major portion in the diaphysis = A2.3
Is there after reduction no contact between the main fragments? If yes = A3
   Subgroups:
      Large, reducible fragments = A3.1
      Smaller, multiple fragments = A3.2
      One fragment with its major portion in the diaphysis = A3.3

Intraarticular fractures (the tibial pilon) = B or C

Is there still some anatomic connection between the articular surface and the diaphysis? If yes = B

Is there complete disruption between the joint and the diaphysis? If yes = C

Questions in B-type fractures:

Articular split only = B1
Subgroups:
    Evident on the lateral view = B1.1
    Evident on the AP view = B1.2
    Multifragmentary in the metaphysis = B1.3

Is there a depression (combined with a split) of the articular surface? If yes = B2
Subgroups:
    Evident on the lateral view = B2.1
    Evident on the AP view = B2.2
    Multifragmentary in the metaphysis = B2.3
Is there a complex fracture of the articular surface itself (disintegration)? If yes = B3
Subgroups:
    Posterior wall intact (lateral view) = B3.1
    Medial or lateral wall intact (evident on the AP view) = B3.2
    Additional metaphyseal or diaphyseal multifragmentation = B3.3

Questions in C-type fractures:

Is there a simple fracture of the articular surface and the metaphysis (Y or T shape)? = C1
Subgroups:
    Pure split = C1.1
    Split-depression = C1.2
    Extending into the diaphysis = C1.3
Is there a simple articular fracture (split or depression) combined with metaphyseal impaction or multifragmentation? = C2
Subgroups:
    Metaphyseal impaction = C2.1
    Metaphyseal multifragmentation = C2.2
    Extension into the diaphysis = C2.3
Is there disintegration of the articular surface (complex)? = C3
    Disintegration confined to the joint and distal metaphysis = C3.1
    Disintegration includes the proximal metaphysis = C3.2
    Disintegration extends into the diaphysis = C3.3

Examples

To provide some practical help in classification, three examples taken from our case material are analyzed:

Example 1 (Fig. 68, p. 82)

The center of the fracture lies in segment 43. The AP radiograph reveals a fissure of increased translucence possibly extending into the joint. According to the AO classification [132], a pure fissure is not considered an articular fracture. Thus it is an extraarticular A-type fracture. At the metaphysis, multiple small fragments are seen. But on the lateral projection, some posterolateral contact is preserved between the main fragments *(arrow)*. The fracture must therefore be assigned to group 2 and not to group 3. There is no impaction. No fragment extends with its major portion into the diaphysis. Thus the fracture must be assigned to subgroup 2. It is classified as A2.2. There is a slight drift into valgus angulation and recurvation and a transverse fracture of the fibular diaphysis.

Example 2 (Fig. 116, p. 127)

The fracture is articular. We see a sagittal and dislocated lateral fracture line extending into the joint. A second, oblique fracture line adjacent to the medial malleolus appears to take a posterolateral course. The fracture is circular at the metaphysis (on the AP view, it is oblique and passes upward from medial to proximal laterally; it is T-shaped on the lateral view). Thus it is a C-type fracture. The AP radiograph reveals a trap-door depression of the articular surface. If the fracture were only partially articular, the depression in combination with the lateral and sagittal split would be allocated to subgroup B2.2. Since it is complete, planes are disregarded. Although the articular surface shows a double split and a depression, it is not disintegrated. Hence, it is either a C1- or C2-type fracture (split or split-depression of the joint). There is a lateral metaphyseal wedge, but no crushing or impaction. The fracture is therefore a circular articular fracture with depression and metaphyseal wedge: it is classified as C1.2. There is no angular deformity. The fibula is intact, and the medial malleolus appears to be an independent fragment.

Example 3 (Fig. 129, p. 136)

We find a lateral, sagittal split and a steplike incongruence of the articular surface; probably one fragment extending posterolaterally (posterior fragment demarcation on the lateral view?); no depression is visible. The fracture becomes circular in the metaphysis; hence it is a C-type fracture. The fracture is multifragmentary in the metaphysis. There is no impaction. The fracture is assigned to group C2. Two fragments extend with their major portion into the diaphysis determining subgroup 3. The fracture is classified as C2.3. There is a neutral axis, and the fibula shows a barely displaced transverse fracture at the level of the syndesmosis (the radiograph does not show the second, subcapital, fibular fracture). There appears to be a slight upward impaction of the articular surface.

■ *Chapter 4*

Operative Technique

1. HISTORICAL REVIEW AND PATIENT SELECTION

The history of medicine has seen frequent changes and even complete reversals of opinions and beliefs governing the treatment of choice for certain injuries. These developments are driven not only by basic research and technical innovations but likewise by the purpose and skill of the treating physician.

Closed reduction and plaster immobilization will only produce acceptable results if there is no displacement of the fracture. The method continues to be used [32] but has the following shortcomings: the rate of secondary dislocation, trophic impairments (osteodystrophy) associated with joint immobilization, and skin necrosis. In displaced fractures, better results were achieved as early as 1956 by Rieunau and Gay [165], who performed internal fixation of the concomitant fibular fracture (medullary wiring) in combination with plaster immobilization of the lower leg. The school of Böhler developed calcaneal traction as a technique involving accurate positioning of the pin or wire, and as the astonishing results of Jahna et al. [84] show, have brought it to a high degree of perfection.

The preference given to operative management of the main tibial fracture emerged quite early. Internal fixation of pilon split fractures was first demonstrated by Albin Lambotte in 1905. Lambotte used a combination of screw fixation and cerclage wiring [93] (Fig. 79). Further case reports were provided by Couvelaire and Rodier in 1937 [33] and by Trojan and Jahna in 1956 [196]. Another operative procedure of early times consisted in screw fixation of posterolateral fragments, which are particularly common in malleolar fractures. In French-speaking countries, these are still classified as pilon fractures [13, 20, 32, 159, 215].

Most authors, however, recommend open reduction and fixation of single, irreducible fragments instead of stable internal fixation of the fracture as a whole. The procedure is also recommended by Jahna et al. [84] as a supplement to accurate calcaneal drill traction.

Gay and Evrard [46] were the first to advocate operative stabilization of the complete tibial fracture and not of individual fragments only. The recommendation, however, was limited to simple fractures with large fragments. Even today we find some authorities still favoring this solution [19, 123, 149, 160]. From its beginning, the young AO-ASIF group was well aware that anatomic reduction and fixation of articular fractures were crucial for the prevention of secondary osteoarthrosis. Stable internal fixation should enable the patient to perform functional exercises and early motion without plaster immobilization, both of which are essential for nutritional bone requirements and cartilage regeneration.

The concept was expanded to include fractures of the tibial pilon, which, for operative and tactical reasons, were more difficult to approach. The tactic of the four-step procedure had been described in 1963 [1]. With the experience of the first 10 years, the AO operative technique was elaborated and defined in more detail. It is explained below [173].

The first publications of the AO aroused international attention and enthusiasm, and the treatment recommended was widely adopted. But soon it was realized that the results achieved in young patients with sports accidents could not be obtained in all cases. The standard set by the pioneering work of a few highly skilled surgeons working in comparatively small hospitals could not be equaled at major teaching hospitals where several surgeons shared the operative work [67, 168]. The rate of 80% to 90% of a favorable outcome was also regarded with skepticism.

The 1970s marked a significant change regarding the mechanism of accidents: there was an increase in traffic accidents, in open fractures, in patients with multiple injuries, and in falls of mentally ill patients. The associated soft tissue lesions came to the fore [116–118, 126, 192, 194]. In particular, in complex articular fractures the question arose whether well-positioned calcaneal traction, as suggested by Jahna et al. [84], would not achieve comparable functional results without entailing the risks of a technically demanding internal fixation. Subsequent research leading to the development of traction methods has led to the use of the external fixator. It combines the advantages of minimal soft tissue trauma with stabilization, and while no physical restrictions are imposed on adjacent joints, these may be mobilized to meet nutritional bone requirements. Well-known clinics worldwide have adopted this procedure. We refer here to the works of Lechevallier [103], Nordin [141, 142], Mast [116–118], Rüedi [170], Muhr [126], and Bone [17] and their co-workers.

The external fixator is also increasingly used to facilitate operative reduction and provide additional stabilization in the tissue-protecting, so-called minimal internal fixation of the tibia performed in complex fractures (see also sections 6 and 7). With regard to damage to the medial soft tissues, Vivès et al. [203] recommended the lateral approach for the tibial fracture and anterolateral plate fixation. In this procedure, the anterolateral muscles must be detached, which we consider precarious for biological reasons.

The experience of recent years has shown that the original AO technique must be modified to fit local circumstances. But the objectives remain unchanged, and the principles are rarely questioned [123, 126].

Anatomic restoration of the tibial articular surface should be attempted in simple as well as complex fractures. Only then will there be some prospect of proper healing with no or little arthrosis developing. This is of particular importance in younger patients. With the worldwide spread of AO techniques, we have, unfortunately, observed some decline in discipline.

The choice of treatment procedure for the individual patient is best described by Mast [118] and in Tile [192], whose algorithm is shown in Figure 140. Mast concludes with the observation that "problems resulting from this fracture can be divided in two categories: those related to the surgeon and his environment and those related to the severity of the fracture itself."

Only experienced and skilled surgeons should be entrusted with internal fixation of a complex pilon fracture. It is not only thorough preoperative planning that matters but purposeful and timely intervention. We firmly believe that this will lead to a decrease in infections, which in recent publications have been shown to have reached unacceptably high and alarming figures [20, 21, 127].

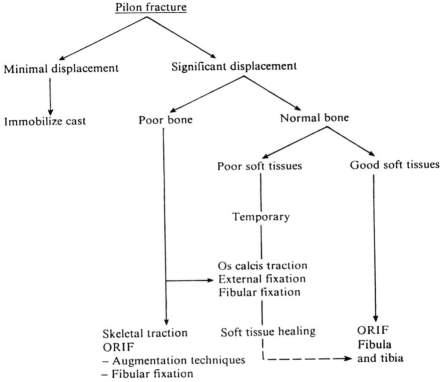

Figure 140. Algorithm for decision making in pilon fractures. ORIF, open reduction with internal fixation. [Adapted from Schatzker J, Tile M (1987). *The Rationale of Operative Fracture Care.* Heidelberg, Springer, p. 354.]

2. OPERATIVE TACTICS OF THE AO-ASIF

The surgeons of the AO-ASIF group are convinced that the best chances for functional recovery are achieved by operative reduction and stabilization, even in complex fractures of the distal tibia. While the operative techniques have evolved over time with the growing understanding of biological issues, the operative techniques defined in 1968 and repeatedly confirmed since then are beyond question for fractures without major soft tissue damage (see Figs. 141 and 142).

In *Technik der operativen Frakturenbehandlung* [129] ("Technique of Operative Fracture Care'') published in 1963, the operative techniques were outlined on the basis of individual case reports. The relevant chapter was written by M. Allgöwer. The experience gained on more than 80 cases led to a review and a codification of these basic AO principles in 1968 by Rüedi, Matter, and Allgöwer [173]. Today, they are well-established. They are explained and interpreted below and comprise the following steps:

1. Internal fixation of the fibula
2. Reconstruction of the tibial articular surface
3. Autogenous cancellous bone grafting of the defect
4. Medial buttressing

Figure 141. Stabilization of the fibula: schematic showing its indication and function. **A.** The initial dislocation: distal tibial fragments are impacted and pushed apart by the upper tibial cylinder. Lateral tibial fragments are attached to the distal fibula through the intact syndesmosis. Shortening and axial malalignment of the fibula. **B.** Axial and rotational realignment is achieved by reduction and stabilization of the fibula. The lateral fragment of the tibia allows determination of the accurate position of the articular surface.

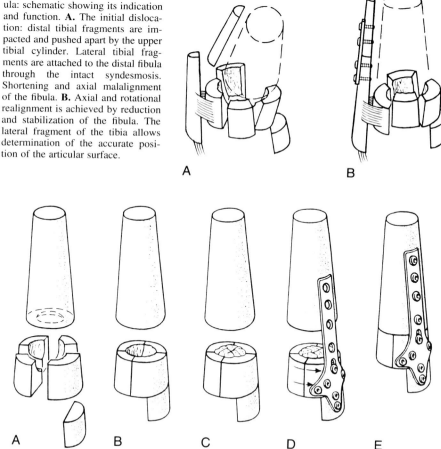

A   B

A   B   C   D   E

Figure 142. Schematic of various stages of surgery of the tibia. **A.** Fragmentation and dislocation with cancellous bone defect. **B.** Reduction of the epimetaphyseal elements. **C.** Packing of the defect with cancellous bone. **D.** The implant with its broad lower end clasps the fragments, pulling near them. **E.** The shaft of the plate will connect the epimetaphyseal block to the diaphysis.

Internal Fixation of the Fibula

The importance of reducing the fibular fracture for angular alignment and position-ing of the tibia was first recognized by Rieunau and Gay [165] in 1956. The significance of this initial phase is explained in Chapter 2, sections 1.3 and 3.2. For the main intervention on the tibia, the reduced and stabilized fibula serves as a useful indicator of angular alignment, rotation, and the articular level of the tibial joint surface. Another effect is the provisional reduction and fixation of the tibia. Once the tibia has been stabilized, the fibula is subject only slightly to bending and torsional forces, but much more to compression and tension. The mechanical relevance of internal fixation of the fibula is a key factor in complex and multifrag-mentary fractures of the tibia with a bone defect [14, 88, 175].

Unfortunately, we have occasionally observed some negligence toward these requisite operative techniques. Typical examples taken from our series are docu-mented in Figures 187, 189, and 202. Primary fixation of the concomitant fibular fracture is, with rare exceptions [21, 126], also recommended in fractures with medial soft tissue damage. It goes without saying that definitive management of the tibial fracture must follow as soon as possible. Achieving interfragmental axial compression, however, is technically realistic only in the simple forms.

Accurate reduction of complex diaphyseal fibular fractures is compounded by considerable technical difficulties [57]. It is for this reason that for such cases, Rüedi et al. [173] recommended in 1968 that the tibia be stabilized prior to internal fixation of the fibula. But with the techniques of indirect reduction now widely adopted (Fig. 154), the contraindication of primary fibular internal fixation has probably become obsolete, even in complex fractures.

Reconstruction of the Tibial Articular Surface

The technique of anatomic restoration of the articular surface in complex pilon fractures is highly demanding. The precision of the restoration will largely deter-mine the long-term prognosis of the joint, unless the joint doomed by damage to the cartilage [20, 29, 94, 100, 146]. The procedure is described in section 3.

If severe and inoperable disintegration is present, acceptable long-term results may be achieved by traction, particularly when it is combined with external fixation [84, 103].

In closed and open fractures with concomitant soft tissue damage, almost always on the medial side, one should try to reconstruct the tibial articular surface and to hold the fragments in place, whenever possible.

Autogenous Cancellous Bone Grafting of the Defect

Defects in cancellous bone are common in pilon fractures. They are located beneath the cartilage under trap-door or pestle-shaped depressions and become apparent after the latter have been reduced. Cancellous defects are regularly found once impactions and metaphyseal areas of multifragmentation have been reduced. Packing of these gaps is mandatory for mechanical reasons (risk of secondary collapse with angular deformity) and for biological reasons (risk of pseudarthrosis). Recently, the use of corticocancellous bone chips to provide additional buttress has been recommended by some authors [17, 170]. Details of this procedure are given in section 3.6.4.

If in an open fracture the soft tissues cannot be safely approximated, a primary cancellous bone graft should not be performed, as this would endanger its incorporation. The intervention for the cancellous bone graft will then be scheduled together with the skin-covering techniques of plastic surgery (see also sections 6 and 7).

Medial Buttressing

Medial fracture stabilization was first considered as a buttress [1, 129]. One was still influenced by the high incidence of secondary varus deformity or bony collapse on the anteromedial side of the tibial metaphysis that was seen after conservative treatment. It was Heim [55] who pointed out that complex fracture elements should be first reassembled into a closed block. He used the French term *assembler et embrasser* ("assemble and embrace"). In terms of tibial stabilization, this may be considered as the first step in the work sequence. In the second phase, the block of epiphyseal and metaphyseal fragments is joined to the diaphysis. This will only give the necessary mechanical support if the articular components are either comparatively simply structured and thoroughly fixed, or if the block can be anchored in the medial malleolus as a solid body.

Various implants may be used to accomplish reconstruction and stabilization of the tibial fracture (see section 3.6.4). Because of the soft tissue damage, however, there is increasing reluctance to use the plates initially employed. Under the designation of "minimal internal fixation," these are being replaced by Kirschner wires or individual small screws and combined with temporary application of an external fixator for additional support [21, 117, 127, 145, 150, 189, 211]. For details, see the explanations given in section 6.

3. STANDARD INTERNAL FIXATION OF THE PILON FRACTURE WITHOUT SOFT TISSUE DAMAGE

> Standard internal fixation is strictly reserved for fractures without significant soft tissue damage. It must be performed by an experienced surgeon.

The experiences gained from skiing accidents (closed fractures in young patients) provided the groundwork when in the late 1960s a group of young AO-ASIF surgeons attempted to standardize internal fixation of a pilon fracture. The model soon became well-established and has also proved suitable for the treatment of complex fractures in which there is no manifest soft tissue damage. Extraarticular fractures are managed with the same technique, particularly if a short distal main fragment, axial malalignment, fibular fracture, and fracture of the medial malleolus are present. Opening of the joint, however, should be avoided. An alternative technique recommended for this site consists of an unreamed interlocking nail. Its advantage is that there is no need to open the center of the fracture, thereby avoiding devitalization of comminuted areas. It may also be used in closed fractures with medial soft tissue damage. But the shorter the distance between the center of the fracture and the ankle joint, the greater the risks with this technique, namely, axial and rotatory malalignment, compartmental syndromes, and so forth [181].

So far the practical approach of the AO technique has not been laid out in detail, and we repeatedly observe that many surgeons are not familiar with all aspects of the method. Therefore it is appropriate to include a detailed description explaining the technique of reduction and some well-tested surgical skills.

3.1. Technique Used in Simple Fractures (Type B1)

Simple fractures are generally associated with only minor soft tissue damage. The approach then generally corresponds to that used in displaced fractures of other joints. Split fractures are reduced under vision and fixed with lag screws. The use of other implants is seldom indicated.

Because of the thin soft tissue envelope in this region, we must carefully select the appropriate approach. Considering circulatory aspects and innervation, and because of the difficulties involved, it is recommended that internal fixation be performed through the incisions described below. Of course, these may be extended slightly. To minimize tissue trauma with devitalization, connections between fracture fragments and the periosteum or the vascularized joint capsule should be spared by placing longitudinal incisions [2].

In fractures without fibular involvement, sufficient access is generally obtained by an anteromedial incision (Fig. 158). The presence of a fibular fracture or lateral tibial fragments usually requires a double incision unless percutaneous reduction of the lateral tibial fragments with pointed forceps is feasible. In these cases, the soft tissues may be spared by inserting a compressing screw (e.g., a cannulated screw over a Kirschner guidewire) through a laterally placed stab incision.

3.2. Diagnosis

A thorough diagnosis must precede any decision on the approach. The clinical examination must first assess the condition of the skin. Predominantly, this concerns the region around the medial malleolus. It must be noted that immediately after a trauma contusions may not be readily evident and abrasions may be difficult to evaluate in terms of their clinical significance. Of vital importance but hard to assess is the degree of local swelling. Swelling is crucial to the course and prognosis of the injury and is responsible for the most frequent complication after conservative as well as operative treatment: skin necrosis, which in turn leads to the dreaded infection of deep structures (see section 5.3). Swelling may be produced by directly acting external forces (contusion) and by internal fragment pressure or fracture hematoma.

Contrary to malleolar fractures, where the swelling presents as a hemarthrosis, this is not the case in pilon fractures. In the former, immediate evacuation is performed. Thus direct reduction of internal pressure is achieved with subsequent skin relief. Skin blisters and the development of necrosis are prevented. In pilon fractures, the situation is different. The joint contains little blood. Blood is carried upward through the fragments and the pierced periosteum and enters fascial and subcutaneous spaces. A collarlike imbibition of the distal lower leg ensues, which is composed of a mixture of blood and edema fluid. Because of the poorly distensible soft tissue envelope at this site, this tends to be a specific preoperative complication in pilon fractures (Fig. 143).

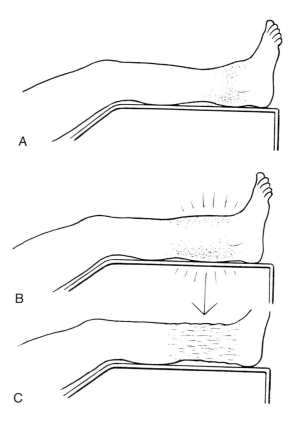

Figure 143. Posttraumatic swelling at the ankle and around the distal tibia. **A.** The swelling in malleolar fractures is typically limited to the ankle joint (hemarthrosis). An early operation will relieve tension. **B.** The typical swelling in pilon fractures involves the distal third of the leg and produces tension and shining of the skin. **C.** Once the tension has subsided, the skin has a dim appearance with fine creases.

A

B

C

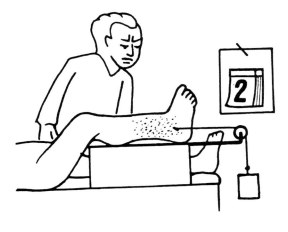

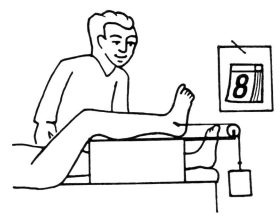

Figure 144. The surgeon assessing the condition of the soft tissues. The swelling usually reaches its maximum after 2 days. Eight days later, tension and swelling have died down.

Figure 145. The time required (P.M.) for the study of multiple radiographs when planning the details of the operation.

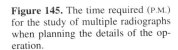

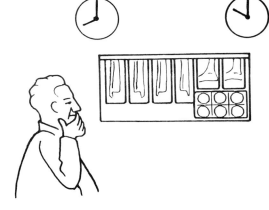

Swelling may develop with or without delay, depending on individual factors. We assume that temperature differences between indoors and outdoors play a role. Our observation is that swelling appears particularly pronounced after skiing accidents where the patient is moved quickly from the cold into a heated hospital room. It is important to know that the broad imbibition of the subcutis cannot be removed efficiently by an operative incision. Its spontaneous resorption should be awaited. When the hematoma extends into muscle spaces, compartmental syndromes are menacing. These may become manifest within hours after the accident [30, 194, 201]. Dorsal flexion of the hallux is an indication of an impending anterior tibial compartment syndrome. On clinical examination, imminent posterior compartment syndromes easily go unnoticed in recently injured patients because the pain is less severe, and clinical testing is impracticable before operative stabilization.

It goes without saying that the clinical examination must also include evaluation of the peripheral arterial circulation and innervation. The swelling may be so pronounced as to preclude palpation of the foot pulses. This is why the assessment must primarily be based on the microcirculation (toes). Sensorimotor disturbances of the foot are rare in pilon fractures and are confined to open fractures with marked displacement.

Appropriate testing is pivotal in patients in whom concomitant injuries proximal to the fracture are present (see Chapter 2, section 2.1); this concerns especially fractures of proximal tibial segment 41 or the spine. In patients with multiple trauma, examination may be difficult or even impossible. Motor function may only be tested by active movement of the toes, particularly the hallux. The metatarsus and calcaneus are too close to the pain radiating from the fracture site.

The test for sensory function includes both the plantar and the dorsal parts of the foot. The lateral and the medial sides must be examined separately, and special attention is given to the interdigital space I-II (early manifestation of an anterior tibial compartment syndrome; see section 5.2.2).

It is essential to report all findings of the clinical examination, even those that are normal. Only then will it be possible to differentiate between traumatic and iatrogenic lesions in the event of later impairments. The physician should also be wary of more remote concomitant injuries, which are especially common in traffic accidents. They may bear a considerable influence on the approach to the pilon fracture. Faultless radiographs are vital for the diagnosis of injuries to bones and ligaments. Standard films in two projections are often insufficient. Axial deviations may complicate adequate focusing. The first radiographs are often of poor quality and repeat films are required. Additional oblique films may provide useful information.

Conventional tomography [118], available today in almost all major hospitals, has proved useful when depression is suspected, and complements the CT scan [170].

3.3. Preoperative Guidelines

In this discussion we concentrate on the technical details of more complicated fractures (A2, A3, and in particular, B3, C2, and C3). Experience has shown that these fractures may pose extra problems at operation.

3.3.1. General Remarks

When the patient is admitted to hospital, the question is whether the definitive operative reconstruction should be carried out as an emergency and single-stage-procedure, or whether a two-stage-procedure (limited emergency measures and planned internal fixation) should be performed. Often, the decision depends on external circumstances (patients with multiple injuries, open fractures). Emergency measures may be inevitable because of gross dislocations and severe pain. Both approaches, i.e., emergency internal fixation and the two-stage procedure, have well-known advantages and disadvantages. These will be briefly reviewed:

Advantages of the Emergency Intervention

1. Psychological advantage for the patient who experiences the accident and the operation as one chronological entity (only one period of pain and anxiety).
2. No nosocomial infections.
3. The risk of thromboembolism is lower.

Advantages of the Operation in Two Stages

1. Reinforcement of the relationship between the physician, the patient, and the family; the patient is mentally prepared for the main intervention and is encouraged to actively cooperate during the postoperative period.
2. A comprehensive evaluation of the patient's general state of health, concomitant injuries, and local findings (additional radiographic examinations if necessary) is possible.
3. No time pressure with the preoperative preparation of the patient.
4. The optimal surgical team will be available.
5. If the swelling has subsided, the incidence of impaired wound healing is lower [21, 30, 67, 121, 211].

Currently, most authors favor delay of the main intervention [17, 79, 170, 192]. Emergency operation of a closed fracture should only be carried out under highly favorable circumstances (fresh injury, experienced surgeon). The distal lower leg shows some local features requiring consideration:

1. The swelling reaches its maximum between the second and the fourth day. In the absence of primary skin contusions or abrasions, we have not observed skin

blisters if calcaneal traction had been applied. Should skin blisters occur, this would necessitate further delay of the internal fixation.

> Posttraumatic swelling is unpredictable. It may jeopardize the result.

2. The ligamentous complex is almost always intact in pilon fractures. In consequence, realignment as well as reduction of major tibial fragments (ligamentotaxis) may be effected by simple traction. The excellent results obtained by accurately placed traction and manual reduction are demonstrated in the comprehensive series of Jahna et al. [84].

3. The bony structures have a significantly better blood supply than the skin and subcutaneous tissues [2]. Conservative treatment will never lead to fragment necrosis [46, 84].

The best approach is probably to make decisions based on the circumstances of the individual case and not to adhere to rigid principles. The following options are available:

- Primary internal fixation
- Primary application of traction alone (Kirschner wire or external fixator) with delayed internal fixation
- Primary internal fixation of the fibula combined with provisional measures on the tibia (see section 3.3)
- Transfer to a specialized clinic

If the decision is made to perform delayed internal fixation of the tibia, the timing for the operation must be determined by a daily clinical examination. According to our experience, the operation may be performed when the swelling starts to subside. This is indicated when the shiny appearance of the skin turns mat, and very fine creases appear (Figs. 143, 144).

Undue delay jeopardizes the vitality of the articular cartilage and complicates anatomic restoration, which is most successful when done before granulation tissue has formed. A maximum of 2 or 3 weeks should be allowed for the healing of manifest soft tissue damages [17, 79, 192].

If a two-stage procedure has been chosen, the following emergency measures must be carried out:

1. A traction or distraction system is set up to achieve provisional reduction (correction of angular deformities, distraction of grossly displaced fragments) and immobilization (alleviation of pain). Calcaneal traction (Kirschner wire with loop or Steinmann pin) or the external fixator is generally used.

2. Elevation of the leg to control swelling. As this may favor the development of compartmental syndromes, close observation for early recognition is mandatory (cf. section 5.2.2).

3. Immediate initiation of drug therapy to prevent thromboembolism. Differ-

ent regimens are used in various institutions. Prior to the intervention, adjustment of the dosage is required.

4. Evaluation and, if necessary, therapy of preexisting conditions and diseases.

5. The following are required during the days preceding the operation: additional radiologic investigations (oblique projections, tomograms, CT scan) (Fig. 145), designation of the surgeon allowing him or her time for adequate preparation; daily examination of the patient; and choosing the optimal time for the internal fixation (Fig. 144).

6. Informing and motivating the patient with regard to active functional exercises after the operation. Encouragement with regard to the main intervention.

7. Antibiotic prophylaxis is routine in many hospitals today. It begins just before the operation itself.

Choose the date of the planned operation in accordance with soft tissue conditions and prepare all particulars carefully.

3.3.2. Preparation of the Operative Site

1. Disinfection and draping of the iliac crest for bone harvesting prior to the main intervention (the iliac crest is the preferred donor site).

2. A tourniquet is applied to the upper leg. Tourniquet time should be kept to a minimum; if possible, it should be confined to the time needed for reduction and provisional fixation.

3. The position of the injured leg corresponds to that of the malleolar fracture. External or internal rotation of the patient's lower leg may be achieved when the leg is elevated, the knee partially flexed, and the operating table slightly tilted. Almost all posterior structures and in particular the posteromedial tibial wall are then brought into view from the side (Fig. 146). Disinfection and sterile draping should include the knee joint, thereby enabling the surgeon to harvest cancellous bone from the tibial plateau (second choice of donor site) during the operation, if necessary.

4. The following disposition of the operating team has proved efficient for internal fixation of complex fractures (Figs. 147, 148): The operator sits at the lower end of the operating table. He or she will repeatedly shift from the lateral to the medial side and back again, using a stool on castors. Accordingly, the instrument nurse will take his or her position either on the operator's right or left side. Two assistants are needed, one placed medially and the other laterally. Both remain standing and keep their place. The more experienced assistant takes the lateral side.

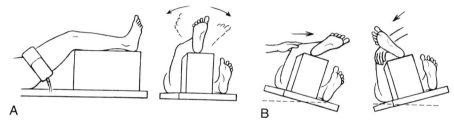

Figure 146. Positioning of the patient for internal fixation in the region of the ankle joint. **A.** The lower leg is elevated on a firmly padded rest. The uninjured leg below allows free access to the medial side. The knee in flexion permits adequate rotational movement of the foot. **B.** Rotation of the foot may be improved by tilting the operating table and by one assistant applying manual pressure onto the knee so that undisturbed visualization of the posterolateral and posteromedial aspects of the fracture is obtained.

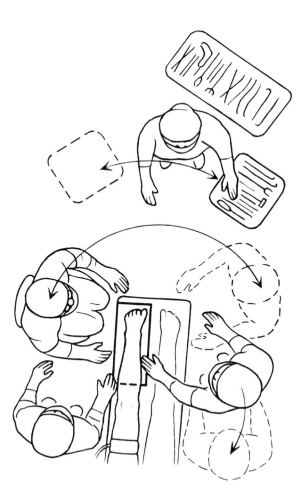

Figure 147. The surgical team viewed from above and the changes of positions during the operation *(dashed lines)*. The surgeon sits on a mobile chair which is moved alternately to the lateral and medial sides. The two assistants stand, and the scrub nurse shifts her table with the instruments.

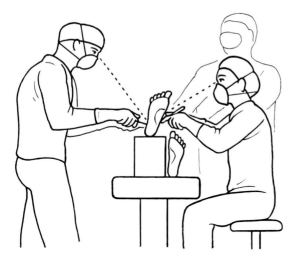

Figure 148. The surgical team standing, viewed from distally.

3.4. Harvesting Cancellous Bone (Preliminary)

The majority of complex tibial fractures require a cancellous bone graft: it serves either to pack defects produced by the reduction of cancellous impactions or articular depressions, or for the biological reinforcement of comminuted areas. To promote rapid integration of the graft, it is best to use only high-quality autogenous cancellous bone. Biological and mechanical considerations make the pelvis the preferred donor site. If the lesser intervention is carried out as a separate and preliminary operation, tourniquet time may be limited to the tibial phase of the operation. The patient's informed consent to this additional intervention must be obtained before the operation. If the defect is expected to be significant, remove cancellous and corticocancellous grafts from the iliac bone as the first step of the planned operation.

Technique of Bone Harvesting (Fig. 149)

A longitudinal incision is made over the iliac crest. The bone is exposed by dissecting the muscles. Hemostasis is obtained. The iliopsoas muscle is retracted from the inner wing of the ileum using a wide raspatory. The lateral cutaneous nerve of the thigh passing in the muscles close to the pelvic wall must be spared during preparation. A deeply inserted bone lever retracts the muscles toward the abdomen. Corticocancellous bone chips are harvested from the inner table of the iliac wall or the iliac crest using a gouge or a curette. The amount of cancellous bone required is estimated. If during the intervention it proves to be insufficient, it may be supplemented by cancellous bone from the upper tibia.

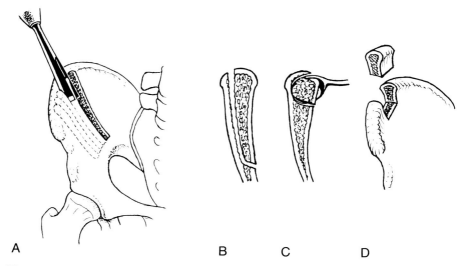

Figure 149. Harvesting cancellous and corticocancellous bone from the pelvis. **A, B.** Corticocancellous chips are obtained from the inner side of the iliac bone using a hollow chisel. **C.** Cancellous bone is taken from the iliac crest with a curette. **D.** A corticocancellous block is removed from the ilaic crest.

Hemostasis is usually unsatisfactory. Absorbable, hemostatic gauze may be pressed into the donor site. The muscles detached from the iliac crest will have to be fastened back again. The use of a suction drain is precluded, because aspiration from the cancellous wound would result in enormous loss of blood. This is why a closed, nonsuction drain is inserted in most cases or no drainage at all is performed. Hematomas frequently develop, but infections are rare. Local pain may persist for some time, and may be troubling. The wound is closed, a protective dressing is applied, and instruments and operating gowns are changed. Until the time of implantation, the graft material is stored separately in a gauze soaked in Ringer's solution.

3.5. Internal Fixation of the Fibular Fracture

3.5.1. Patient Selection

The indication of internal fixation for a fibular fracture is undisputed. Even in open fractures or in fractures with medial soft tissue damage, it is generally recommended. Internal fixation is the initial step in the operative approach according to the AO [173]. This rule applies primarily to pilon fractures, but also holds true for unstable extraarticular fractures with displaced fracture of the fibula.

Anatomic reduction of the fibula restores axial and rotational malalignment. It provides an indicator for the correct orientation of the tibial articular surface. Because the ligamentous apparatus is preserved, the fibula remains bound to the tibia and is displaced along with the latter. It is referred to as a "lateral pillar" [185], "buttress to the lateral joint" [16], or as *attelle péronière* ("fibular splint") [203]. It absorbs the asymmetric forces acting on the tibial articular surface and the metaphysis. From our series it is clear that these are most commonly valgus forces. If the dislocation drifts into varus angulation, the stabilized fibula will assume a tension band function. If a malleolar fracture is stabilized, the plate is supposed to neutralize comparatively weak bending and torsional forces, but here the construction must resist axial compression.

No special benefits are achieved by internal fixation of the fibula if the main tibial fracture consists of simple and large fragments. This holds true, e.g., for extraarticular wedge fractures, where a broad contact is present between the main fragments. In such cases, bending forces are neutralized by a strong medial implant (e.g., a straight 4.5-mm plate). Bending of the tibial plate will then exert a tension band effect on the laterally acting valgus forces (Fig. 150A).

The situation is similar to that of the classic tibial plate in diaphyseal fractures. Torn syndesmotic ligaments or irreducible dislocations are then the only indications requiring additional stabilization of the fibula [72].

> Reduction and internal fixation of the fibula must consider the future axial load on this lateral pillar.

3.5.2. Technique

In the literature available so far, the technique of fibular fixation is not described. Apparently, it is falsely assumed to be identical with the procedure in malleolar fractures. We have discussed the different biomechanical aspects, but peculiarities must also be observed regarding the approach.

Incision, Approach, and Reconstruction

Consistent with the operative plan to start with fixation of the fibula, we begin with the lateral incision while carefully planning the location of the large, medial incision to be made later. From the outset, access to the fibula is restricted because we must keep a skin bridge of at least 6 to 7 cm between the two incisions. The Basel school [130] recommends making the fibular incision slightly more posterior, as they place the tibial incision more to the anterior side ending it at the medial malleolus in a slight curve (Fig. 151B). Heim [55] recommends placing the tibial incision more closely to the edge of the medial malleolus. This opens the possibility of starting the lateral incision behind the fibula, making it cross the fibula above the malleoli, and finishing it below anteriorly (Fig. 151A), thereby facilitating access to anterolateral tibial fragments, as is frequently required.

Immediately beneath the skin the sensory branch of the superficial peroneal nerve must be identified and spared. Its course is highly variable. In most cases it emerges from the fascia of the anterior tibial muscle, but in some cases from the peroneal compartment.

Exposure is initially confined to the fibular fracture, and is extended as needed for reduction and trial fitting of the plate. If subsequently the approach allows control of the anterior syndesmotic ligament and reduction of the anterolateral tibial fragments, the cruciform ligament must be incised and the long extensor muscles retracted medially (Fig. 152).

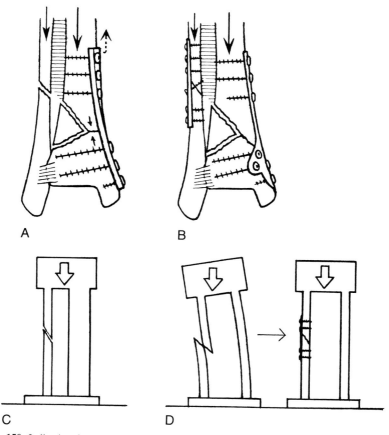

Figure 150. Indication for internal fixation of the fibula in an extraarticular fracture. **A.** There is no need to stabilize the fibula when the assembly on the tibia is of optimal stability: a strong medial implant and interfragmentary compression. The implant will also absorb bending forces. **B.** A loadbearing internal fixation of the fibula is essential for fracture patterns in which meticulous interfragmentary compression is precluded. The same holds true when a weak medial implant would fail to withstand bending forces. **C.** Diagram showing two columns: a strong and a fractured, thin column. The strong column will tolerate asymmetric compression forces without deformation. **D.** Diagram showing two thin columns: asymmetric pressure will bend and break the intact column. To resist this force, stabilization of the fractured column is necessary.

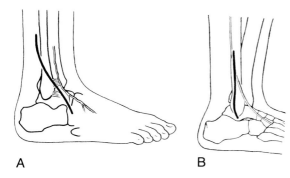

A   B

Figure 151. The lateral incisions. **A.** As recommended by Heim and Pfeiffer [70]: the incision crosses the fibula and is terminated below anteriorly. This approach also provides adequate exposure of the anterolateral tibial metaphysis. The terminal branch of the superficial peroneal nerve is shown. **B.** Incision of Müller et al. [130]: the incision runs parallel to the fibula and is placed slightly more posteriorly so that the skin bridge to the tibial incision is larger.

Figure 152. The lateral approach to deeply situated structures. After incision of the cruciform ligament, the long extensor muscles and the terminal branch of the superficial peroneal nerve are pulled medially with the blunt retractor. The joint capsule has not yet been incised. The fibula, anterior syndesmotic ligament, distal interosseous membrane, and anterolateral tibial metaphysis are exposed.

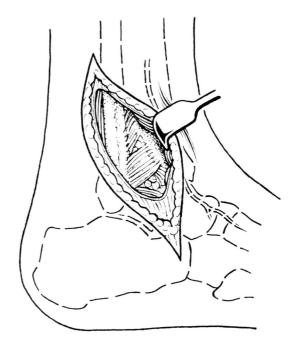

Figure 153. The inclination of the lateral surface of the distal fibula changes its angle from proximal to distal. The plate must be precisely adapted to the anatomy by bending and contouring. [From Heim U, Pfeiffer KM (1973). *Small Fragment Set Manual.* Heidelberg, Springer, p 205.]

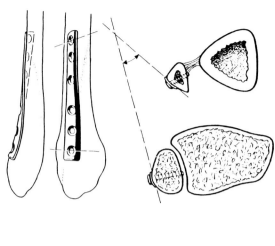

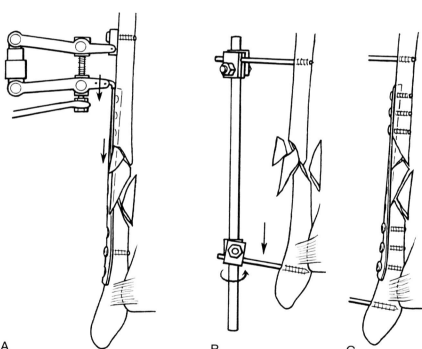

A   B   C

Figure 154. Indirect reduction of a multifragmentary fibular fracture to avoid devitalization. **A.** A long, one-third tubular plate partially attached distally and twisted for trial fitting. Reduction is achieved by pulling with a tension device on which the hook has been reversed. **B.** Indirect reduction using the small external fixator: threaded Kirschner wires 2.5-mm (or fine Schanz screws) are inserted as far away from the fracture as possible to avoid axial dislocation while pulling. Reduction is achieved by means of distraction. Rotational adjustments may be made. **C.** Finished plate assembly in which fixation of both main fragments has been carried out; the area of multifragmentation has been left untouched without attempting anatomic reduction.

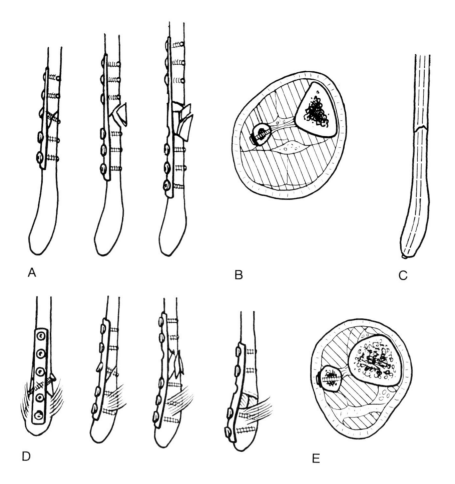

Figure 155. Assemblies used for various forms of fibular fractures. **A.** Around the diaphysis, a five-hole one-third tubular plate is used to exert interfragmentary compression for a simple oblique fracture; a six-hole plate is used for a wedge fracture without attempting to reduce the wedge; and an eight-hole plate is used for a multifragmentary fracture. **B.** Diaphyseal cross section: musculature surrounds the fibula completely. **C.** A thin medullary nail is only suitable with a combination of lateral soft tissue damage, simple transverse fracture, and valgus position. Under such conditions, the buttress is stronger than with a plate according to Tile [192]. **D.** Fractures of the metaphysis: for a simple oblique fracture, a five-hole plate and separate interfragmentary lag screw or interfragmentary lag screw applied through the plate; a six-hole plate to bridge an area of multifragmentation at the metaphyseal-diaphyseal junction which deliberately has been left without anatomic reduction; a five-hole plate to bridge a metaphyseal bone defect (interposition of a corticocancellous bone chip). **E.** Metaphyseal cross section: only the anteromedial and posterolateral aspects of the fibula are covered by musculature.

Reduction and Stabilization

A thorough knowledge of the fracture patterns described in Chapter 2, section 1.3, is essential for adequate internal fixation of the fibula. A simple fibular fracture may easily be reduced and stabilized. In an oblique fracture, interfragmental compression is achieved by a lag screw applied through a plate, less frequently by inserting a separate lag screw between the fragments (Fig. 155). Attention should be paid to the following situations:

INTERNAL FIXATION OF THE FIBULAR DIAPHYSIS

In simple fractures, splinting of the medullary cavity continues to be used in some places [192], but it is important to preserve the physiologic valgus curvature of the lower fibula (Fig. 155C).

When a fracture of the diaphysis is present, the wedge or a complex fracture pattern predominates. The standard technique, i.e., initial screw fixation of the wedge to one main fragment, is often precluded in wedge fractures. A good view is often obstructed by the circular muscle envelope, but if fragments are embedded in the muscle, these maintain their vitality. Forced reduction by the insertion of cerclage wires would then produce undue additional trauma.

Our experience has shown rapid consolidation of diaphyseal fibular fractures even though wedge fragments have not been reduced or only incompletely reduced. If the fragments maintain their vitality, an early callus bridge is formed. Management consists in application of a buttressing device linking the two main fragments. In comminuted fractures, it is best to bridge the comminution with a plate of adequate length, leaving the fragments untouched if possible. Fracture union is remarkable if four, or better, six cortical threads are used to attach the plate to each main fragment (see Fig. 155A). We ascribe this to the circular muscle envelope. The technical difficulty encountered in complex fractures is determining precisely the length and rotation of the fibula. In such cases, the method of indirect reduction is of special value:

Distraction may be achieved with the reversed tension device in combination with a plate temporarily applied to the lower fibula (Fig. 154A), but then rotation must be previously adjusted by twisting the plate.

Alternatively, distraction is achieved with the small fixator. The Schanz screws must be inserted as far away as possible from the fracture site, and they must be placed so as not to impede the final positioning of the plate. Using the small fixator as a distractor with only two Schanz screws provides the advantage of correcting rotational malalignment (Fig. 154B).

FIXATION OF THE FIBULA WHEN THERE IS
MULTIFRAGMENTATION OR IMPACTION ABOVE THE
MALLEOLI

Again, the plate is recommended as a buttressing device. In this region, assessment of fibular length and rotation tends to be easier than at the diaphysis, and may be achieved with simpler means.

At this level, the muscular envelope comprises only two sides of the fibula (Fig. 155D). Fracture union is generally good. Bone defects require a cancellous graft. Impaired fracture healing (delayed consolidation, nonunion) was found in a few cases where a plate had been attached to the anterolateral aspect of the tibia (deterioration of the vascular supply to the fibula as a result of detaching the anterior muscle envelope?). Vivès et al. [203], who use the technique routinely, do not comment on this point.

IMPLANTS

The one-third tubular plate is the implant used in the vast majority of diaphyseal, metaphyseal, and segmental fractures of the fibula. A medullary wire may be superior to the plate in cases where lateral soft tissue damage is combined with a simple transverse fracture of the diaphysis. Simple supramalleolar torsional fractures or long oblique fractures are rarely managed with screw fixation alone (20 cases in our series). In the distal area of cancellous bone, Kirschner wires are occasionally found.

3.5.3. Results

The 1-year follow-up results of our series are probably the best proof of how important internal fixation of the fibula is (cf. Appendix, section 3). We summarize:

1. Failure to perform internal fixation resulted in ten cases in secondary valgus deformity in groups A2, A3, and C2 (Fig. 187). The tendency to drift into valgus angulation could be halted or, in two other patients, corrected only by secondary internal fixation of the fibula (Fig. 202).

2. All segmental fractures healed without complication. Management consisted either in one long or two short one-third tubular plates.

3. Delayed consolidation was found in 15 plated fibulas. In ten cases, this concerned multifragmentary and complex fractures, and in only two cases simple fractures. The diaphysis was affected in four cases, the diaphyseal-metaphyseal border in four cases, and the area above the syndesmosis in seven cases. Eight patients developed valgus deformity, and two developed varus deformity (cf. Chapter 2, section 3). Rupture of the mortise was not observed in any of these cases, which demonstrates once again the amount of axial compression an intact syndesmosis is able to resist. With secondary displacement, loosening of the plate associated with bending or fracture of plate screws occurred. The buttressing one-third tubular plate, however, always remained intact (Fig. 185).

4. In two cases an atrophic pseudarthrosis was found which was located above the malleoli and occurred after a simple fracture (in one case following infection).

5. Of 20 screw fixations, 19 healed without complications. In one case secondary valgus deformity developed as a result of pressure induced by delayed consolidation of the tibia.

6. Following Kirschner wiring, one case of delayed consolidation in valgus position was observed.

Examples

Radiographs illustrating the technique of internal fixation of the fibula and the postoperative course are given in Figures 174–187, 190, and 204.

Complications resulting from inadequate fibular stabilization or failure to perform internal fixation of the fibula are shown in Figures 175, 176, 185, 187, 189, 202, and 205.

3.6. Internal Fixation of the Tibia (Type C2)

3.6.1. Skin Incisions

The incisions must be selected for the way in which they provide adequate visualization of the important fracture elements. These are identified on preoperative radiographs. Each approach requires consideration of the vascular supply to bone, subcutaneous tissue, and skin [2].

The lateral incision was described above. A skin bridge of at least 6 cm or, better, 7 cm must be left between the incisions so as not to compromise skin perfusion. Sufficient distance must be kept from the tendon of the anterior tibial muscle, whose gliding system must be spared [118].

The Basel school has opted for a fairly anterior tibial skin incision ending in a curve below the medial malleolus (Fig. 156C). Consequently, the lateral incision must be placed relatively posteriorly (Fig. 151B). Heim [55] recommended placing the lateral incision nearer the medial malleolus, continuing it in a gentle curve, and extending it far distally (Fig. 156A) instead. The intention is to avoid the creation of dangerous skin flaps. With the extension, posteromedial fragments and fissures may be exposed without tension if the tendon sheath of the posterior tibial muscle has been incised.

After incision of the skin, the medial periosteum is exposed directly without dissecting the subcutaneous tissues. The anterior border of the medial malleolus serves as a landmark. Occasionally, it is necessary to separate the greater saphenous vein between two ligatures. The joint is opened with a moderate longitudinal incision. Anterior fragments remain attached to the joint capsule (Fig. 158B). A synovial margin is preserved at the medial malleolus since this will facilitate suturing at wound closure. Vivès et al. [203] recommended making only one anterolateral incision in cases with medial soft tissue damage. From this approach, internal fixation of both fractures is carried out (anterolateral position of the tibial plate).

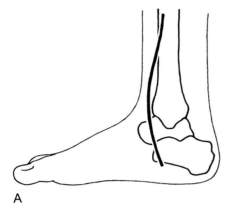

A

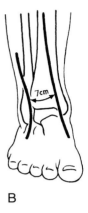

B

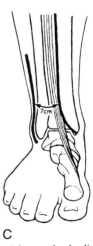

C

Figure 156. Tibial incisions for standard internal fixations of pilon fractures. **A.** A long and only slightly curved incision extending far distally, as recommended by Heim [55]. **B.** Anterior view of the relation between the medial and the lateral incisions. The skin bridge in between (supplied by the anterior tibial artery) should measure, whenever possible, 7 cm. **C.** The tibial incision according to the *Manual of Internal Fixation* [130] is placed more anteriorly; it is shorter and ends in a curve. The distance wanted between the two incisions amounts to 7 cm.

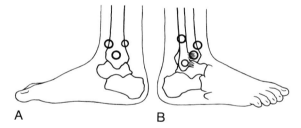

Figure 157. The critical sites *(circled)* to be exposed at revision. The order in which they are listed below indicates their practical significance. **A.** Medial approach: (1) anterior tibial metaphysis, (2) medial malleolus, (3) the posterior wall (if necessitated by the course of the fracture line). **B.** Lateral approach: (1) fracture of the fibula, (2) anterior syndesmotic ligament and tubercle of Tillaux-Chaput, (3) anterolateral tibial metaphysis, (4) distal lateral ligamentous complex (if necessary).

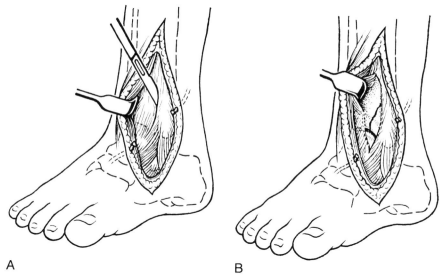

Figure 158. The medial approach to deep structures. **A.** The greater saphenous vein is divided between ligatures. The soft tissues are carefully retracted laterally. Incision of the joint capsule is made close to the medial malleolus with proximal extension. **B.** Exposure of the anteromedial fracture lines. The soft tissues are retracted laterally at the level of the syndesmosis; a possibly required visualization up to the lateral incision may be accomplished at this site. The joint capsule maintains its continuity with the anterior articular fragments.

Massari et al. [115] occasionally employed an additional posterolateral incision giving access to posterolateral fragments.

> The important rule to be observed with the medial incision is to place it at sufficient distance from the lateral incision.

Special Features of Exposure

1. Regarding the lateral incision, the reader is referred to the explanations given above.

2. Free dissection of the anterior tibial tendon is to be avoided to prevent a postoperative bowstring effect (bowing of the tendon is seen under the skin). This point is also mentioned by Mast et al. [116].

3. Marginal fragments mostly remain attached to the joint capsule. Thus, devitalization will not occur. When the joint is opened, the anterior capsule must be very carefully handled (Fig. 158).

3.6.2 Review of Bone Injuries

The systematic examination of the fracture must consider the following injuries (Fig. 157):

- From the lateral approach: the anterior syndesmotic ligament, anterolateral fragments in the region of the tubercle of Tillaux-Chaput, and lateral aspects of the talar trochlea (cartilage damage).
- From the medial approach: anteromedial articular and metaphyseal fragments and the medial trochlea of the talus (cartilage damage); deeply situated depressions and centrally located, deep incongruences are easily missed from the anteromedial view (see below).
- Posterior fragments are exposed by incising the tendon canal of the posterior tibial muscle behind the medial malleolus (Fig. 161F).

> Periosteal and capsular attachments to anterior fragments should be carefully preserved during reduction.

3.6.3. Reduction and Provisional Fixation

Study of the preoperative radiographs determines the strategy of reduction and allows identification of the ''key fragments,'' the central points of fragmentation. They serve as guiding posts for reduction and provisional fixation.

Figure 159. Anterior view of a complex fracture. **A.** Before internal fixation of the fibula; it is uncertain how the numerous elements relate to one another. **B.** Following internal fixation of the fibula; because the anterior syndesmotic ligament has remained intact, the anterolateral tibial fragment may serve as a guide indicating the level and position of the remaining articular fragments. [From Heim U (1972). Le traitement chirurgical des fractures du pilon tibial. *J Chir (Paris)* 104:307–322.]

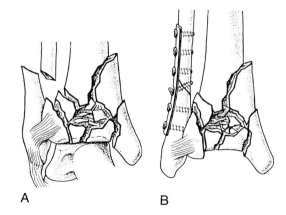

A   B

Reduction Tactics

All reduction maneuvers are performed under direct vision. The anteromedial view is the most important, followed by the anterolateral view (Fig. 152). Even though radiographs are time-consuming and often unsatisfactory because of poor focusing or exposure, they are essential as final records. During reduction, short observation periods with the image intensifier may be helpful, but adequate focusing of the ankle joint tends to be difficult.

Fragment reduction is facilitated by the manual application of traction to the foot. The assistant appointed to carry out this maneuver will be thankful when a Steinmann pin inserted preoperatively into the calcaneus is left in place. This makes traction as well as dorsiflexion of the foot easier, but the forces applied are irregular and uneven. Recently, the use of the external fixator or a distractor applied to the medial side has been recommended as an aid to reduction [117] (Fig. 198). Schanz screws are inserted in the tibial diaphysis as well as in the neck of the talus or in the calcaneus. Distraction may be slowly and gradually increased, and the subsequent reduction maneuvers are carried out under controlled conditions. These traction maneuvers, however, increase tension in the soft tissues, especially the skin, and may complicate visualization of deeper structures.

Any reduction maneuver might lead to displacement of previously reduced opposing fragments. The effects of each step on the total fracture and soft tissues must therefore be continuously monitored. While the operator is working on one side, the assistant on the opposite side takes on these responsibilities (Fig. 148).

Observing a definite sequence while performing the various steps of the complicated reduction procedure has proved to be efficient. The main articular finding is tackled first: start with removal of depressions, then restore anatomic congruence of the joint surface, and finish by managing any remaining diastases. In most cases, the last-named have been spontaneously corrected during the earlier two maneuvers. During reduction of the metaphyseal components, most problems are encountered on the anterolateral side. Here, visualization is limited proximally, and the preliminary stabilization of the fibular fracture may have caused a slight drift into varus position with irreducible fragments.

Instruments That Should Be at Hand (Fig. 160)

- Variously curved elevators for retraction or elevation of fragments.
- An awl or thick Kirschner wire mounted in a holder. The pointed tip of these instruments allows poking and levering without slipping.
- A bent retractor with one prong which allows pulling without slipping.
- A fine and sharp raspatory to expose fragment edges.
- An impactor that allows pressure to be applied without sinking into the bone (in French-speaking countries, a highly practical instrument is available, the *fouloir* with four fine prongs).
- Assorted reduction forceps, which can be operated with one hand; the most important type is the pointed, widely grasping reduction forceps. The wide pelvic reduction forceps, of which one branch may be fixed percutaneously to the bone, allows even better grasping and careful handling of the soft tissues.
- Bone spreaders (both small and large) to allow careful separation of fissures and splits.
- A compressed air machine ready to drive Kirschner wires of 1.6-mm diameter for temporary fixation of reduced fragments. If cannulated screws are to be inserted, Kirschner wires of 1.2-mm diameter must be used.

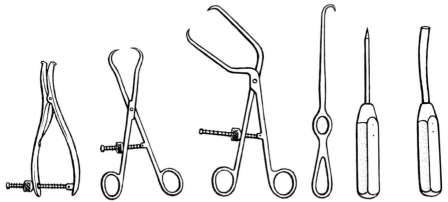

Figure 160. Some useful instruments for the reduction of pilon fractures. *From left to right:* small distraction forceps; angulated forceps with points; pelvic forceps; sharp hook; awl; impactor.

Reduction Maneuvers and Tricks

- Jammed pestle-form depressions: the first step in releasing these is to separate adjacent fissures with the elevator or bone spreader (Fig. 161A). Subsequently, they are reduced with the impactor using the trochlea as a buttress, if necessary. Pestle-form depressions do not always produce a cancellous bone defect (Fig. 109B).
- The same procedure is used to reduce trap-door depressions in order to prevent the development of axial deviations or additional fragmentation during reduction.
- To correct medially or centrally located steplike incongruences, it is recommended that the fractured medial malleolus be opened and turned aside (Fig. 161C). This maneuver was described by Weber in 1967 [207].

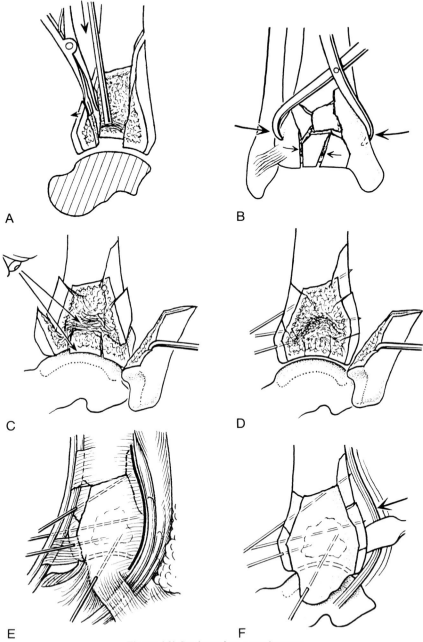

A

B

C

D

E

F

Figure 161 *See legend on opposite page*

- If posterior and anterior impactions occur in combination, the posterior fragments tend to be large and only slightly displaced. In these cases, the posterior wall may be held temporarily by applying gentle pressure with a bone lever inserted along the posterior aspect of the tibia while the anterior fragments are being reduced. Occasionally, an elevator or pointed reduction forceps is required to accomplish anteroposterior compression (Fig. 161F).
- Persistent diastasis raises the suspicion of interposition or impaction, especially when it occurs in the sagittal plane. Pointed reduction forceps secures fragments that have been reduced (Fig. 161B).

During this serial reconstruction, the reduced fragments are temporarily held by drilled-in Kirschner wires (1.6 or 1.2 mm) while sparing those areas where a plate will be attached (Fig. 161E).

> The best way to learn the tricks of atraumatic reduction is to assist and observe skilled surgeons.

3.6.4. Cancellous Bone Graft

Defects in cancellous bone may be evaluated after reduction. If depression of the joint surface is present, the defects may be epiphyseal (Fig. 162), but in most cases they are in the metaphysis. Very often, however, defects are created further proximal, at the junction between cortical and cancellous bone. Here, the cortical shell is extremely thin and small fragments break off and enter the medullary cavity. In such cases, adequate packing of the medullary cavity with cancellous bone serves as a mechanical aid to reduction. As outlined in section 3.4, pp. 170–171, we prefer to take cancellous bone from the pelvis in a separate and preliminary operation. In the early years, the AO recommended taking cancellous bone from the greater trochanter, but this has been abandoned owing to the occurrence of fatigue fractures. Another donor site that has proved suitable is the proximal tibial metaphysis of the injured leg [65]. Because the procedure and its technical details are little known, a comprehensive description is given here.

Figure 161. Reduction maneuvers and tricks. **A.** Reduction of depressed fragments using the impactor: first the surrounding fragments are separated with the bone spreader. This aids visualizaton and avoids additional trauma to the released interposed fragment at reduction. **B.** Gaping splits in the sagittal plane are compressssed by large pointed reduction forceps while carefully preserving the soft tissues. **C–E.** Reduction of central steps from an anteromedial approach under visualization; the large fragment of the medial malleolus is turned back and retracted with a pointed hook. The reduced fragments are secured temporarily with Kirschner wires. **F.** In posterior fractures, a flat-bladed bone lever is inserted along the posterior wall after the tendon canal of the posterior tibial muscle has been incised. Slight pressure with the bone lever helps to reduce or avoid displacements in this area. At this stage, the medial malleolus has already been reduced and is held temporarily with Kirschner wires.

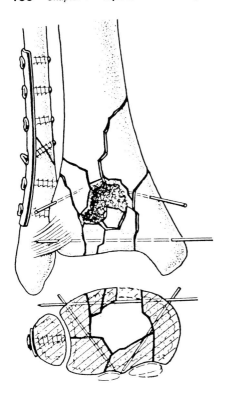

Figure 162. End appearance of a reduced tibial fracture. Anterior view and cross section. Restoration of the articular surface with reduction of the metaphyseal splits. Assessment of the bone defect becomes possible. The provisional Kirschner wires present no obstacle when applying the medial plate.

Harvesting Cancellous Bone From the Upper Tibia

The cancellous bone of the tibial head has proved to be ideal autologous cancellous bone material for situations in which an unexpected defect is encountered intra-operatively and filling material is required, or more cancellous bone is needed than what had been previously obtained from the pelvis. The cancellous bone of the upper tibia consists of finely textured trabeculae interspersed with fat, and is highly compressible.

The harvesting technique is simple. A longitudinal incision is made over the medial aspect of the upper tibia; a cortical flap is chiseled out which remains attached to the periosteum on one side, and the cancellous bone is obtained with a curette. A considerable volume is available (up to 40 cc). It can be measured by filling the donor cavity with irrigation fluid. The wound is closed by separate sutures of the periosteum and skin; a drain is not inserted (Fig. 163).

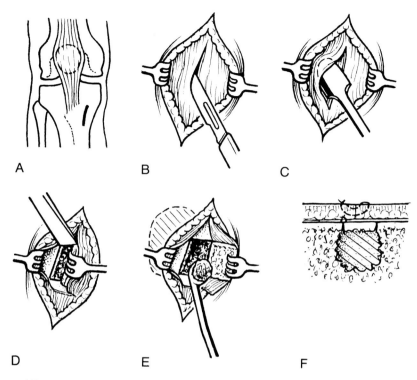

Figure 163. Harvesting of cancellous bone from the proximal tibial metaphysis. **A.** Topographic relations: The donor site is located medially, about 5 cm distal to the knee joint. Spare the terminal branches of the saphenous nerve and avoid injury to the filaments of the pes anserinus. **B.** Incision of the periosteum. **C.** A raspatory is used to separate the periosteum from cortical bone. **D.** A cortical window is chiseled out. Medially, it remains attached to the periosteum and is turned back around that hinge. **E.** Cancellous bone is obtained with a curette. **F.** Wound closure: first, the cortical window is replaced; then separate suturing of the periosteum and the skin is performed.

Weightbearing on the leg is restricted after the operation to allow healing without complications. Healing of the distal tibial fracture is neither delayed nor compromised, because the two areas have separate blood supplies.

> The proximal tibial metaphysis is a suitable donor site for a cancellous graft, but its quality does not match that of iliac bone.

Harvesting of Cancellous Bone in the Vicinity of the Defect

When there is only a simple depression in a partial fracture, only small amounts of cancellous bone are needed. Provided that the intact portion of the metaphysis is large, the removal of a small amount of cancellous bone will do no harm. It would serve, e.g., for the packing of a subchondral defect following reduction of a trap-door depression [69] (Fig. 164).

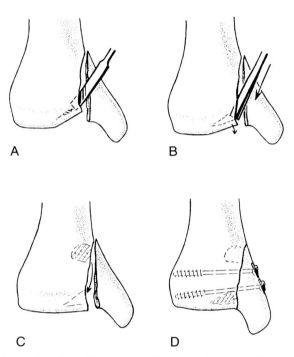

Figure 164. Local harvesting of cancellous bone. **A, B.** A trapped anteromedial impaction is released with the raspatory and reduced with the impactor. **C.** The small volume of cancellous bone required is taken from the metaphysis of the proximal fracture area and pressed firmly into the distal defect. **D.** Compression is achieved with cancellous screws and washers.

Implantation

The graft material is filled in through a preexisting or specially created cortical window and the cancellous bone is firmly pressed in with the impactor so that all recesses of the cavity are filled. Fragments which have been reduced may dislocate again due to the pressure of the implant. During this maneuver, the fracture must be carefully monitored by the assistant on the lateral side (Fig. 148). In cases with an extremely delicate assembly, it may be reasonable to fill cancellous bone in the defect only after the medial implant has been partially screwed into place. Fracture stability will then be considerably increased when compared to the temporary fixation with Kirschner wires.

3.6.5. Definitive Stabilization of the Tibial Fracture

A biomechanically correct, definitive stabilization requires advance planning. Of prime importance are the postoperative functional exercises of the joint. The construction must be strong enough to allow active exercise. At the same time, careful handling of soft tissues is required. Stripping of fragments or separating tibial surfaces from the periosteum is to be avoided, if at all possible.

Apparently, only minor forces act on the reconstructed articular surface. We rarely see secondary dislocations of articular fragments. Posttraumatic osteoarthrosis results from an inadequate reduction or primary damage to the cartilage. Postoperative stress affects predominantly the metaphysis. It is only at this site that delayed consolidation, eventually leading to secondary deformity or pseudarthrosis, occurs.

Because the distal tibia has no compartmental structure, its epimetaphysis must be looked at as a whole. A fixation that stabilizes only one side of the epimetaphyseal block is inadequate. The AO technique emphasizes the function of the medial buttress to prevent secondary collapse into varus position. The early concept was strongly influenced by the impression of anteromedial impactions and comminutive areas [129, 173]. The effect of the fibula giving lateral support and thereby preventing a drift into valgus position was discussed above.

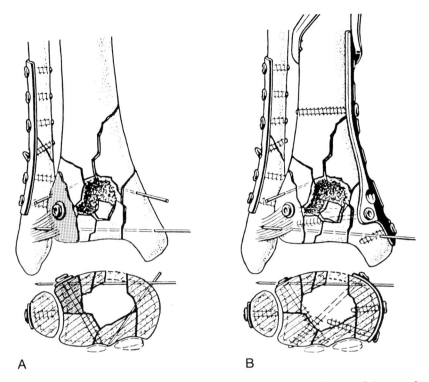

A   B

Figure 165. Definitive reconstruction and fixation, first stage. **A.** Screw fixation of the anterolateral tibial fragment. **B.** Following contouring of the medial plate, it is attached temporarily with individual screws while optimizing the reduction. The provisional Kirschner wires are removed successively. The wide contact established between the plate and the metaphysis and the screws engaging in various planes provides clearly improved stability when compared to construction with Kirschner wires.

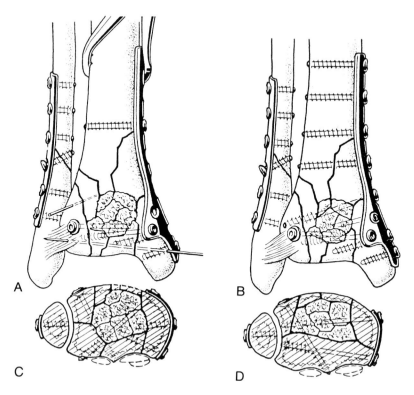

Figure 166. Completing the medial stabilization with the cloverleaf plate (anterior view and cross section). **A.** The defect has been packed with a cancellous bone graft. The remaining Kirschner wires are removed. **B.** The screws fixing the plate in the metaphysis are inserted; 3.5-mm cortical screws are used to join the metaphyseal block to the shaft. Note that screws applied through the plate should only be inserted at sites where they are required for mechanical reasons. Not every hole of the plate takes a screw. **C.** Cross section through the metaphysis in fractures of the posterior tibial wall: the cloverleaf plate stabilizes the medial side; the screws cross and engage in various planes. **D.** An alternative when the posterior tibial wall is intact: the posterior tab of the cloverleaf plate has been removed, and plate contact is restricted to one side; crossing of the plate screws is not required for stability.

In complete articular fractures, particularly in cases where the articular surface itself is badly damaged, the first step is to establish an epimetaphyseal block and to join this to the diaphysis. The objective is therefore not restricted to buttressing, but involves an all-embracing fixation of the entire circumference of the tibia (see section 2). Once this has been accomplished, the proximal connection may be effected in a way similar to that used in extraarticular fractures. To form the epimetaphyseal block, on the other hand, fixating tools must be employed which hold in all planes. The strength of the construction will be improved if, in addition, a large fragment of the medial malleolus has been stabilized.

3.6.6. The Anterolateral Tibial Fragment

Clinical experience has shown that in complex fractures an anterolateral tibial fragment (Fig. 165A) is almost always present. Because it remains attached to the intact anterior syndesmotic ligament, spontaneous reduction is prevented. It requires separate screw fixation (often supplemented with a washer to prevent sinking of the screw head into bone or disruption of the fragment). Sufficient lateral support is achieved by stabilization of the fibula. Lateral plating (perhaps in combination with a medial implant or as the sole stress bearer) is recommended only by Weber [208] and Vivès et al. [203]. When we analyzed this series, we recognized that even with a less-than-optimal reduction of the anterolateral fragment, it was unusual for arthrosis to result. We believe that shearing of this fragment only insignificantly affects the stability of the syndesmosis as a whole. The tibiofibular disk and the posterior syndesmotic ligament would then be preserved as stabilizing factors.

> Definitive stabilization of the tibial fragments begins on the anterolateral side.

3.6.7. Medial Implants and Their Positioning

Implant selection is of prime importance in these complex fractures. Personal preferences and dislikes are marked in each clinic and in the various schools, and are discussed with verve. But in recent years, the dogmatism has appeared to ease up a little, which is also reflected in our case data. Recent trends and developments are dealt with in section 7.

The tools used for definitive fixation consist of screws, a considerable selection of plates, and—a recent addition—the external fixator.

Screws

There is a clear trend to abandon the 6.5-mm cancellous screw and the 4.5-mm cortical screw because of their large size and prominent heads. The preferred screws for the whole distal tibia are the small 4.0-mm cancellous screw and the 3.5-mm cortical screw. These provide adequate stability in every respect and cause far less trauma. If axial stability is problematic, the external fixator is added to provide extra support until bony union has occurred (see section 6).

Plates

The main objective with plates is whether they permit shaping to fit the various anatomic situations found after reduction. Strength is also important. The narrow, straight AO plate (4.5-mm), still used occasionally, was the implant originally recommended. In the metaphysis, 6.5-mm cancellous screws are inserted. The plate is especially suited for extraarticular fractures in which the distal main fragment is sufficiently long, or for fractures where a simple and solid epimetaphyseal block has been established (Fig. 180). When straight implants are to be used, the trend today is toward plates of the 3.5-mm configuration, which have a narrower and thinner design (dynamic compression plate [DCP], reconstruction plate, or low contact dynamic compression plate [LCDCP] made of titanium). These implants are attached with small screws.

The T-plate (4.5-mm) is predominantly suited for fractures with a short distal main fragment, and where two screws must be inserted at the same level. Since the plate is less thick, contouring to the metaphyseal shape is easier (Fig. 189).

Semitubular plates are also used together with screws of 6.5-mm or 4.5-mm diameter. They are chiefly recommended by Weber [208]. At the end, the plate is cut and bent to a right angle to form a double hook. This is driven or hammered into the distal fracture area, pulling the plate proximally. These implants are often inserted in pairs (see Fig. 180).

The spoon plate is also employed with screws (6.5-mm and 4.5-mm). It is a massive implant and requires extensive exposure of the anterior tibial aspect. The upper end of the plate has a groove that engages the anterior tibial margin. The plate has proved useful in fractures in which the posterior aspect of the tibia has remained intact or consists of long, large fragments [43] (Fig. 185).

The cloverleaf plate (Figs. 167, 168) was designed by Heim, introduced in 1968, and described in 1970 [54]. It widens at the lower end, where it shows three processes which extend onto the medial malleolus and clasp comminuted areas like ''a protective hand'' [109]. The implant has a symmetric design (for use on either side), and it is thin, allowing easy contouring of the plate to the various anatomic conditions. The distal processes may be detached with a strong pair of cutting pliers. In one way the plate resembles an extended washer. It should be used with small screws only, even when applied to the shaft. If it is attached anteriorly, the distal process must be removed (Fig. 183). Many surgeons who use the implant fail to appreciate all aspects of its concept. Most errors are the result of inadequate contouring, so that the plate does not fit snugly against the metaphysis or medial malleolus. The result is less-than-optimal stability, and even the creation of valgus forces (Fig. 202). Repeated requests have been made to reinforce the plate in the region around the shaft, since secondary angular deformity or malunion always occurs in the metaphysis. The cloverleaf plate has therefore been produced in stronger thicknesses, but then the distal processes cannot be detached, and contouring the plate becomes more difficult.

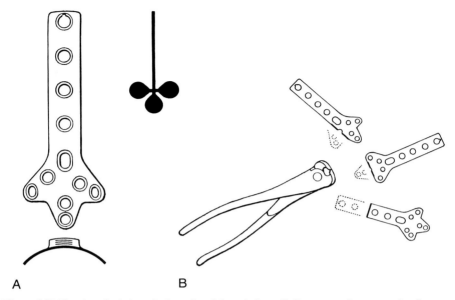

A   B

Figure 167. The cloverleaf plate. **A.** Overall and frontal views. **B.** By means of strong cutting forceps, the plate itself may be shortened or any of the tabs removed.

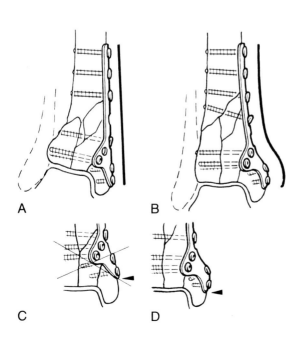

A   B

C   D

Figure 168. Faulty and correct adaptation of the cloverleaf plate to the medial aspect of the tibia. **A.** Failure to shape the plate creates a valgus angulation. **B.** Correct adaptation of the plate. **C.** The distal tab of the plate has been placed too far proximally. **D.** Correct position of the distal tab of the cloverleaf plate. The medial malleolus is held well.

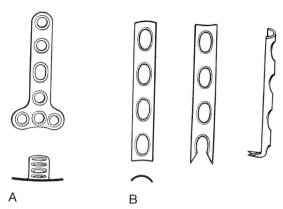

Figure 169. The small plates for the tibia. **A.** The radius T-plate viewed from above and in cross section. **B.** One-third tubular plate. Two terminal double hooks may be formed by means of a cutting forceps. See also Figures 170E and 180C.

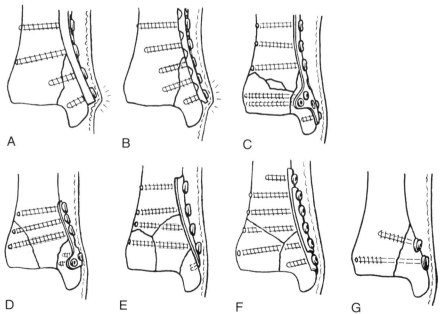

Figure 170. Soft tissue problems encountered at the medial malleolus. The tips of the 4.5-mm straight plate (**A**) and the 3.5-mm limited contact dynamic compression plate (LCDCP) (**B**) may interfere with the skin. The cloverleaf plate (**C**), the radius T-plate (**D**), the one-third tubular plate with distal hooks (**E**), two superimposed one-third tubular plates (**F**), and isolated screws with washers (**G**) are much thinner and do not bulge.

The small T-plate for the distal radius is another plate that takes small screws (bone cortex, 3.5-mm, and cancellous bone, 4.0-mm). It is especially suited for small fractures involving the joint and can be placed medially, anteriorly, or posteriorly. Because it is short and thin, it is preferred for these sites instead of the spoon plate (Figs. 169 and 186). It is also increasingly used in the presence of soft tissue damage (see section 6).

Medial stabilization may be achieved with plates of various designs. Currently, the trend is to choose small screws and an additional external fixator as a buttressing device.

3.6.8. Wound Closure

Before the wound is closed, the result of the reduction is recorded radiologically (on the image intensifier). Special attention is given to the reduction and the correct length and siting of the screws. The strength is checked clinically, and is decisive for planning postoperative management.

Suturing of the fascia is dispensed with completely. To prevent the development of a compartmental syndrome, the fascia of the anterior tibial compartment is be incised as far as the wound permits. The same applies to the deep posterior fascial compartments, provided that access is feasible. The joint capsule is sutured to the anterior edge of the medial malleolus sealing the joint. Suction drains are placed medially and laterally in the vicinity of the fracture area. The suturing of the skin must be atraumatic, completely free of tension, but leakproof (suction drain).

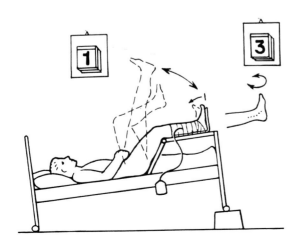

Figure 171. Early postoperative mobilization of the patient in bed. The injured leg is elevated on a fracture cradle; the ankle is held at 90 degrees with a plaster splint permitting active extension and flexion exercises of the hallux. In open wound management, dorsiflexion exercises of the foot can be supplemented on day 3 by rotatory movements.

There is virtually no other site where the quality of skin suturing is so crucial for wound healing. Only when the surgeon himself or herself carries out the whole of the wound closure, including the stitching of the skin, is it possible to prevent skin necrosis and keep septic complications to a minimum (see sections 5.2.6 and 5.2.7).

If the skin approximation is not completely free of tension, the wound must be left open. Wound closure is then performed stepwise as the swelling subsides, and under local anesthesia. Alternatively, the lateral wound may be left open. When in doubt, it is recommended that the medial wound be closed first [118, 192] (see Fig. 195A [45]).

The skin is dressed with a nonadhesive gauze. Subsequently, a well-padded, absorbent gauze and a light bandage are applied. Any pressure on the wound is to be avoided.

To prevent footdrop, the foot is elevated on a padded plaster splint placed posteriorly with the ankle flexed at 90 degrees. This is worn in the early postoperative days. Later, the leg is raised on a fracture splint, and the peripheral circulation is regularly checked (by observing the toes) (Fig. 171).

> Never close a wound under tension. Skin necrosis is the worst of all complications. It is almost always preventable.

3.7. Postoperative Management

Postoperative management is similar to that following internal fixation of malleolar fractures, but the onset of mobilization tends to be slightly delayed. The leg is elevated on a fracture splint with the knee partially flexed, while the ankle joint is held in resting position by a right-angled plaster splint. The circulation, motility, and sensation in the toes are checked regularly. Active movement of the toes, knee, and hip joint is started on day 1 (Fig. 171). Draining of the wound is maintained until the tubes are removed, after about 36 hours.

The first change of dressing is done after about 48 hours. Subsequently, the wound may be left open or be protected with a light bandage. After the change of dressing, active functional exercises are intensified. Dorsiflexion exercises are supplemented with rotatory movements. The patient is allowed to walk on crutches if healing of the wound is established (after about 5–7 days) and if postoperative swelling has subsided.

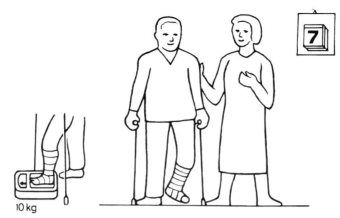

Figure 172. Mobilization and walking classes start after wound healing is established. After about 1 week, walking on crutches is supervised by a physiotherapist. Note the bandaged leg for walking. See p. 201. Depending on the strength of the assembly achieved by the operation and the surgeon's instructions, either no foot-to-floor contact or partial weightbearing (checked on scale) is permitted.

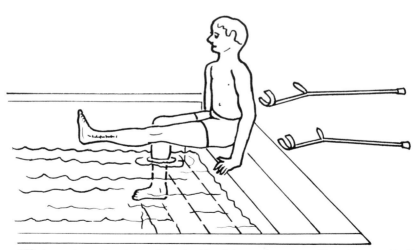

Figure 173. Access to a swimming pool is gained by sitting on the stairs and lowering oneself without bearing weight on the injured leg. The same procedure is used in reverse when getting out of the pool.

When the patient gets up for the first time, an elastic bandage is applied to the foot and lower leg to counteract the hemostatic pressure that develops with the leg dependent. Even diffuse and small petechiae may develop, and the foot may swell up again. The wound must be examined after the first walking exercises. If necessary, postoperative management is modified accordingly.

Walking classes are conducted according to the surgeon's instructions and, (depending on stability, without weightbearing, with foot-to-floor-contact and heel-and-toe walking, or with partial weightbearing of 10 to 15 kg (Fig. 172). Stitches are generally not removed before day 14.

Drug therapy to prevent thromboembolism is started preoperatively and is continued until full weightbearing of the injured leg is achieved. The patient may leave the hospital as soon as he or she is mobile on crutches. Discharge from hospital will often depend on other injuries and on social circumstances (living conditions, nursing situation, etc). In many patients, a detachable plaster or synthetic splint has proved useful to protect the leg. When the patient performs regular functional exercises, it is removed. It presents no obstacle to walking on crutches or to heel-and-toe walking and provides valuable protection of the leg and the foot especially during sleep.

Recommendations for postoperative management form part of the surgeon's report. They include the proposed delay for loadbearing.

Fracture consolidation is monitored by monthly radiographs. The timing of initiating or increasing weightbearing depends on these films, but it should always be in line with the postoperative management plan. The clinical situation (edema, pain, etc.) must be taken into consideration. In complex fractures, an increase in weightbearing generally starts at week 12, and full weightbearing (walking without crutches) at about week 16. It may be necessary to delay this scheme for some weeks if large defects requiring extensive cancellous bone grafting are present. At week 20, bony union of the fracture should have occurred, and the patient should be able to walk without pain. Persistent swelling and pain at this time indicate delayed consolidation.

When the wound is closed, hydrogymnastics and swimming have proved to be useful. But the patient must be taught how to get in and out of the pool to avoid undue stress on the leg (Fig. 173). Following fracture consolidation, walking on sand in knee-high seawater has proved to be a valuable aid to mobilization. In patients with multiple injuries, this regimen is modified as required.

Implant removal is different for fibula and tibia. The fibular fracture heals earlier. At this site, the implant may be removed after 6 to 8 months. On the tibia, the implant should be left in place until month 14. Medial implants, depending on their size, are more or less troublesome. Plates are large foreign bodies. They lie directly beneath the skin, are felt through the skin, and may interfere with the wearing of sport shoes. We generally recommend their removal, a wish often expressed directly by the patient. The technical procedure is simple: only the lower end of the scar needs to be reopened. Proximally, the screws of the plate may be removed in pairs through a stab incision. Laterally, damage to the branch of the superficial peroneal nerve is to be avoided (see Fig. 151).

Remove the implants only if the patient complains, but respect the timing carefully in order to avoid refracture.

---

4. CLINICAL RADIOGRAPHS ILLUSTRATING OPERATIVE TECHNIQUE, POSTOPERATIVE COURSE, AND RESULTS

We present Figures 174 through 187 to illustrate the operative technique as far as this can be done by means of a radiograph. Further details are obtained from the surgeon's reports, and the subsequent course is documented in the patient's record. These provide the necessary information regarding details of postoperative management, course, and results. When additional particulars were needed, these were obtained by questioning the respective surgeon. These examples do not attempt to cover the whole variety of our case material. For this, we refer to the detailed analysis in the Appendix, section 3. But they enable us to show the essential operative techniques as well as some postoperative complications which may be recognized radiologically. The case reports were chosen on condition that a follow-up of at least 1 year was available. Straight plates on the tibia have not been included in our selection, because this technique hardly differs from internal fixation of tibial fractures located further proximal. Some examples have been depicted by slightly stylized drawings. With regard to the technique of reconstructing the tibia, our examples focus on fixation with screws and plates. Minimal internal fixations and in particular the application of the external fixator are discussed in sections 6 and 7. The same applies to cases illustrating secondary internal fixation. With regard to the fibula, our examples of internal fixation are particularly characteristic.

Text continued on page 219

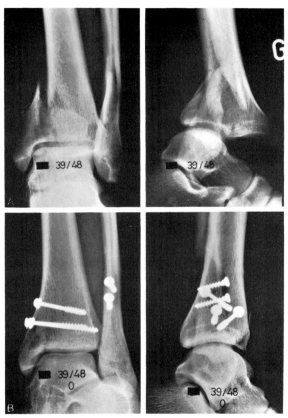

Figure 174. Screw fixation of the tibia and fibula in a partial articular split fracture (18-year-old with a closed injury sustained in a traffic accident). **A.** Posteromedial split of the tibial articular surface in the frontal plane (running obliquely) including the medial malleolus; long oblique fracture of the fibula at the junction between diaphysis and metaphysis. The same case is depicted in Figure 100 to illustrate the classification. **B.** Internal fixation of the tibia was performed with small cancellous screws and washers and of the fibula with two small cortical screws. Following accurate reduction and stabilization, functional postoperative exercises were initiated with partial weightbearing. The postoperative course was uneventful with full weightbearing at 6 weeks and full rehabilitation at 8 weeks.

Illustration continued on following page

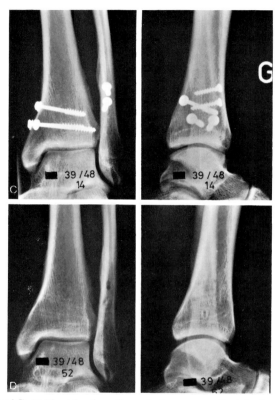

Figure 174 *Continued* **C.** At 14 weeks, the radiograph shows uncomplicated primary bone healing and a fine seam of callus on the fibula. **D.** At 52 weeks, the radiograph shows a normal joint. The patient recovered with full function and no muscular atrophy.

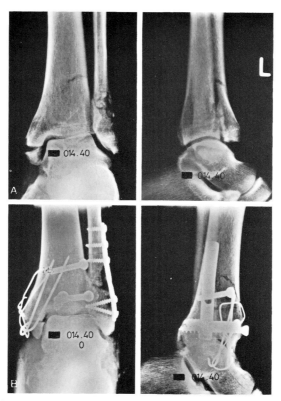

Figure 175. Screw fixation of a partial split in the tibia; impaction of the fibular metaphysis (a 39-year-old sustained a closed injury without concomitant injuries after a fall). **A.** Anterolateral sagittal split of the tibia with dislocation into valgus deformity, impaction of the fibular metaphysis, and a small avulsion fragment of the medial malleolus. The presence of a small anterolateral depression could not be excluded. In Figure 40, the same case is shown to illustrate the classification. **B.** The reduced tibial fracture was fixed with screws inserted from the anterolateral side. A lateral, six-hole one-third tubular plate was applied to the fibula which was shortened because of the impaction. The persistent dislocation of the medial malleolus was fixed with a tension band assembly composed of Kirschner wires and a wire loop. Wound healing was uncomplicated. Following initial functional exercises, the patient was placed in a circular cast for 8 weeks.

Illustration continued on following page

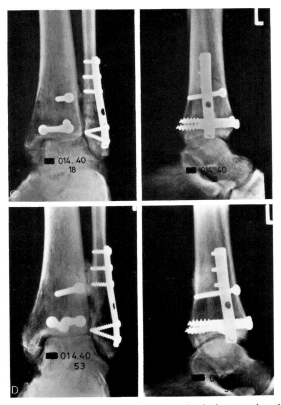

Figure 175 *Continued* **C.** Follow-up at 18 weeks: fracture union had occurred, and a callus bridge was beginning to form at the upper margin of the fibular fracture. Full weightbearing at 18 weeks; the patient was unable to work for 8 months. **D.** At 1-year follow-up (53 weeks), moderate narrowing of the lateral joint space was found, and the callus bridge was established. There was slight limitation of motion, and the patient complained of pain during exercise. *Comment:* No attention was paid to the typical morphology of the fibular fracture. The shortening of the fibula was not serious owing to the intact syndesmosis, so that at 1 year, only prearthrosis was observed. The slight lateralization of the talus as a result of inadequate reduction of the medial malleolus contributed to this development.

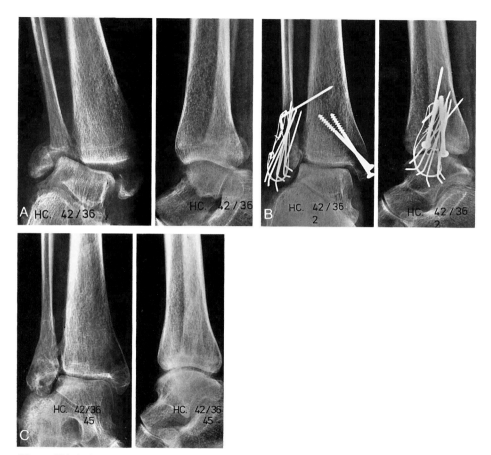

Figure 176. Arthrosis due to shortening that developed after a distally impacted fibula associated with lateral depression. (This 69-year old woman fell during a mountain tour in a remote locale and surgery could only be carried out after a delay of 4 days.) **A.** Lateral subluxation of the talus with small depression of the lateral articular surface (recognized in retrospect). There was an important dislocation into valgus angulation and a cancellous defect in the distal fibula. **B.** Instead of realigning the fibula and packing the defect with a graft, a tension band assembly with compression was performed through which the fibular shortening became fixed. Standard screw fixation of the medial malleolus was carried out. The course was uneventful following initial functional exercises that were replaced by a walking cast worn for 8 weeks. **C.** At 1-year follow-up (45 weeks), early signs indicated narrowing of the lateral joint space and subluxation of the talus into valgus angulation. There was local swelling without pain. *Comments:* If the initial treatment had consisted of interposition of a corticocancellous bone chip while restoring the fibular length, this would have probably compensated for the small lateral depression. The case shows the extreme rare incidence of a lateral depression without a visible split in front.

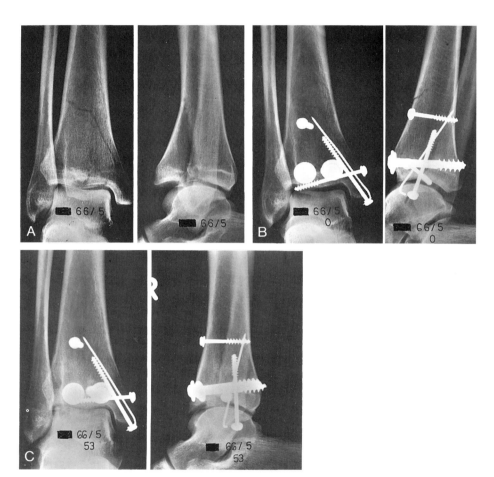

Figure 177. Screw fixation of a partial fracture with centrally located pestle-formed depression (a 40-year-old fell and sustained a closed fracture which was treated in an emergency operation). **A.** Anterior split in the frontal plane with a small, centrally located pestle-formed depression which is evident on both radiographs. A second sagittal split is beside the depression. The fibula has remained intact, and there is an oblique fracture of the medial malleolus. Classified as B2.3. **B.** Internal fixation was performed from the anterior and anteromedial side with screws and washers (compression of the reduced depression and of the sagittal split was effected with a small cancellous screw). The medial malleolus was fixed with a screw and a Kirschner wire (to stabilize rotation). **C.** At 1-year follow-up (53 weeks), the joint appeared normal and the patient had full motion. The implants were left in place. *Comment:* Perfect healing was brought about by the screws compressing the reduced depressed fragment.

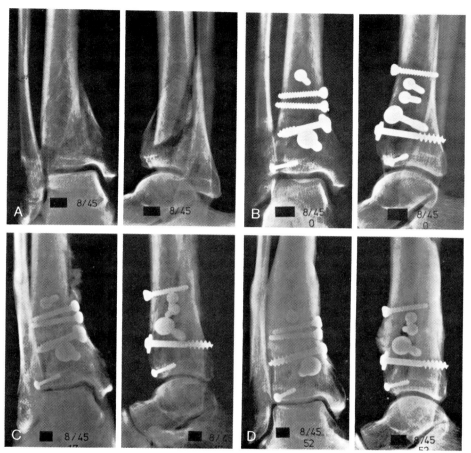

Figure 178. Screw fixation of a complete split fracture. Secondary dislocation (some clinical data were missing for this 43-year-old who sustained an open fracture managed by an emergency operation). **A.** Circular articular fracture. There was a large frontal split with a long posterior wall fragment, and an additional anterolateral split; varus angulation; typical, undisplaced fracture of the fibular diaphysis. The distal talofibular ligaments were torn, and there was a small avulsion fracture of the talus (visible only on radiographs **C** and **D**). Classified as C1.3. **B.** Internal fixation of the tibial fracture was carried out with multiple screws. In retrospect, the second and the third screws from above were found to have been placed into the frontal split. **C.** When seen at 4 months (17 weeks), the patient presented with varus deviation, formation of an irritation callus, and partial loosening of the metaphyseal implants. **D.** At 1-year follow-up, fracture union had occurred (following temporary immobilization?). The articular contours appeared normal, and the deviation of tibia and fibula had not progressed. *Comment:* Obliquely running fractures cannot be adequately stabilized by screw fixation alone. The unfavorably placed implants were not the only cause of delayed union in the metaphysis. This led to recurrence of the original displacement while dragging along the fibula. At this site, where the use of a plate appeared to be contraindicated, an external fixator providing additional support would have been the optimal solution as primary treatment. The articular splits healed without sequelae. The pathologic process took place exclusively in the metaphysis.

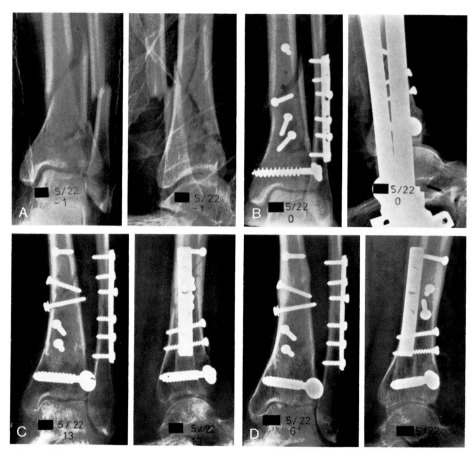

Figure 179. Long fracture of the tibia stabilized with screws and buttressed by external fixation (a 25-year-old woman involved in a traffic accident; closed fracture without concomitant injuries). **A.** Complete split fracture of the tibia with anterolateral depression and extension into the diaphysis; oblique fracture of the fibular diaphysis. Classified as C1.3. In Figure 128 the same case is depicted to illustrate the classification. **B.** Management of the fibula consisted of standard internal fixation with a six-hole one-third tubular plate. The sagittal split and the depression on the tibia were fixed from the lateral side by means of screws, and the remaining fracture elements were reconstructed stepwise by inserting individual screws. An external fixator device applied between the tibial shaft and the calcaneus provided extra support. Because the radiograph showed dehiscence between the main proximal fragment and the lateral wedge, the screws were replaced at this site. The postoperative course was uneventful, and the external fixator was removed at 9 weeks. **C.** At 3-months follow-up, fractures were consolidating. On the AP radiograph, the second and third screws from above inserted at the end of the intervention may be clearly distinguished. Full weightbearing at 14 weeks; partial rehabilitation 2 weeks later. **D.** At 1-year follow-up, the joint appeared normal, and fracture union had occurred; some proximal fixation callus was present. Motion of the ankle joint was still slightly limited. Implant removal was proposed. *Comment:* Careful construction of the tibial stabilization with screws alone, buttressed by an external fixator device. Favorable development after an initially unsatisfactory proximal reduction had been corrected (replacing the screws did not lead to devitalization).

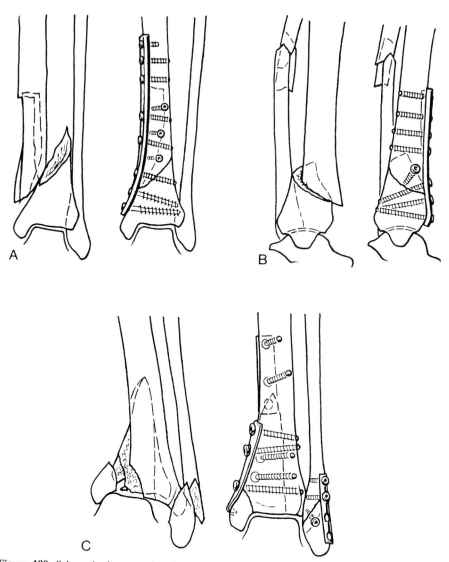

Figure 180. Schematic demonstrating the use of straight plates in distal tibial fractures. **A.** Medial application of a 4.5-mm dynamic compression plate (DCP) with an extraarticular wedge fracture. **B.** Anterior application of a 4.5-mm DCP with a simple oblique fracture. **C.** Stabilization of a complete depression fracture of the tibia by means of two semitubular plates; the distal plate is placed medially. Its lower end has been bent and cut with reduction forceps to form a pointed hook by which it may be anchored in the large fragment of the medial malleolus. The upper plate is applied as a so-called antigliding plate to the posterior side where it compresses the proximal end of the long posterior wedge fragment. The distal oblique fracture of the fibula is stabilized with a one-third antigliding plate and fixed with an additional screw.

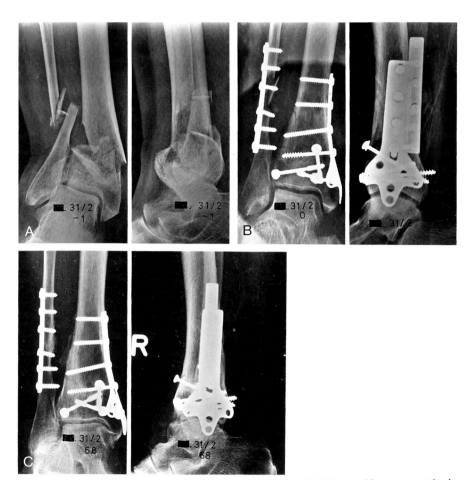

Figure 181. Plating of tibia and fibula in a typical C2.2 fracture. (This 73-year-old woman sustained a closed fracture with skin contusions after a fall. Planned operation was performed at day 7; the implants were left in place.) **A.** Double articular split (*sagittal lateral* and *sagittal frontal*); area of multifragmentation in the metaphysis, typical complex fracture of the fibular diaphysis with valgus position. **B.** The fibula was stabilized with a six-hole one-third tubular plate without anatomic reduction of the multifragmented area; management of the tibia consisted of a cloverleaf plate and additional separate screws; cancellous bone grafting was performed. Functional exercises were initiated postoperatively. The course was uneventful; no external fixation; full weightbearing was achieved at 10 weeks. **C.** Follow-up at 1 year and 4 months (68 weeks); the articular lines appeared normal and fracture union had occurred. Full function was achieved. *Comment:* Perfect fracture healing in an elderly patient; a typical case of planned internal fixation.

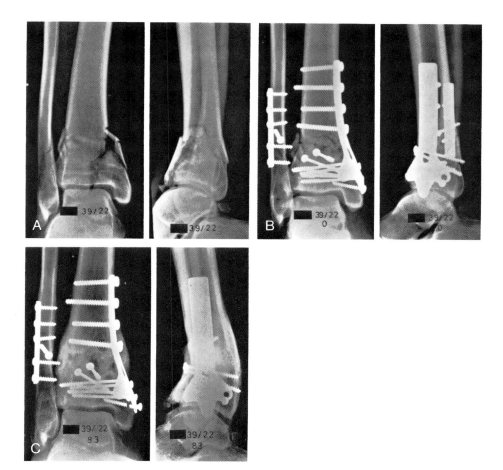

Figure 182. Tibial plate for impaction of the metaphysis, secondary deviation (a 23-year-old fell while skiing; closed fracture). **A.** Sagittal articular split. In addition, a cortical shell was expelled anterolaterally; impaction of the metaphysis in recurvation and slight varus position; typical, varus-type fracture of the fibula above the malleoli. The same case is depicted in Figure 123 illustrating the classification. **B.** Primary internal fixation: a cloverleaf plate was attached medially, and separate screws were inserted. A cancellous bone graft was carried out; the fibula was stabilized with a plate and lag screw. Neither the recurvation nor the varus position of the fibula was fully corrected. With functional postoperative management replaced by a plaster cast, the course was uneventful. Full weightbearing was achieved at 18 months. **C.** Follow-up at 1¾ years (83 weeks): considerable callus formation at the metaphysis partly incorporating the plate; 15% recurvation; screw fracture distally. Apart from small osteophytes that had developed anteriorly and posteriorly, the joint structure appeared normal. The patient had slight limitation of motion in the ankle and tibiotalar joint, probably resulting from too early weightbearing against medical advice. *Comment:* Secondary deviation (predominantly recurvation) without major functional impairment. The development of fracture consolidation shows that secondary deviation will always follow the direction of the original angulation. The morphology and course of the fibular fracture lines allow the conclusion that the initial malalignment was dominated by recurvation.

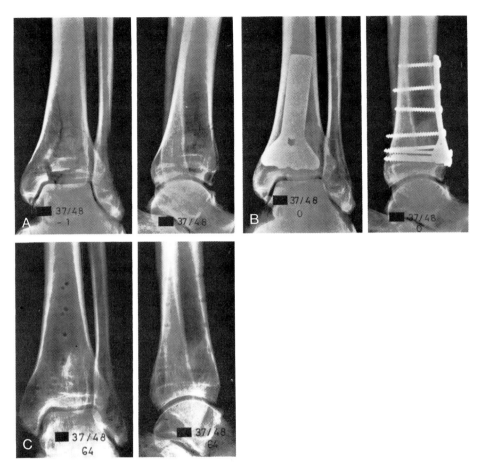

Figure 183. Anterior plating of the tibia with a pestle-formed depression. (A 48-year-old man with a closed injury after a fall presented with fracture of the calcaneus on the same leg which was treated nonoperatively.) **A.** Partial articular fracture with preserved posterior wall. The centrally located, pestle-formed depression is better evident on the AP radiograph (it is only suggested on the lateral projection; see Figure 97). Multiple splits in the metaphysis; intact fibula; osteophytes are seen at the tip of the medial malleolus and the neck of the talus (preexisting). Classified as B2.3. **B.** Following reduction and a cancellous bone graft, the fracture was stabilized with an anterior cloverleaf plate, the distal tab of which had been detached. Following functional postoperative management, the course was uneventful. Full weightbearing was achieved at 14 weeks, rehabilitation at 4 months. **C.** Late follow-up at 1¼ years (64 weeks) following implant removal: no signs of arthrosis, no progression of the preexisting exophytosis; mild osteoporosis; slight limitation of motion in the ankle and tibiotalar joint. *Comment:* The anterior plate secured perfect compression of the reduced depression which had been buttressed by means of a cancellous bone graft; the plate was selected because of the multiple splits in the metaphysis. The still marked osteoporosis may be assumed to be associated with the concomitant fracture of the calcaneus.

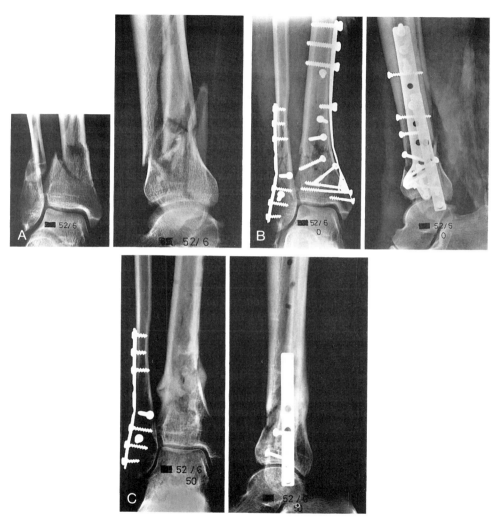

Figure 184. Long plate in a complete articular split fracture extending into the diaphysis (a 33-year-old sustained a closed injury after a fall; treated by emergency operation; developed a late infection that was cured; 100% disability for 8 months). **A.** The fracture had its center in the metaphysis and a wedge extended into the diaphysis. Frontal split into the joint (evident on the lateral radiograph); area of multifragmentation in the metaphysis; distal wedge fracture of the fibular diaphysis; valgus position. **B.** Reduction and stabilization was accomplished by means of a long cloverleaf plate and separate screws. Management of the fibula consisted of an eight-hole one-third tubular plate and two separate screws. No cancellous bone grafting; perfect reduction and stability. Postoperatively, infection developed with a fistula. The patient was hospitalized for 3 months; closed suction drainage. Infection was cured. Early removal of the tibial plate. **C.** At 1-year follow-up (50 weeks), the articular lines were normal, there was mild osteoporosis; a fixation callus had developed in the metaphysis (secondary cancellous bone graft). *Comment:* The initial management did not include a cancellous bone graft for the multifragmented area in the metaphysis. At this site, infection developed. However, it did not spread to the joint, and was cured following early implant removal. Prolonged disability and restriction of articular function resulting from the period of immobilization remained as unfavorable outcomes.

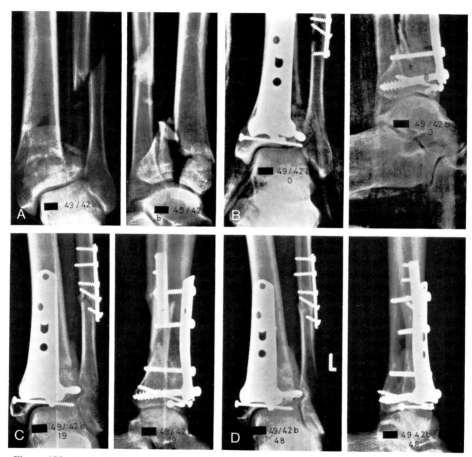

Figure 185. Anteriorly applied spoon plate; secondary shortening of the fibula with valgus deformity. A 50-year-old man involved in a traffic accident sustained a closed fracture of the tibia and a double open fracture of the facial bone; healing proceeded without further complications after emergency internal fixation (temporary disability for 6 months). **A.** Dehiscence in the frontal plane with anterior impaction; wedge fracture of the fibular diaphysis; valgus angulation and antecurvature. Classified as C2.1; Figure 122 illustrates the classification. **B.** Emergency operation was carried out: a spoon plate was attached anteriorly. In addition, small screws were inserted to secure fissures which could not be safely identified on the radiography. The selected one-third tubular plate at the fibula held the distal main fragment with only one screw, which was too short. Following functional postoperative management, the postoperative course was uneventful. **C.** At 5 months' follow-up (19 weeks), irregularities are seen in the posterolateral part of the tibia where an osteolytic ring has formed around a plate screw. Shortening of the fibula was associated with loosening of the implants. Both phenomena promoted the recurrence of the initial drift into valgus angulation. **D.** When seen at 1 year (49 weeks), the fractures had consolidated without progression of the deviation. Motion in the ankle joint was restricted, and implant removal was planned. *Comment:* The stabilization of the fibula failed to provide adequate buttress to withstand the postoperative load. The strong implant attached to the anterior aspect of the tibia could not prevent secondary deviation into valgus angulation.

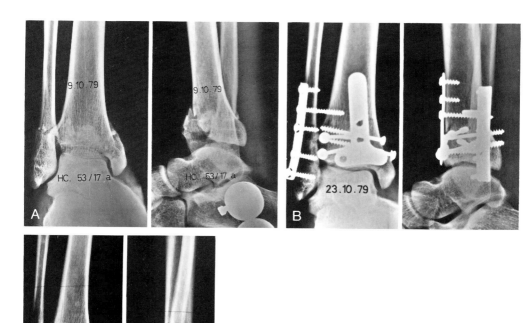

Figure 186. Anterior radius T-plate in a partial complex articular fracture (B3). A 25-year-old involved in a traffic accident sustained concussion of the brain and bilateral fractures of the tibial head; managed by internal fixation together with the pilon fracture. Walking pool exercises were started at 8 weeks, and by 3 months the patient could walk normally again. **A.** Partial disintegration of the anterior articular surface with trap-door depression. Preserved posterior wall, and transverse fracture of the fibular metaphysis; oblique fracture of the medial malleolus, initially treated by traction. **B.** A small-radius T-plate effecting compression was attached to the anterior aspect of the tibia which was additionally fixed with screws; a cancellous bone graft was performed, and the fibula was stabilized by means of a one-third tubular plate and a positioning screw. Postoperative management was functional. **C.** Partial rehabilitation by 6 months, and full rehabilitation by 8 months. When seen 7 years later, the patient had no limitations in walking distance, no pain, no muscular atrophy, and only moderate arthrosis. *Comment:* The small-radius T-plate is especially suited for partial fractures of limited extension. This case demonstrates that adequate technique and functional postoperative exercises may keep the arthrosis within acceptable limits even when the articular surface has disintegrated.

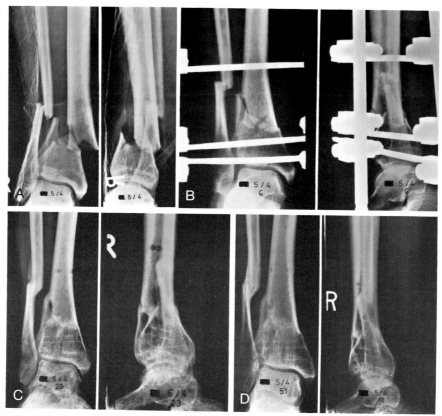

Figure 187. An extraarticular open fracture that was initially treated with an external fixation device (38-year-old driver with a third-degree open fracture sustained in an accident). Initial incision of the skin to achieve decompression was followed by open wound treatment; free movement of the joints. **A.** Extraarticular wedge fracture of the tibia; some contact between the main fragments was preserved posteromedially; dislocation into valgus angulation; typical, oblique fracture of the fibular diaphysis. The same case is depicted in Figure 67 to illustrate the classification (A2.2). **B.** Emergency treatment consisted in application of an external frame: two Steinmann pins were inserted into the distal main fragment. Except for a slight valgus angulation, satisfactory fragment reduction was obtained. The postoperative course was uneventful, and the patient received functional postoperative management. **C.** The external fixator was removed at 8 weeks; at 5-month follow-up, the radiograph showed fracture union, osteoporosis, and 10 degrees of deviation into valgus angulation. Full weightbearing was achieved at 14 weeks. **D.** When seen at 1 year (51 weeks), the patient was almost free of pain and fully rehabilitated. On the radiograph, the articular lines appeared normal, the fractures had consolidated, and the osteoporosis had improved. *Comment:* Very rapid consolidation of a widely open, extraarticular wedge fracture was achieved by means of the external fixation device and optimal management of the soft tissue lesions (decompression incisions, open wound treatment). The initial valgus position, which had not been realigned, seems to have had only minor functional consequences. It would have been readily corrected if initial management had consisted of internal fixation of the fibula.

5. COMPLICATIONS

Complications after internal fixation of the distal segment of the lower leg are frequent, and of great variety. Some are specific. Because of the rarity of the injuries, even the most experienced surgeon has not seen all of them. But knowledge of these complications is essential if they are to be avoided. We place special emphasis here on prophylactic measures, since often very ordinary circumstances will have serious consequences. For this reason, it may become necessary to repeat some of the preceding comments on patient selection, pre-operative management, and operative technique (cf. section 3). Treatment is discussed only when the management of these complications is more or less specific.

From the case data filed at the AO documentation center only manifest complications involving the bone may be recognized. The late results of our series have been analyzed (see Appendix), and in Tables 3 to 6, pp. 317–320, they are presented in detail in relation to the classification in Table 4. The figures are indicative and correlate well with those found in the literature. Case records selected for illustration and comment, however, are only individual examples and no statistical conclusions can be drawn. Primarily, they serve as evidence supporting the classification.

If we want to study complications as a whole, we are obliged to refer to further data, primarily one's personal experience [30, 67, 140]. Another forum is the exchange of information, for which the narrow circle of the AO group provides many opportunities. Many statements, which may be taken as a personal opinion because they are given without reference to the literature, actually reflect the experience of other surgeons who have a special interest in this field. We also refer the reader to the Preface to this book.

5.1. Statistics (Table 1)

The first step is to study the recent literature. In Europe, other useful sources of information are also unpublished doctoral theses. Often, these are more precise and detailed than what is published later in a shorter form. By discussing them here at greater length, we express our appreciation for the diligence, perseverance, and power of observation shown by our younger colleagues. Current university regulations do not provide for their early scientific work to appear in print, so that the few copies available are easily overlooked and the knowledge they contain is forgotten. The studies of Songis-Mortreux [184], Hourlier [80], Comminot [30], and Macek [110] merit special attention in this context. To our knowledge, only the work of Hourlier has been published [203].

Large and complete series were analyzed. The causes of accident vary, and also the management concepts. Songis-Mortreux [184] reviewed the patient data from Lille (106 cases) including 35% open fractures. Hourlier [80] studied 84 cases from Amiens, concentrating on aspects of classification (Fig. 94). Comminot [30]

Table 1

RESULTS OF OPERATIVE TREATMENT OF PILON FRACTURES SINCE 1975[a]

Authors	Year of Publication	No. of fractures	Personal Cases of the Clinic	Mixed Methods: Conservative and ORIF	Cases of Other Hospitals Included	No. of ORIF	No. of EF	Late Results: ORIF and EF	Period of Follow-up	Mean Follow-up (Yr)	Remarks
Songis-Mortreux (184)	1975	106	+	+		78	2	78	1966–1974	4.0	Open fractures, 27%; 17 arthrodeses; 5 amputations; first mention of external fixation (2 cases)
Heim and Näser (67, 68)	1976, 1977	128	+	+		128		121	1962–1973	4.0	Published in German and French
Lecestre and Ramadier (101)	1976	40	+	+		26		20	1968–1975		
Hackenbruch (50)	1977	215		+	+	215		84	1972–1976	1.0	Skiing accidents; data from AO documentation center
Stampfel and Mähring (185)	1977	56	+	+		48		48	1969–1975	6.0	Depressions
Rüedi and Allgöwer (171)	1978	99	+			99		75	1968–1973	6.0	
Müller KH, and Prescher (127)	1978	64			+	55		36	1971–1976	6.0	31 osteoarthritides
Pierce and Heinrich (149)	1979	42		+	+			19	1970–1979	2.0	
Kellam and Waddell (88)	1979	26	+	+		21		21	1975–1977	1.5	
Mischkowsky and Dichgans (121)	1980	33	+	+		23		18	1970–1974		

Author (reference)	Year	n	ORIF	EF	No.	No.	No.	Period	Follow-up (yr)	Comments
Hourlier (80)	1981	84	+	+	67		59	1970–1979	4.8	Same patients as Vivès et al. (203)
Tassler (189)	1981	54	+	+	54		54	1977–1980		Only open 3rd-degree fractures
Comminot (30)	1981	221	+		221		221	1962–1980	6.0	Includes Heim and Näser (67, 68)
Welz (211)	1982	77	+	+	67		61	1968–1981		
Börner (14)	1982	102	+	+	102		102	1971–1979		First observation of ligament ruptures
Möller and Krebs (123)	1982	23	+	+	13		13	1976–1980	5.4	
Rogge (166)	1983	27	+	+	27		27	?		
Macek (110)	1984	62	+	+	52			?		
Vivès et al. (203)	1984	84	+	+	67		59	1965–1977		Same cases as Hourlier (80)
Lamprecht and Ochsner (94)	1984	66	+					1970–1979	2.0	15 osteitides, 40 arthrodeses
Ovadia and Beals (146)	1986	145	+	+	80		80	1964–1982	7.5	
Resch et al. (161)	1986	176	+	+			35	1970–1982		
Dillin and Slabaugh (39)	1986	11	+	+	8		8	1979–1981		
Nordin et al. (142)	1988	25	+	+	28		25	1974–1986	3.0	
Schweiberer et al. (181)	1987	28	+			25		1982–1986		
Breitfuss et al. (21)	1988	131	+	+	131		111	1969–1984		Only closed fractures
Mast et al. (116)	1988	37	+	+	37		37	1974–1980		
Ayeni (3)	1988	19	+		12		12	1977–1983		
Lechevallier et al. (103)	1989	28	+	+		28	28	1977–1981		11 delayed union or pseudarthroses
Bourne et al. (19, 20)	1989, 1983	50	+		33		33	1972–1980		Same statistics published in 1983
Höntzsch (79)	1990	50	+	+	50		50	1984–1988		EF partly transitory
Etter and Ganz (43)	1991	55	+		55	24	41	1972–1978		
Massari et al. (115)	1992	110	+	+	65	8		1982–1990	10.0	
Copin and Nérot (32)	1992	706		+	394	70		?		
Perraudin and Nordin (147)	1992	70	+		70		70	?		
Biga et al. (11)	1992	9	+		9		9	?		Additional percutaneous reduction and fixation of displaced fragments
Hochstein et al. (76)	1992	54	+	+	54	32	54	1988–1990		
Welz (212)	1992	171	+	+	143	9	143	1967–1990		Includes Welz (211)
Scheller et al. (178)	1992	58	+	+	52		52	1982–1991		
Waddell (204)	1993	38	+	+	38		38	?		
Beck et al. (7)	1993	380	+		380		256	1972–1985	4.9	56% ski accidents
Bone et al. (17)	1993	20	+	+	20		20	1989–1992	7.5	EF + ORIF with minimal implants
Muhr and Breitfuss (126)	1993	182	+	+	182	47	182	1969–1983 1984–1989	2	Conventional ORIF; EF + ORIF with minimal implants
Rommens et al. (167)	1994	81	+		81		81	1980–1990	4.5	

ORIF = open reduction with internal fixation; EF = external fixation.

continued the observation of 128 cases from Chur, a series recorded by Näser [140] until 1973 and published in 1976 and 1977 [67, 68]. The subsequent 92 patients were then followed until 1980. Comminot was able to trace five of six patients who had been lost to follow-up in Näser's series. He also recorded the long-term results of patients from the Näser series who had developed complications; at 6 years, he checked the results of 36 patients who had been previously included, but in whom the final outcome of the injury could not be assessed at the time. Thus a very homogeneous, complete series from the Kreuzspital Chur was obtained for the years 1962–1980, including 221 fractures in 220 patients with a late follow-up. The series also comprises some metaphyseal fractures of the early years, when the main emphasis was placed on the cancellous bone defect rather than on the clear distinction between extraarticular and articular fracture patterns. The majority of patients discussed by Näser [140] and Comminot [30] had sustained closed fractures while skiing. Virtually all of them were operated on in the Kreuzspital by Heim himself, so in every respect they may be looked upon as selected patients. Macek [110] followed the patients from Mainz during the years 1965–1977 (66 fractures in 62 patients). As in the series from Lille and Amiens, traffic accidents or accidents at work (fall from a height) make up the majority of patients with 31% open fractures. Numerous publications in the last 15 years must be considered in this context. Some of them report on large numbers of patients (Table 1, pp. 220–221). Smaller studies are more homogeneous and reflect the personal experience of the authors. Problems with interpretation arise when percentages are used, a temptation many authors are apparently unable to resist. A summary of these data is given in Table 1. The most relevant figures in our opinion are those concerning patients followed after internal fixation. The direct comparison between the total number of patients, the number of internal fixations, and follow-up probably gives the best insight into how many problems are involved when interpreting patient series with an incomplete follow-up.

Several publications are also available on postoperative results after external fixation [17, 32, 79, 103, 126, 142, 166, 204]. To evaluate the frequency and severity of complications from this material is difficult. Often, the authors fail to differentiate between the patients they personally treated and other cases. Frequently, only a subset of the patients were examined; others were evaluated by means of a questionnaire or other data. Very often, the data file presents a potpourri of closed and open fractures, of patients having received nonoperative treatment, and patients on whom a wide spectrum of operative techniques had been employed. The only exceptions are the following series operated on on the same principles and followed completely: Rüedi and co-workers [171, 173], Comminot [30], Tassler [189], Börner [14], Waddell [204], Bone et al. [17], Ayeni [3], Höntzsch [79], Kellam and Waddell [88], Beck [7], Muhr and Breitfuss [126], and Etter and Ganz [43]. The analysis and tabular arrangement of the complications is not based on frequency and severity. Instead, in analogy to the description of operative techniques, we followed the chronological sequence in which they occurred. To the clinician, the sequence of events is more important, and this is why the chronological arrangement is more appropriate and of greater clinical relevance.

5.2. Complications Involving Soft Tissue

These are by far the most important. We differentiate the complications of the early hours and days from those of the first week. Problems involving bone become relevant only later, and in most cases they are directly related to the preceding soft tissue complication. Between these two events lies infection. Damage to soft tissue includes impaired arterial circulation, compartmental syndromes, postoperative swelling and hematoma, skin necrosis, early infection, and thromboembolic events.

5.2.1. Impairment of Arterial Circulation

In view of the fact that the arterial blood supply to the region of the ankle joint is derived from three sources, and the neurovascular bundle (see section 1.8) is located at a site relatively protected from the operative approach, injury to the arteries only occurs in severe open fractures [19], but it may be so severe as to make amputation inevitable [184, 203].

Valuable information is provided by the complete series of severe open fractures reported by Tassler [189], in which seven amputations had to be performed out of 54 injuries. Arterial reconstruction is rarely accomplished at this site [166].

We are not aware of any iatrogenic injuries to the artery during the operation. However, the vascular supply may be affected by the pressure induced by the retractor or by the protrusion of surplus cancellous bone. At the end of internal fixation, we have also seen arterial spasms leading to menacing disturbances of the pedal perfusion. A possible explanation is application of the tourniquet.

Preexisting vascular occlusions must also be thought of in such situations [203]. Systemic diseases of the arterial vascular system are increasingly seen. Clues may be provided by the history when asking for the walking distance prior to the accident. But patients who do not engage in any sport may be asymptomatic. The swelling around the fracture site often prevents palpation of foot pulses prior to operation, and assessment of the microcirculation at the toes is ambiguous. In any case, one should always examine the pulses of both popliteal arteries and compare auscultation of the femoral arteries.

5.2.2. Compartmental Syndromes

The compartmental syndrome to be feared in a distal tibial fracture is above all the anterior tibial compartment syndrome. It may develop within hours or days. An early surgical series was reported by Heim and Grete in 1972 [66]. In five of seven cases, the distal tibial segment was affected, and in three of these the fracture was intraarticular. The complication is rarely reported in the literature [110]. It must be assumed that this syndrome continues to be frequently missed; a possible explanation is that it is concealed within a range of severe and spectacular soft tissue lesions.

In a patient without further injuries, the diagnosis should be established quickly and on clinical grounds only. Immediate decompression of the compartment is essential. In a patient with multiple injuries, especially when unconscious or in shock, measurement of tissue pressure is recommended provided that no time is lost. There is no doubt that early decompression of the anterolateral fascia may enable a complete cure, and that systematic incision of the fascia during the operation may prevent the anterior tibial compartment syndrome from developing [56]. Among the patients from Chur are three cases with a deep posterior compartment syndrome. Subclinical signs are likely to develop at this site, where the condition progresses less rapidly than it does in the anterior tibial compartment.

The cardinal symptom is a spastic and painful equinus position of the foot. Because the pain is less severe, the diagnosis is often missed. This applies also to our patients whose diagnoses were made only in retrospect [30]. At follow-up, the patient presents with a contracted foot and clawfoot, passive dorsiflexion of the foot is limited, and the tendon of the flexor hallucis longus muscle appears to be shortened (which results from muscle necrosis). The diagnosis of tarsal tunnel syndrome [67, 146] or posterior tibial peritendinitis [23] as well as certain refractory equinus deformities following immobilization [184] points to an earlier posterior compartment syndrome.

Prophylactic incision of the deep dorsal fascia during the operation is advisable if, at reduction, the compartment is accessible. Proximal extension of the medial incision with exposure of the posteromedial neurovascular bundle may become necessary. In the more recent literature, compartmental syndromes are more frequently reported but the affected sites are not further differentiated [7, 32]. The figures given by Höntzsch [79] and Muhr and Breitfuss [126] exceed 10%.

5.2.3. Sensory Disturbances and Complaints of Neuroma

Sensory disturbances on the dorsolateral arch of the foot are caused by injuries to the terminal branch of the superficial peroneal nerve coursing in the lateral wound area [110] (Fig. 151). To avoid damage to this branch, it must be carefully identified. A prolonged or poorly functioning tourniquet (venous congestion) may also result in typical paralysis of the peroneal nerve [30, 32, 110, 146].

5.2.4. Postoperative Swelling

The most frequent complication in pilon fractures is postoperative swelling. The poor distensibility of the muscle envelope, which is subject to bilateral incisions, accounts for the specific character of the swelling here in contrast to other sites, where the process is of little significance. Jahna et al. [84] described this complication after conservative management.

The swelling starts on the first postoperative day and reaches its maximum after 2 to 4 days. Its extent is difficult to predict, but after a delayed operation it is certainly less than after an emergency internal fixation. It may lead to healing by second intention or actual skin necrosis above tension blisters. In its early stages, the swelling cannot be distinguished from hematoma.

5.2.5. Postoperative Hematoma

Postoperative hematoma cannot be avoided in this type of internal fixation where open areas of cancellous bone are often in the direct vicinity of the subcutaneous tissue. Even though the hematoma is bound to provide ideal growth conditions for bacterial organisms introduced into the wound during the operation, this ''banality'' is not mentioned in the literature. Initially, there is a bloody imbibition of the subcutaneous tissue undergoing partial liquefaction after a few days. In the first series at Chur, 19 hematomas (14%) were detected [140].

Every time a fluctuation is palpable, it must be evacuated as fast as possible since the chances for resorption are poor in this muscleless region. A simple aspiration is almost always inadequate to remove the mixture of fluid blood and dissolving coagula. The latter adhere to the subcutaneous tissue in a like fashion. The only treatment is surgical evacuation. This requires opening of individual skin sutures or a separate stab incision. A short general anesthesia and tourniquet are mandatory, and antibiotic cover is recommended. We introduce a curette into the wound, and while turning the spoon against the subcutis, scrape out any remaining adherent hematoma. A relapse can be prevented in most cases by insertion of a suction drain, and immobilization for 2 to 3 days. The extremely low infection rate in the series at Chur [30, 140] (see section 5.3.2.) demonstrates the efficiency of these procedures.

5.2.6. Wound Dehiscence

Wound dehiscence leading to healing by second intention and tension blisters appearing postoperatively as a result of swelling can only be avoided if the decision to reopen skin sutures is made early while the tension is increasing. Wound dehiscence always implies necrosis of the wound edges. Blisters are more likely to lead to a superficial spread of necrosis. These findings are often summarized as ''temporary wound healing impairment'' [14, 171, 211] or as *problèmes cutanés divers* (''miscellaneous skin problems'') [80]. At Chur, we saw seven cases in the first series. In five of these, an emergency internal fixation had been carried out. In the second series, where operation was delayed for several days, wound dehiscence was not observed [30].

5.2.7. Skin Necrosis

Necrosis of the skin may be confined to the superficial area and remain dry, as is occasionally observed after focal contusions. But if it occurs in association with surgical incisions, the necrosis tends to extend onto the bone or the implants where it is more or less specific. In the various studies, the incidence of necrosis generally ranges between 5% and 10% [14, 146, 160, 203, 211], but sometimes higher [32, 149].

Necrosis is virtually limited to the tibial approach, from which the complex main intervention is to be carried out, and where high-volume implants may cause additional pressure from within (Fig. 170). The complication is particularly grave if detected late, e.g., when a plaster cast is being changed several weeks postoperatively.

Necrosis is both cause for and origin of the majority of serious infections. It seems as though skin necrosis cannot be completely avoided in these injuries. Of prime importance is that the patient be assessed by an experienced surgeon at admission and, if the operation is delayed, that the patient receive continuous further surveillance. The timing of the operation is crucial. In our experience, undue delay, i.e., when granulation tissue has formed, will complicate the anatomic reduction (cf. section 3).

5.2.8. Thromboembolic Events

Although prophylactic thromboembolic drug therapy is carried out in every clinic, thromboembolic complications occasionally develop. They may occur early, but in cases of postoperative immobilization they may not develop before the cast is removed. Case reports appear in many papers [14, 19, 32, 43, 110, 140, 160, 173, 211]. Some postoperative pneumonias, often fatal, are another manifestation of this problem [140, 160]. As a whole, however, pilon fractures are not associated with a special thromboembolic risk.

5.2.9. Troublesome Scar Formation

While the physician generally gives little attention to operative scar formation, it is a matter of considerable concern to the patient. The discomfort produced by broad or keloid-like scars is hardly mentioned in the literature, although it may be very troublesome, preventing the patient from wearing normal shoes. Again, we emphasize the necessity of placing skin incisions correctly (see Figs. 151, 152, 156, 158). There are, however, other causes of troublesome scars. Careless suturing increases tension, thereby promoting localized necrosis. Keloids may result from postoperative swelling as well as by second intention. Näser [140] reported three keloids; Comminot [30] described four problematic scars. It should also be noted that scar neuromas may be very painful [32].

5.3. Postoperative Infection

Postoperative infections tend to originate in the soft tissues and to spread down to the bone later. We must look at the infection as an intermediate stage, which is to be analyzed separately in view of the special importance it has in these fractures. Following internal fixation of closed fractures, infections are generally the result of hematoma or skin necrosis that has become infected. At this site, infection appears to be more frequent than in other articular fractures. Various circumstances favor its development: length of operating time and, where applicable, tourniquet time; both contribute to the contamination of the surgical wound [21]. Bacteria adhere tightly to the broad implants situated directly under the skin. Because the region around the ankle joint lacks muscular cover, it compares unfavorably in terms of perfusion in comparison to other peripheral joints, i.e., the joints of the arms and shoulders. In severe open fractures, complete avoidance of postoperative infection is unrealistic [126], but it can be reduced to acceptable limits, as demonstrated by Tassler [189] and Bone et al. [17]. The former observed only six infections out of 54 third-degree open fractures; the latter saw no infections in 12 open fractures.

The literature of postoperative infections, however, is complicated by notorious ambiguities and inaccuracies concerning the time of onset, the severity, and the course of the infection.

5.3.1. Early Infection

Reviewing the literature, it is seldom possible to differentiate precisely between early and late infections [21]. Similarly, the data are inexact with respect to how far the joint is involved. Acute, early infections in the first week associated with high temperatures appear to be uncommon at this site. Songis-Mortreux [184] reported four cases. In the series of Rüedi et al. [171, 173], Näser [140], and Comminot [30], no early infections were observed. The large series of Beck [7] contains only one early infection.

To differentiate a superficial from a deep infection is possible only in retrospect. We call a process a superficial infection if treatment is carried out (including early removal of metal, if necessary) without sequelae. Of the six cases at Chur among 221 internal fixations, five healed without sequelae [30, 140]. In the series of Rüedi et al. [173], four of six cases were treated successfully. In their second series [171], there was no incidence of osteitis.

5.3.2. Osteitis and Osteoarthritis

The dominating infections described in the literature are deep infections in the sense of an osteitis or osteoarthritis. They are characterized by a prolonged course refractory to therapy and consequently have a poor outcome. On the radiograph, they are recognized by osteoporosis; osteolysis, possibly with formation of sequestra; and by secondary displacement, often associated with loosening of the implants.

While it has been demonstrated that osteitis is more frequent when the internal fixation is carried out as an emergency [14, 67], the figures vary considerably. Rüedi et al. [173] observed two infections in 84 cases; Heim and Näser, 1 in 128 cases [67]; and Börner [14], 2 in 102 cases. Where the authors failed to discriminate between closed and open fractures, the situation becomes confusing. In most studies, the frequency of osteitis ranges between 8% and 10% [21, 110, 146, 184, 211]. A higher incidence is reported by Mischkowsky and Dichgans (5 of 33 cases) [121], and K.-H.. Müller and Prescher (6 of 36 cases) [127]. If the infection is life-threatening, amputation may be necessary. Börner [14] reports 2 amputations in 102 cases; Ovadia and Beals [146], 3 in 76 cases; Pierce and Heinrich [149], 1 in 21; Macek [110], 4 in 62; and Songis-Mortreux [184], 3 in 79 cases.

If the joint is involved, and this applies to the majority of patients, arthrodesis may be necessary. Unfortunately, information as to whether arthrodesis was performed for infection or for arthrosis is often missing. Songis-Mortreux [184] reports 7 arthrodeses in 68 cases owing to infection, and Breitfuss et al. [21] report 16 in 131 cases.

What we know for certain is that not every infection originating in the metaphysis will penetrate the joint. Agglutination and encapsulation of articular fragments will occur. Infections of small metaphyseal sequestra may develop comparatively late and remain extraarticular. An illustrative case is depicted in Figure 202.

The case data filed at the AO documentation center analyzed in this study contain 21 cases of osteitis demonstrated radiographically. Of the 615 cases with late follow-up, the percentage is thus 3.4%. But of much greater importance is the clear correlation found between the complexity of the injury or the difficulties encountered intraoperatively, or both, and the appearance of osteitis. Neither groups A1, B2, and C1 nor subgroups B1.2, B1.3, and C3.1 contain any cases of osteitis (see Table 6, p. 321).

Except for a few cases, osteitis starts to accumulate only in groups B3, C2, and C3. In group C2, 10 cases in 119 late follow-ups are recorded; in C3, 4 cases in 23 late follow-ups, and in B3 (very few cases), the highest accumulation is seen with 3 cases in 10 late follow-ups. This means that the number of infections only exceeds 10% in groups with complex articular fractures (B3 and C3). What should be kept in mind is that the infection generally becomes evident within weeks, so that the patient will blame the infection on the surgeon which is not the case with arthrosis developing at a later stage. If a fracture has become infected, documentation is continued until the infection heals (more than 1 year in our patients). For this reason we assume that the majority of cases with postoperative infection are included in our case material; by contrast, cessation of recording is more likely in cases where the postoperative course is uneventful. The only exception would be patients changing their physician when infection appears. We think it legitimate, therefore, to relate the rate of infections to the total number of internal fixations. The percentage so obtained is clearly more favorable.

Another striking finding is that the rate of infections following closed fractures nearly equals the rate after open fractures. Details are given in the systematic analysis of the subgroups (see Appendix, section 3) and are summarized in Table 6, p. 321.

5.4. Aseptic Complications Involving Bone and Joint

Disturbances of fracture healing unrelated to infection are secondary dislocation, delayed and nonunion, malunion, pseudarthrosis, dystrophy, avascular necrosis, and arthrosis. The first four complications take place in the metaphysis, the latter two in the joint itself. With these complications, we must take into account the results of the statistical analysis reported here (see Appendix, sections 3 and 4).

5.4.1. Delayed Union and Secondary Displacement

The effects of asymmetric traction on the soft tissues or weightbearing commenced too early lead to secondary dislocation of unstable fragments and collapse of nonviable comminuted areas. This in turn may cause loosening or rupture of implants (Figs. 182 and 185). Delayed union is a process that takes place exclusively in the metaphysis. In the literature delayed union is difficult to detect and is often confused with true pseudarthrosis. Many studies also include cases that were managed conservatively. The comprehensive series of Jahna et al. [84] contains no such cases. The principal goal of treatment of these authors is healing with the bone shortened, a treatment goal we are unable to share.

Early detection of this problem is important because healing may be obtained almost without exception if reoperation is carried out in time. Moreover, the second intervention is technically much easier than primary internal fixation or an osteotomy, which may be required at a later date. Näser [140] reported 1 reintervention in 121 internal fixations; Comminot [30], 4 in 100 cases (two metal fractures). In the series of Vivès et al. [203], 3 cases occurred out of 70 (dislocation or rupture of the implant), and in the series of Börner [14], in 7 in 102. Examples are shown in Figures 178, 182, 185, and 189.

Among our patients (see Table 3), there were no cases of delayed union after simple, extraarticular fractures (A1). Following a wedge fracture (A2), we find 13 out of 72 cases that had been followed, and after complex metaphyseal fractures (A3), there were 6 out of 33 cases with follow-up. In B-type fractures, i.e., in partial articular fractures, problems involving the metaphysis are, of course, rare (1 case out of 187 with follow-up). After C-type fractures, i.e., complete articular fractures, metaphyseal complications are scarce when compared to arthrosis (see Appendix, Tables 4 and 5). Provided that systematic and close surveillance of the patients is assured, delayed union may heal while the fracture is temporarily immobilized. Thus Etter and Ganz [43] report healing in 4 of 5 cases; Höntzsch [79], 11 in 14; and Waddell [204], 5 in 8 cases. When postoperative treatment includes immobilization problems (trophic problems, perfusion, mobility, and psychological problems) always arise. Experience is required to deal with these problems.

5.4.2. Malunion

When the term *malunion* is used in the literature, its meaning is often extended to include delayed union. In its strict and narrow sense, it should only apply to cases in which consolidation has occurred but with malalignment. Whereas rotatory deformities may occur after conservative management, only valgus and varus deformities and antecurvature and recurvation are observed in patients operated on. In the literature, the number of valgus and varus deformities is about equal. Recurvation is hardly mentioned (Songis-Mortreux [184], one case). A problem repeatedly encountered with the data is the mélange of conservatively and operatively treated cases, which makes a clear differentiation difficult. The data may also include infections. Songis-Mortreux [184] reports 5 in 79 cases; Macek [110], 14 in 62; Stampfel and Mähring [185], 1 in 48; Resch et al. [160], 1 in 35; Pierce and Heinrich [149], 6 in 21; Rüedi et al. [173], 3 in 84; Börner [14], 5 in 33; Ovadia and Beals [146], 27 cases (mixed data file); and Muhr and Breitfuss [126], 3 in 47 cases.

The findings in our patients were reported in detail in section 3.2. The valgus position is dominant. We observed that the secondary malunion always drifts in the same direction as the course of the fracture line.

If and to what extent reoperations become necessary for these deformities remains unclear because of the inadequate length of follow-up periods in our patients and in the literature. Nor can we assess whether late arthrosis will result from the asymmetric loadbearing of the joint.

5.4.3. Pseudarthrosis

Pseudarthrosis is the result of delayed union managed neither by immobilization nor by reoperation and in which healing has not taken place. True pseudarthrosis is not frequent. The figures cited in the literature vary, and are often unreliable when operatively and nonoperatively treated patients are lumped together. In the majority of studies, the incidence is less than 2% [110, 140, 171, 173, 185]. Remarkable figures are provided by Börner [14], 7 in 102; Ovadia and Beals [146], 6 in 76; Bourne et al. [20], 4 in 33; and Songis-Mortreux [184], 3 in 79 cases. In our opinion, these authors failed to differentiate clearly between delayed union and pseudarthrosis. In the series analyzed in this study, we only found 1 case of true pseudarthrosis, namely, in subgroup C2.2 (see Appendix, section 3.4).

In the most recent literature, an increase of pseudarthrosis is reported; a possible explanation is the distracting effect of the external fixator. Bone [17], e.g., reports 3 cases in 12 patients; Waddell [204], 3 in 38; Lechevallier et al. [103], 3 in 27; and Höntzsch [79] 3 in 50.

5.4.4. Synostosis

Another complication involving the bone is synostosis, which may be described as a bridging callus (Fig. 188), and which is occasionally observed between the fibula and the tibia. Vivès et al. [203] report one case. Another case was described by Jahna et al. [84]. The remaining literature is unrevealing. In our data, several cases distributed among all fracture types are found, and they are listed individually in the Appendix, section 3. Two cases are shown in Figures 175 and 189. The synostosis is generally located 4 to 6 cm above the joint, so it concerns the metaphysis and less frequently the diaphysis. The majority of patients affected sustained a suprasyndesmotic comminuted fracture of the fibula plus a fracture of the tibia at the same level. Failure to achieve accurate reduction will more or less induce ossification via contact fragments. Another possible cause is in an interconnecting fracture hematoma when the interosseous membrane is torn. Sometimes one gets the impression that the synostosis was induced by drilling too deeply. A synostosis may lead to functional impairment, but we have also observed patients without any restriction of movement in the ankle joint.

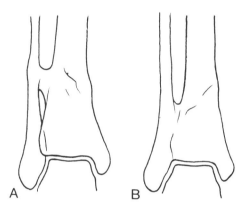

Figure 188. Tibiofibular synostosis at (**A**) diaphysis and (**B**) metaphysis. The drawings show radiologic contours.

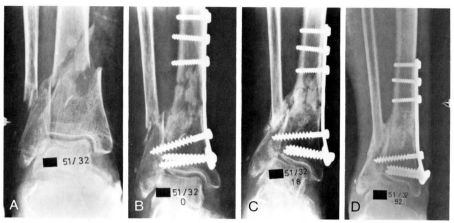

Figure 189. Valgus deformity following an extraarticular wedge fracture. This 74-year-old woman sustained a closed injury in a traffic accident; she walks without discomfort. **A.** Extraarticular fracture of the oblique type with a multifragmented wedge (A2.2); signs of osteoporosis; wedge fracture of the fibula above the syndesmosis; deviation into valgus position. **B.** Internal fixation of the tibia alone using a medial T-plate. Because the bending of the implant was insufficient, the valgus deviation persisted. **C.** When seen at 18 weeks, there was delayed fracture union and increased malalignment; a callus bridge had developed. **D.** At 1-year follow-up, the fractures had consolidated without progression of the deviation; the callus bridge was established; the implants were left in place. *Comment:* The decision against internal fixation of the fibula was responsbile for the poor assessment of the distal tibial angulation. Failure to prebend the implant as needed increased the valgus position and stimulated bridging callus formation.

5.4.5. Avascular Necrosis of Articular Fragments

This complication does not occur after conservative management of closed fractures, a phenomenon pointed out by Gay and Evrard [46], and confirmed by the large series of Jahna et al. [84]. Marginal fragments remain attached to the joint capsule—their source of blood supply. Depressions which remain unreduced are rapidly revitalized from the surrounding structures in which they are trapped.

Necrosis is, without exception, caused by devascularization of fragments during internal fixation. The approach to and reduction of articular fragments should always be carried out through a moderate longitudinal incision of the joint capsule and periosteum (see section 3.4.1).

In the attempt to accomplish accurate anatomic restoration of the articular surface, little attention was given to this problem in the past. Intraoperatively, however, the surgeon may encounter situations preventing restoration. Evidence of such necrosis is difficult to procure, but it is suspected by many authors [7, 88, 127, 146, 160, 184]. An early developing arthrosis following anatomic reduction of a complex fracture suggests this mode of origin [94]. A typical example from our personal case material is depicted in Figure 190, p. 233.

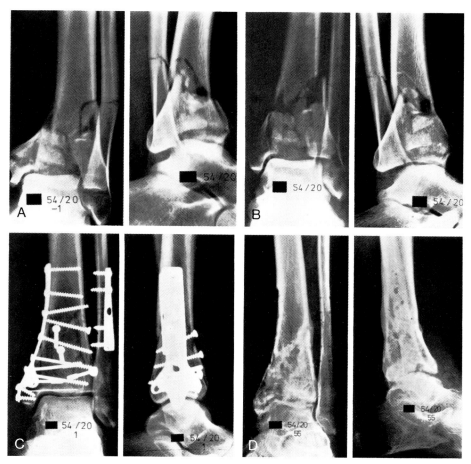

Figure 190. Early arthrosis following anatomic reconstruction of a complex C-type fracture (a 29-year-old fell from a platform; a closed fracture was the only injury). **A.** Complex complete fracture of the articular surface; centrally located pestle-formed depression with comparatively large fragments. The fibula shows a typical transverse fracture of the diaphysis with varus angulation. The distal, lateral ligaments were ruptured. Double fracture of the medial malleolus and anteromedial dislocation of the talar trochlea. Classified as C3.2. **B.** Realignment and partial reduction of the cortical shell fragments were performed while applying traction to the calcaneus. The dislocation of the talus persisted, and the depression became more evident. **C.** Internal fixation after a delay of 7 days: anatomic reconstruction by means of a one-third tubular plate for the fibula, and a cloverleaf plate and small screws for the tibia. After reduction, the depressed fragment is held by a single horizontal Kirschner wire. Because the lateral incision was under tension, it had been left open at first, and was closed in stages a few days later. Uncomplicated wound healing; heel-to-toe walking; full weightbearing was achieved at 14 weeks. **D.** When seen at 1 year (55 weeks), the patient showed severe arthrosis with cyst formation. He complained of problems and pain when walking, and arthrodesis was indicated. *Comment:* The early arthrosis is assumed to result from intraoperative fragment devitalization.

5.4.6. Reflex Dystrophy

Sudeck's atrophy has a subacute onset and is characterized by pain at rest, torpid swelling of soft tissue, restricted mobility, and patchy osteoporosis. The arms and shoulders are predominantly affected. It is rare after internal fixation and functional postoperative management of distal tibial fractures [110]. As a temporary finding treated successfully, it has been observed at Chur [30]. It has also been reported by Hourlier [80], Pierce and Heinrich [149], and Ovadia and Beals [146], but it is not clear whether these patients had been treated operatively.

When immobilization is prolonged, patchy osteoporosis and corresponding trophic impairment of the soft tissues are very common [39, 123]. A particularly high incidence of such is given by Copin and Nérot in their large series [32]. Unfortunately, the authors do not describe the postoperative management, and we must assume that the majority of patients were immobilized with plaster casts. Because casts restrict mobility, the outcome is generally some measure of disability. We must keep in mind, however, that osteoporosis is only one sign within a manifold and complex clinical picture.

5.4.7. Posttraumatic Arthrosis

The goal of treatment in articular fractures is to achieve a functional recovery free of pain. In a joint with a small surface area subject to heavy load—and this applies to the ankle joint—the task becomes particularly challenging. There is consensus among authors [11, 17, 29, 32, 100, 115, 118, 160, 192, 203, 204, 211] that proper healing requires reconstruction of the articular surface with realignment of any steps, and an infection-free postoperative course. Early motion improves cartilage nutritional requirements and promotes regeneration [176].

Besides the state of the tibial articular surface, cartilaginous lesions of the trochlea of the talus must also be taken into account. It is surprising that the classic literature on pilon fractures contains no information on this problem. Only recently, Lantz et al. [96] have pointed to the frequency of such lesions in malleolar fractures.

The clinical picture of arthrosis is multifarious. Thickening of the joint develops with restriction of mobility. The initial pain on motion evolves into continuous pain with limitation of walking distance. Osteophytosis is the first radiologic sign; narrowing of the joint space follows. It may be compared with the normal side when stress films are obtained [10]. The disease may progress to subchondral sclerosis, deformity, and widening of the epiphysis, less frequently to formation of cysts. In the end, the joint space may be completely obliterated. The corresponding clinical picture consists of ankylosis.

As is the case in other joints, we often find a discrepancy between the clinical and the radiologic picture. In particular, when the arthrosis appears to be moderately severe on the radiograph, it may produce amazingly little discomfort [11, 60, 62, 161].

The problem of arthrosis was thoroughly analyzed in 1979 by Jahna et al. [84] in their large series comprising predominantly conservatively treated cases. It was shown that the degree of severity could be reliably assessed only 4 to 5 years after the accident. Later changes were minor. This concept is consistent with the investigations of Rüedi et al. in 1968 [173] and Comminot in 1981 [30], in which complete postoperative series were followed for more than 6 years. These data were also confirmed by Waddell [204]. As early as 1 year after the operation, one may clearly recognize on the radiograph whether the joint is free of traumatic arthrosis [62, 168]. If at this time, incongruences are seen, the prognosis is uncertain. This applies also to patients who are free of complaints. Severe cases of postoperative arthrosis manifest clinically as well as radiologically after 1 year [94, 161].

Progress was less rapid in the nonoperative series of Jahna et al. [84]. Studying the case material, one gets the impression that after conservative management osteoarthrosis starts at a later date and advances more slowly, being on the whole more benign than postoperative arthrosis. Apparently, this applies also after use of the external fixator [10, 17, 79, 103, 126, 141, 142, 147]. The situation resembles that found in malleolar fractures where the arthrosis takes a less disabling course when the reduction has been incomplete or the treatment nonoperative than is the case with internal fixation, after which incongruences persist [213, 214].

The data in the literature on the frequency of posttraumatic arthrosis after internal fixation are inconsistent. The terms are ill-defined, observation periods differ, and only some of the original patients have been followed up. Most authors generally report an incidence of arthrosis between 20% and 50% [19, 21, 110, 121, 211]. The figures given by Heim and Näser [67], Comminot [30], Rüedi [171, 173], and recently by Beck [7] are lower, but were obtained in selected patients (mostly closed fractures with skiing accidents prevailing).

In our series, the assessment was based on purely radiologic criteria (see Appendix, section 3, Tables 3 to 5). The follow-up period was generally 1 year, rarely longer. Our main intention was to determine how frequently and in which types of fracture the joints remained free of arthrosis. In the detailed analysis, the number of patients developing alterations in the joint is indicated for each subgroup. These have been classified as prearthrosis, established arthrosis, and post arthrodesis.

Prearthrosis is defined as a condition in which radiologic abnormalities of the articular contours are evident at 1 year. These patients may be expected to develop minor or moderate arthrosis. In an attempt to organize the material more coherently, cases of prearthrosis and arthrosis are considered collectively in the Appendix (see section 4), and cases in which arthrodesis had been carried out are listed in a separate column. The development of an extremely severe and early arthrosis is rare and confined to complex fractures.

Prearthrosis and arthrosis are almost completely absent (below 1%) in extraarticular fractures. Among pure partial splits, they are still uncommon; they increase considerably in depressions, and concentrate in certain forms of C2- and C3-type fractures. With our case data, the figures computed are given in the following list. If prearthrosis, arthrosis, and early arthrodesis are considered collectively (all postoperative cases showing pathologic changes involving the joint), the following picture is obtained (total number of patients with long-term, at least 1-year follow-up: 615):

1. Extraarticular fractures (type A): 215 with follow-up, 3 cases with changes involving the joint (1 technical fault)
2. Partial articular fractures (type B): 187 cases with follow-up
   - Partial articular split (B1): 138 cases with follow-up, 10 articular changes (7.2%)
   - Partial articular fracture with depression (B2): 39 cases with follow-up, 14 articular changes (about 33%)
   - Partial complex fracture (B3): 10 cases with follow-up, 7 cases with articular changes (about 67%)
3. Complete articular fractures (type C): 213 cases with follow-up
   - Complete, simple fracture (C1): of 71 patients with follow-up, 14 showed articular changes (19.7%); 11 of these were observed among the 19 fractures with depression
   - Articular split with metaphyseal impaction or multifragmentation (C2): of 119 cases with follow-up, there were 59 with articular changes (54%); 11 of these concerned the 14 cases where additional depression was present
   - Complex articular fracture (C3): of 23 cases with follow-up, 15 showed changes in the joint (about 60%)

In summary we may conclude that the severity of the fracture as assessed for classification from the postinjury radiograph, i.e., on purely morphologic criteria, correlates with its further course and final outcome. See also Tables 3 to 5.

Examples

Radiographs illustrating complications are depicted in Figures 189 and 190.

Examples of malunion are given in Figures 175, 176, 178, 182, 185, 187, 189, and 205.

Examples showing arthrosis or prearthrosis at 1-year follow-up are given in Figures 175, 176, 185, 186, and 190.

Radiographs illustrating the finding of synostosis are given in Figures 175 and 189.

6. TACTICS AND TECHNIQUES IN SOFT TISSUE DAMAGE

> The presence of soft tissue damage necessitates a change of operative tactics. This concerns mainly the medial side of the tibial fracture.

Damage to soft tissue is the dominant topic in the recent literature on pilon fractures. Sometimes one gets the impression that the simple fractures at this location to be treated in line with classic AO principles as outlined in section 3 have disappeared. This assumption is, of course, not realistic, especially in view of the fact that in the early studies and publications, most injuries were caused by a fall from a height. Then skiing accidents, undoubtedly associated with less soft tissue damage, became prevalent. In addition to falls from a height, traffic accidents are now coming to the fore. The term *high velocity* is commonly used for both falls and traffic accidents, and the corresponding fractures are referred to as *explosion fractures*. In our opinion, this terminology is debatable. In all mechanisms of accident, including many skiing accidents, a sudden deceleration takes place that is subject to well-known physical laws. In traffic accidents, however, external forces are generally involved.

They are many aspects to soft tissue damage. With the anatomic conditions found in the lower leg, with its scanty skin envelope and fairly precarious blood supply, the damage is of much greater importance, and consideration from three different angles is required.

6.1. Closed Injuries

Closed fractures are characterized by the increase in pressure from within, produced either by dislocating fragments, by initial axial deviation, or by hematoma. Even though the accident itself rarely produces manifest ischemia, compressions and, in particular impairment, of venous return must be thought of. Contusions frequently occur in traffic and work accidents. They are readily overlooked immediately after the accident, skewing the overall assessment. The first two lesions favor the development of posttraumatic swelling or compartmental syndromes (see section 5.2.2).

6.2. Operative Trauma

The second form of soft tissue damage to be discussed is operative trauma. Necrosis of the skin and, under unfavorable conditions, of fragments may be produced by gross manipulations or inadequate approaches.

6.3. Open Fractures

The early data contain numerous open fractures. Open fractures require an emergency procedure to reduce and stabilize the bone, and debridement of devitalized soft tissue must be carried out. The precarious circulation limits the extent to which plastic reconstruction may be performed.

The preceding paragraphs indicate the difficulties encountered with the evaluation of soft tissue trauma. It requires the skillful realization and perhaps modification of previously described tactical and technical steps and of aftercare concepts. Only a surgeon with extraordinary clinical expertise is able to meet these demands.

Most of the skin lesions affect the medial side of the distal lower leg. Local perfusion can be assessed only after gross reduction of the fracture and its temporary fixation. Local conditions permitting, the typical internal fixation of the fibula is carried out as the first step of the procedure [79, 192] (see section 3.3.2 and Fig. 155). Afterward debridement and temporary fixation of the tibia may be accomplished. It is advantageous to reduce the articular surface of the tibia at this stage since when this step is performed at a later time, it is often impossible to obtain the desirable precision.

Temporary fixation is accomplished under traction (calcaneal traction or external fixator), with the aid of individual Kirschner wires and occasionally with individual small screws. Trentz and Friedl [194] recently described a technique adjusted to the conditions of the soft tissues: in a first-degree open fracture and minor soft tissue lesion, they prefer to attach the plate at a site distant from the injury (anteriorly or posteriorly). With increasing damage to the soft tissues, or in second-degree open fractures, buttress is provided by an external fixator; and if the soft tissues are badly damaged, the authors recommend primary shortening to relieve the soft tissue (combined with arthrodesis) and secondary callus distraction. Except for the last-named, fixation of the fibula is always carried out as the first step.

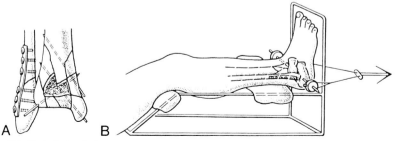

Figure 191. Technical solutions suggested with medial soft tissue damage. **A.** Fibular plate, reduction of the tibial articular surface, and fixation with Kirschner wires. **B.** Fibular plate combined with calcaneal traction.

Stabilization with the external fixator has become a mainstay of this type of pilon fracture. Variations in the assembly are possible (see Fig. 192). Steinmann pins are anchored either in the talus or calcaneus and in the tibial shaft. Some authors prefer the one-plane, unilateral fixator applied medially with Schanz screws, while others favor a triangular frame construction [79] (Fig. 193A). The objective is to bridge both the ankle joint and the tibiotalar joint. According to Bone et al. [17], articular lesions do not occur if the leg is immobilized for less than 2 months.

The use of the external fixator has certainly brought about a significant reduction in the risk of infection. However, an increase in delayed union, pseudarthrosis, and reportedly in malunion [126] has been noted (see section 5.4.2). Welz [212] was the first to describe how to insert Steinmann pins or thick, threaded Kirschner wires into the tibia close to the joint in patients with a simple articular component. This has the advantage of permitting at least some movement of the ankle joint (Fig. 194).

In any case, when stabilization with an external fixator is compared to classic calcaneal traction, the former has the great benefit of allowing free movement in the knee and hip joints, thereby allowing ambulation, and often also earlier discharge from hospital. The use of the external fixator confers positive effects on nutrition and circulation and also on the psychological state of the patient. There is some reluctance to primary packing of defects in open fractures with cancellous bone, since the ambiguous circulatory conditions of deep structures may jeopardize incorporation of the graft. Instead of cancellous bone, some authors prefer to fill the defects with small antibiotic cement beads until definitive reconstruction of the bone and soft tissues becomes possible in a second intervention [118].

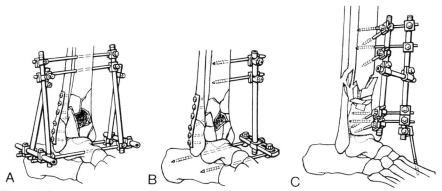

Figure 192. External fixation: systems used with soft tissue damage. **A.** Frame construction with Steinmann pins (on tibia, talus, and calcaneus). **B.** Fixation assembly with a medial rod and a distal T-piece bridging the joint. **C.** Anteromedial V with two rods; additional fixation in the first metatarsal bone.

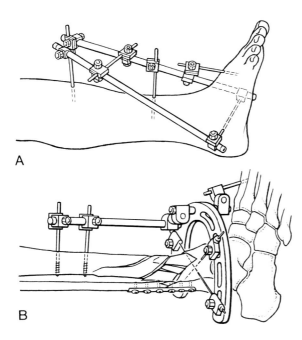

A

B

Figure 193. Other applications of the external fixator. **A.** Triangular frame between the calcaneus and the tibial shaft with two rods. The first metatarsal is included to ensure a right-angle position of the foot. **B.** Rod assembly at the tibial shaft combined with a half-frame in a second- to third-degree open fracture with multifragmentation of the metaphysis. The Kirschner wires are placed through the already reduced articular split fracture. A plate has been previously applied to the fracture of the fibula (see Figure 201).

Figure 194. Use of the small external fixator according to Welz [211]. The distal pin is introduced into the tibial epiphysis after reduction of a split fracture. **A.** Sagittal plane. **B.** Frontal plane. The two devices may be combined by connecting the bars.

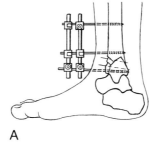

A

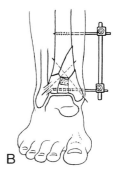

B

In third-degree open fractures associated with injuries of tendons and neuro-vascular bundles or large cutaneous defects, the initial management relies on tem-porary measures. Large cutaneous defects require plastic reconstruction. There is no doubt that the cross-leg flap has superseded the technique of free flaps trans-ferred by the use of microsurgery. Close cooperation from the outset with the microsurgeon and the plastic surgeon is mandatory in these situations.

A second-look operation and a second debridement may become necessary after a few days. Definitive stable fixation of the fracture, cancellous bone grafting, and plastic reconstruction of the defect are then scheduled together as a single procedure.

It should be recalled in this context that in the case of medial soft tissue damage Vivès et al. [203] reduce the tibial fracture from an anterolateral approach, where they also place the implants.

The same procedure has recently been recommended by Ganzoni and Jiricek [45]. They leave the medial incision open wide to reduce the tension on the soft tissue, and cover the fibula with muscles mobilized from the posterior and anterior aspects (Fig. 195A). The lateral defect is covered in a second procedure with a mesh split-thickness graft [126]. Further technical alternatives are:

- Tibiofibular transfixion with screws from the lateral side according to Judet et al. [85], referred to as *en peigne,* i.e., like a comb (Fig. 195B). Tibial fragments may be stabilized by long screws applied through a fibular plate. This requires main-tenance of both tibial threads in the fibula as a safeguard against collapse or varus angulation. Trentz and Friedl [194] also mention this technique.
- Transplantar medullary nailing with Steinmann pins (Fig. 196). In extreme situa-tions, this may be valuable in achieving a simple temporary fixation [27].
- The reported percentage of open fractures of the tibial pilon actually lies between 20% and 30% of the total [17, 32, 126, 204].

The case material filed at the AO documentation center and analyzed in this book shows a relationship between soft tissue damage and the morphology of the fracture:

- Among extraarticular oblique fractures (A1.2), open fractures amount to 12%; in wedge fractures (A2.2), 28%; and in the complex A3-type fractures, almost 50%.
- Open fractures are rare in partial fractures (B) except for those of the complex B3 type.
- The rarity with which open fractures occur in simple C1 fractures (about 4%) and in impacted fractures (C2.1) is striking. With the latter, only valgus fractures are open (see Appendix, section 3.4). In C2.2 fractures (metaphyseal multifrag-mentation) by contrast, almost half of the fractures are open. Surprisingly, the proportion decreases to 26% in the complex C3-type fractures, and on the whole, it tends to be lower in extensive fractures with involvement of the diaphysis.

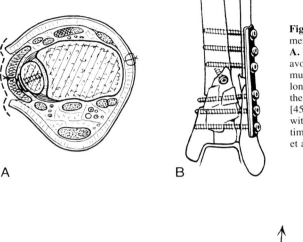

A

B

Figure 195. Alternative in the treatment of medial soft tissue damage. **A.** The lateral incision is left open to avoid tension. The short peroneal muscle and the extensor digitorum longus muscle are mobilized to cover the fibular plate (Ganzoni and Jirecek [45]. **B.** The fibular plate is provided with long screws which at the same time hold the tibial fragments (Judet et al. [85].

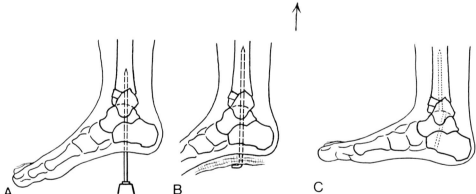

A

B

C

Figure 196. Provisional transplantar fixation of the distal tibia for complex pilon fractures with severe soft tissue damage using a Steinmann pin, according to Childress [27]. **A.** The pin is introduced in slight plantarflexion. **B.** The end of the pin is bent above the dressing. **C.** When the pin has been removed and the foot re-dressed in dorsiflexion and in the right-angle position, the holes in the articular surfaces will not meet.

7. PILON FRACTURES: WHAT'S NEW?

T. Rüedi

The four classical principles of treatment that have been described extensively have proved their applicability and efficiency and have been published in a number of well-documented series [14, 30, 67, 171, 173]. However, recent publications on the operative treatment of pilon fracture [21, 121, 127] report a rather high incidence of complications (20% to 30%), mostly concerning wound healing problems in conjunction with ORIF of the distal tibia. A breakdown of the delicate skin cover at the lower end of the leg or over the metal implant is usually synonymous with a deep infection or osteitis as well as a bad functional outcome.

Compared with the original series of Rüedi and Allgöwer [173] and Heim [67, 68], which consisted of mostly low-energy skiing accidents, it appears that today the majority of these severe injuries are caused by different, more violent mechanisms with much higher energies involved (motorbike, hang-gliding, jumpers, etc.). This is reflected in the fracture patterns (more type C3 fractures) on one side, but especially in more severe soft tissue injuries in both closed and open fractures on the other.

Postoperative complications, poor reduction, and unsatisfactory results may, however, be attributed not only to the severity of the initial injury but also to the experience or rather inexperience of the surgeon. Factors such as timing of surgery, gentleness of the reduction maneuver, handling of the soft parts during surgery, choice of implant, technique of skin closure, and the duration of the procedure are all extremely relevant for the final outcome. Very careful planning of the surgery is therefore just as mandatory as considerable experience and dexterity of the surgeon. Pilon fracture surgery is not for beginners and not for the middle of the night. Emergency surgery should be performed only under optimal overall conditions.

Of course, the question arises, what may and can be done by the junior resident who usually sees these patients at odd hours or in conjunction with other major trauma? The classical closed reduction and calcaneal traction is used less and less frequently, as there always remains some instability with rather slow soft tissue recovery and considerable discomfort for the bedridden patient. The method of choice to temporarily stabilize a pilon fracture in our experience consists in the application of a triangular or unilateral external fixator between tibia shaft and calcaneus or talus with radiolucent carbon fiber bars. In case of a simple fracture of the fibula and no lateral soft tissue problem the use of a third tubular plate on the fibula in combination with an external fixator placed medially proves to be a valuable first step as wel (Fig. 198C). While waiting for the soft tissues to recover, conventional tomograms (anteroposterior and lateral) are requested for easier planning, as these seem to give more information than the computed tomography scan.

In a few exceptional cases with minimal displacement or no involvement of the articular surface (type A) the joint-bridging external fixator may be kept for as long as 6 weeks, when a cast will replace it. The recuperation of joint movement will, however, take rather long.

For definitive stabilization—usually within 8 to 10 days after injury—the external fixator is left in place or is substituted by the distractor, to help for gentle "indirect" reduction maneuvers (Fig. 198A, B). In case the fibula has already been plated initially, we directly approach the tibia; if not, the fibula should be fixed first. The implant of choice for the fibula is the one-third tubular plate or rarely the heavier 3.5-mm DCP or LCDCP. As a routine, all patients with pilon fracture should get a single-dose prophylactic antibiotic, usually a first- or second-generation cephalosporin.

Alternative Techniques of Fixing the Tibia

The classic way to stabilize the distal tibia consists of applying a 4.5-mm T-plate or, more recently, the clover-leaf plate designed by Heim, with a buttress function on the medial or anterior aspect of the bone. While generally providing adequate stability to the fracture fragments, the rather large metal surface may give rise to wound healing disturbances in this area of very delicate skin cover. In patients with good bone stock and large fragments that are anatomically reducible, we have gone back to using lag screws only (3.5 mm cortical, 4.0 cancellous, and/or 3.5 and 4.5 mm cannulated screws) (Figs. 197A, B to 200C).

To support the impacted articular surface after it has been elevated more securely, it appears advisable to harvest a bicorticocancellous wedge graft from the iliac crest rather than simple cancellous bone chips. This bone block combines good biological with excellent mechanical properties and it can easily be shaped to fit into the metaphyseal bone defect. If used with "screws only" the fixation is usually such that early motion and even partial weightbearing may be permitted in a cooperative patient without any additional protection.

In some rare instances there is no room for a secure placement of a screw or plate into the distal articular fragments or the soft parts are so badly contused that no internal fixation should be attempted initially. As an alternative to a temporary joint-bridging external fixator, some authors have advocated the use of the Ilizarov-type ring fixator with rather thin transfixation pins. More recently the so-called hybrid frame has been described and prototypes developed (Fig. 193B). In this technique, 1.8- to 2-mm K-wires are drilled through the larger fragments of the distal tibia and are then anchored under tension within the half ring device. Finally this half ring is fixed to a unilateral external fixator with tube-to-tube clamps (Fig. 201). In order to stabilize the foot in a neutral position, an additional Schanz screw is placed in the first metatarsal and fixed to the frame.

Besides the unconventional and alternative ways of stabilizing the bone, much attention must be given to the soft parts. Any skin defects larger than a few square centimeters should be covered within a few days by a free tissue transfer with microvascular anastomosis as there are no possibilities for any pedicle muscle or skin flaps at the lower end of the leg. As soon as the soft tissue cover appears consolidated, any external fixation device may be substituted by open reduction and internal fixation (Fig. 200).

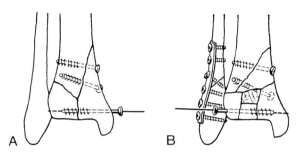

Figure 197. The use of small cannulated screws near the articular surface. **A.** In case of a simple fracture with an intact fibula, the screws are inserted from the medial side. **B.** Screws are introduced from the lateral side, anterior to the already stabilized fibular fracture.

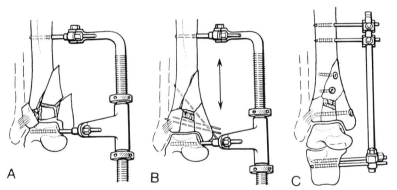

Figure 198. The use of the distractor for indirect reduction at the tibia. **A.** The Schanz screws are inserted in the talus and the tibial diaphysis, and the distractor is then attached to the screws. **B.** Tension applied slowly by the distractor will then correct the shortening. This procedure allows painstaking and careful reduction and temporary fixation with Kirschner wires. **C.** External fixator applied medially for temporary buttressing of a minimal internal fixation of the tibia with small screws. The Schanz screws are inserted in the calcaneus.

Text continued on page 252

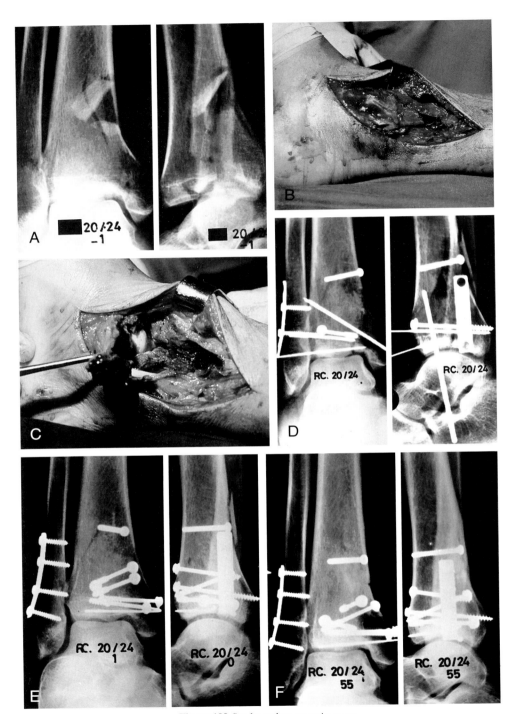

Figure 199 *See legend on opposite page*

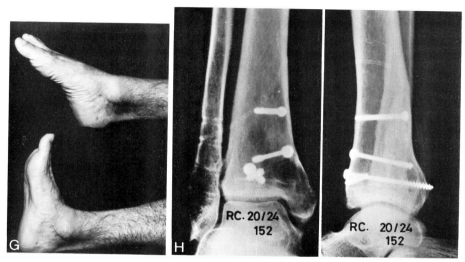

Figure 199. See Color Figure 199. Internal fixation of a depression fracture with small screws in a 29-year-old who sustained a closed fracture without concomitant injuries after falling from a 6-m-high scaffolding. Because of swelling and early blister formation, traction was applied primarily and internal fixation performed 8 days later. Active mobilization was started on day 6. The patient was discharged from hospital on day 20 with a crutch to allow partial weightbearing. Partial rehabilitation as a construction worker was gained after 18 weeks, full rehabilitation at 20 weeks. **A.** Partial fracture; anterior wall remained intact. Oblique, pestle-formed depression posteromedially. Multiple splits of the posterior metaphysis; subluxation of the talus; typical valgus fracture of the fibula. Vertical fracture of the medial malleolus; classified as B2.3. **B.** An atypical, posteromedial incision is made; the fracture line comes into view; cortical fenestration is carried out. **C.** Intraoperative view: the fragments and the depression are clearly recognizable; the medial malleolus is retracted distally. Posteriorly, the tendon of the posterior tibial muscle is visible. **D.** Intraoperative radiograph: temporary stabilization of the fibula. The tibial fracture is reduced, the depression corrected. The large, posterior articular fragment and the corticocancellous shell extending upward are fixed with small screws and washers. The defect is packed with cancellous bone, and the depression and the medial malleolus are held by Krischner wires. The fracture lines are still clearly evident. **E.** Radiologic control at completion of the internal fixation. A Kirschner wire near the joint was left in place. The fracture lines have almost disappeared. **F.** The radiograph at 1 year (55 weeks): fracture union, no arthrosis.

   G. At 3 years, there was full dorsi- and plantarflexion. **H.** Radiograph at 3 years (152 weeks): partial removal of implants (palpable implants). No signs of arthrosis. *Comment:* Optimal reconstruction of a depression fracture. Stabilization was achieved with small screws only. At 3 years, the patient was free of arthrosis.

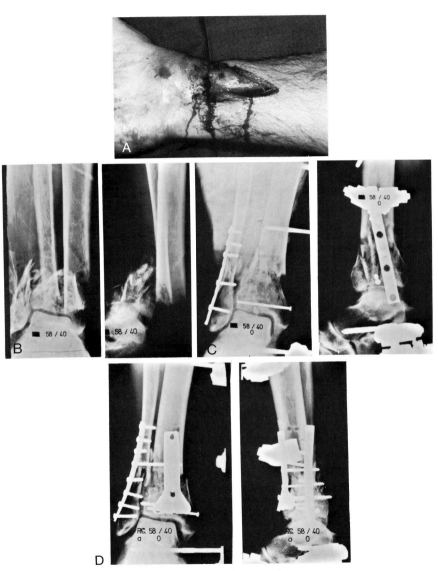

Figure 200 *See legend on opposite page*

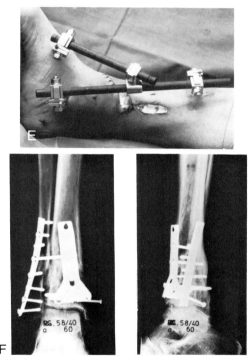

Figure 200. See Color Figure 200. **A, B.** This 42-year-old man fell from a scaffolding and sustained a second-degree open right pilon fracture. (C2.2-type morphology). **C.** Emergency operation: approximate reduction of the fracture by the application of traction with the external fixator followed by open reduction with internal fixation (ORIF) of the complex fibular fracture with an eight-hole one-third tubular plate. This allows better realignment of the tibia and fixation of the sagittal articular split with an isolated cannulated 3.5-mm screw. **D.** External fixator bridging the talus, the calcaneus, and the tibial shaft (carbon fiber bars). Partial adaptation of the wound. Ten days later, ORIF of the tibia. Access is gained by slightly prolonging the existing wound. A cloverleaf plate is placed anteriorly to fix the reduced fracture line in the frontal plane. Cancellous iliac bone graft. Transfixing screw from the fibular plate onto the tibia. **E.** The external fixator is left in place for 6 weeks. No complications. **F.** At 14 months (60 weeks), the fracture has consolidated, and there is satisfactory function to the ankle joint. There are no signs of early arthrosis.

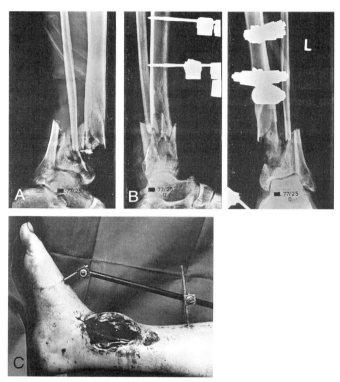

Figure 201. See Color Figure 201. **A.** This 33-year-old patient ran into a car and sustained a third-degree, open and very soiled pilon fracture of the left leg (C2.2-type morphology). **B, C.** An emergency operation was performed 2 hours after the accident under antibiotic cover. **D.** Debridement, lavage, approximate reduction. An external fixator is applied to the calcaneus and the tibia including the first metatarsal. Open wound treatment. Traction on a suspension apparatus. **D–G.** ORIF at day 13: fixation of the fibula with a 3.5-mm titanium limited contact dynamic compression plate. Transfixation of the articular fragments with two Kirschner wires fixed in a half-frame prototype and connected to the Schanz screws in the tibial shaft with carbon fiber bars. Iliac cancellous bone graft into the huge metaphyseal defect. No complications. The fixator was removed at 3 months. **H.** At 5 months, the tibial fracture seems to have consolidated. There is satisfactory ankle function with some osteoporosis. The patient is still under treatment.

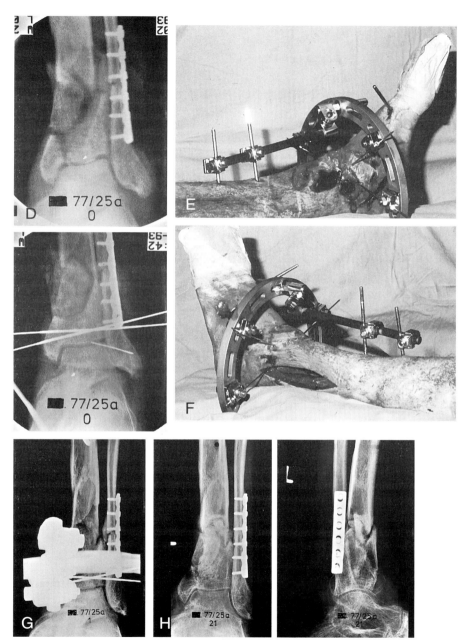

Figure 201 *Continued*

8. SECONDARY INTERVENTIONS

8.1. Secondary Internal Fixation of the Fibula

The circumstances allowing one to refrain from primary internal fixation of the fibula have been outlined in section 3.3. Predominantly, this is the case in extraarticular fractures where contact between the main tibial fragments has been preserved. Furthermore, the biological and mechanical conditions of the tibia must be straightforward, but this is unusual.

If early signs of axial deviation become evident after the operation, secondary stabilization of the fibula is imperative. It is carried out following the technique described in section 3.3.2, and in most cases it will halt the beginning drift into valgus position of the distal lower leg. Healing of the fibular fracture is then uneventful (an example is given in Fig. 202).

Loosening of the fibular fixation indicates delayed union of the tibial fracture. In such cases, a reintervention on the fibula will prove to be insufficient for mechanical reasons, and secondary intervention on the tibia is called for (Figs. 185 and 205).

8.2. Secondary Internal Fixation of the Tibia

Reconstruction of the articular surface is accomplished by primary internal fixation where it presents the second step of the operative technique. Gross dislocations have also been realigned during the first intervention. Minor irregularities or cartilaginous lesions are beyond surgical repair. The only effective management promoting their regeneration consists in intensive exercises without weightbearing. This is often successful in keeping posttraumatic arthrosis within radiologically and clinically acceptable limits. The same holds true for minor depressions [30, 168].

While reconstructive, secondary corrections are feasible in major joints, this is rarely the case with the small articular surface of the distal tibia. When cartilage damage leads to rapidly progressing arthrosis, the pain can only be managed by secondary arthrodesis (see section 8.4). The results with endoprosthetic devices have not been convincing up to now [114].

Delayed consolidation of the distal tibia is always localized in the metaphysis. This is the region where a defect or devitalized area may have been present but which escaped detection. Cancellous bone grafting was not performed, or the graft was compromised as a result of poor stability. The delayed consolidation brings about either axial deviation, with bony union, or pseudarthrosis. If the trouble spot is located laterally, the leg drifts into valgus angulation. If it is on the medial side, varus angulation ensues. The implant material is subject to increasing load (changing loads). Loosening of screws follows, and possibly fracture of the implant.

If consolidation of a tibial fracture has remained incomplete at 20 weeks, and if complaints continue and swelling persists, delayed union must be assumed. Once the suspicion has been confirmed, one should not hesitate to proceed with the reoperation. Immobilization will deteriorate the trophic condition of the leg, and weaken the morale of the patient. Another aspect is that the reintervention is quite simple technically, because it may be confined to a single area. The main problem is reassuring the patient who naturally is anxious about a further operation.

The planning of the intervention must aim at both consolidating the fracture and correcting the deformity. Another cancellous bone graft (with an additional corticocancellous chip, when needed) is inevitable. The approach is always through the existing scars, even if these are less than ideally placed. By extending the former incisions proximally or distally, adequate access can usually be obtained.

Necrosis may result when new incisions are made in this skin area with its precarious blood supply. Moreover, they may favor the development of atrophic skin areas under which bony union is known not to take place.

The loose or fractured implant is exposed and removed. Outside the site of the implant, parallel Kirschner wires are inserted proximally and distally. They allow measurement of the desired angles. The pseudarthrosis is exposed, and the fibrous callus is removed with a curette. Again, a distracting device (external fixator or distractor) has proved a useful aid for axial correction. Sometimes it is possible to accomplish distraction with a plate already attached distally using the reversed tension device [117] (Fig. 210B). The adequately processed autologous cancellous graft is filled in the defect under pressure. While any further devitalization is to be avoided, a stronger implant is now placed in the position of the first one, and pulled upward with the tension device.

Postoperative mobilization of the patient must be vigorously encouraged. As a rule, complete consolidation and full weightbearing capacity is achieved at 2 to 3 months. Typical examples illustrating such cases are given in Figures 203, 204, and 205.

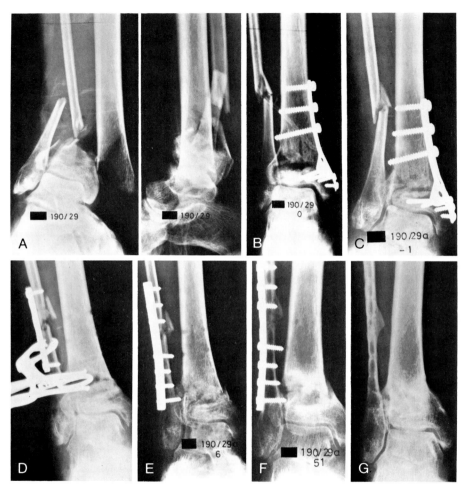

Figure 202. Secondary internal fixation of the fibula and lateral osteotomy of the tibia in a 37-year-old woman who sustained an open fracture after a fall from a platform. Early pregnancy with spontaneous abortion. An infection medially accounted for a protracted postoperative course, and only partial functional recovery was achieved. **A.** Complete articular fracture (lateral split) with an area of multifragmentation in the metaphysis. First-degree open fracture grossly displaced into valgus; medial wound; typical multifragmented fracture of the fibular diaphysis. Classified as A2.2. **B.** Emergency operation: the wound was debrided and medially plated, but no cancellous bone graft was performed. Wound closure was free of tension. The patient received no antibiotics and the postoperative course was uneventful. She left the hospital 3 weeks later with a circular plaster cast. **C.** Increasing drift into valgus angulation resulted from delayed consolidation of the lateral tibial metaphysis and the fibular fracture. **D.** Three months later, secondary internal fixation of the fibula was performed using an eight-hole, 3.5-mm DCP. The tibia was osteotomized laterally and a corticocancellous block inserted. The medial plate was removed, and the intraoperative radiograph confirmed alignment. **E.** Six weeks later, medial infection of the metaphysis and osteoporosis. **F.** Status at 1 year: consolidation of the fibula; infected pseudarthrosis which did not involve the joint but would require several interventions. **G.** Final radiograph following consolidation and implant removal. *Comment:* Initial internal fixation of the fibula would probably have prevented the secondary deviation. Realignment was achieved by the secondary stabilization of the fibula and the corticocancellous graft. It led to rapid consolidation. This intervention did not influence the medial infection that manifested after the plate had been removed.

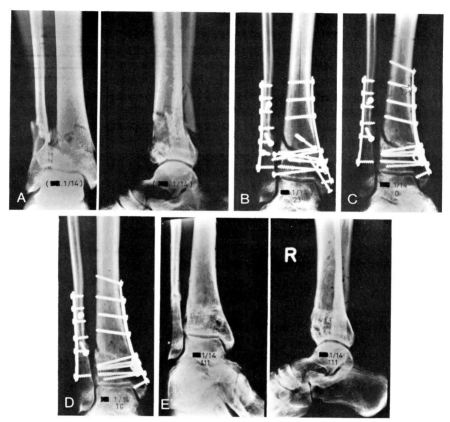

Figure 203. Bilateral revision of internal fixation for delayed consolidation in a 39-year-old who fell while skiing and sustained closed pilon fractures (see also Figure 204). The initial internal fixation was performed in a local hospital. After reintervention, the patient received crutches for both legs and swimming exercises were initiated after wound healing had occurred. Full weightbearing was achieved at 3 months, partial rehabilitation (50%) at 6 months, and full rehabilitation at 14 months. Complete functional recovery of the right leg was obtained. In the left leg, slight functional impairments persist in the ankle and tibiotalar joints, especially when walking on uneven terrain. [From Heim U, Pfeiffer KM (1988)]. *Internal Fixation of Small Fractures,* ed 3. Heidelberg, Springer.)] Right leg: **A.** Complete pilon fracture with articular split laterally and metaphyseal impaction; valgus position. Typical multifragmented fracture of the fibula above the malleoli associated with an oblique fracture of the medial malleolus. Correct classification would be C2.1. Emergency internal fixation of the fibula with a seven-hole one-third tubular plate. The tibia was fixed with a cloverleaf plate and small screws; cancellous bone graft. **B.** By 4½ months (23 weeks), delayed consolidation in the metaphysis became apparent; there was a tendency of a drift into valgus angulation. **C.** Revision of internal fixation of the tibia: through the previous incision, two cloverleaf plates of different lengths were applied one over the other and attached under strong compression (proximal tension hole in the tibia). Another cancellous bone graft. **D.** Consolidation after 3 months. The implants were removed after 1½ years. **E.** At 2-year follow-up (111 weeks), only slight irregularities of the tibial articular surface were seen, and the joint was virtually free of arthrosis. See *Comment*, Figure 204.

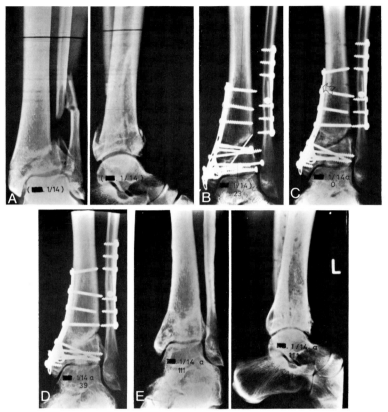

Figure 204. Revision of internal fixation in the same patient as in Figure 203. Left leg: **A.** Complete pilon fracture with articular split laterally; the metaphysis was impacted near the joint. Depression was assumed anterolaterally; dislocation into valgus and fibular wedge fracture of the diaphysis. Correct classification would be C2.1 (with depression). Emergency internal fixation using a seven-hole one-third tubular plate for the fibula, and a cloverleaf plate and small screws for the tibia; cancellous bone graft. **B.** At 4½ months (23 weeks), delayed consolidation in the metaphysis and increasing drift into valgus angulation. **C.** Revision of internal fixation of the tibia; fixation through the same incision with cloverleaf plates of different lengths placed one over the other and attached under strong compression (proximal tension hole in the tibia). Another cancellous bone graft, correction of the axis. **D.** Consolidation was not yet complete at 7 months, but weightbearing was possible. The implants were removed after 1½ years. **E.** When seen 2 years later (after 111 weeks), early signs of arthrosis were found. *Comment:* The revision of internal fixation of the tibia required a stronger implant, a new cancellous bone graft, and intensive functional exercises postoperatively. The less favorable outcome of the left leg is thought to result from an unrecognized small depression.

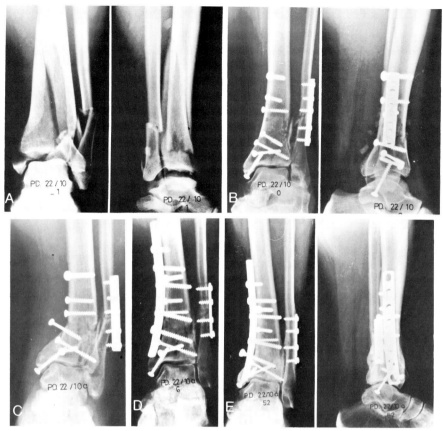

Figure 205. Revision of internal fixation following secondary displacement of the metaphysis in a 38-year-old woman who sustained a closed fracture with skin contusions in a car accident; no concomitant injuries. The patient, who is obese, is assumed to have initiated premature weightbearing against medical advice. **A.** Complete pilon fracture with two laterally displaced articular fragments; an area of multi-fragmentation in the metaphysis and extension into the diaphysis; transverse fracture of the fibular diaphysis. Displaced transverse fracture of the medial malleolus; classified as C2.3. **B.** Initially treated by traction because of skin contusions; internal fixation after a delay of 10 days: the fibula was fixed with a five-hole 3.5-mm DCP (the screws selected were somewhat too short); the tibia was fixed with screws alone; cancellous bone graft was taken from the pelvis. The postoperative course was uneventful, and the patient was discharged from hospital with a plaster splint at 20 days. **C.** Two months later, a varus deformity was observed, as well as secondary displacement of the lateral articular fragment with loosening of the screws. The fibular plate was detached. **D.** Revision of internal fixation of the tibia using a straight plate and a shorter one-third tubular plate for the fibula; cancellous bone grafting was repeated. Uneventful course and rapid consolidation of the fibula. **E.** At 1-year follow-up (52 weeks), in spite of the thick plate, there is a varus deviation of about 14 degrees. The fracture has consolidated. The varus deformity caused discomfort and was subsequently corrected by osteotomy. *Comment:* Detachment of the fibular plate was probably caused by the inadequate (too short) screws. The shorter plate led to rapid consolidation. In tibial fractures, fixation with screws alone is insufficient to resist stress. Buttress with external fixation (see Figure 179) would probably have led to consolidation.

8.3. Corrective Surgery after Malunion in Pilon Fractures
A. Gächter

A correct internal fixation may usually be expected to provide good results in terms of pain and functional recovery. In fractures of the tibial pilon, however, additional factors are involved: in addition to the bony lesions, more precisely the loss of subchondral substance, an important role must be attributed to the destruction of cartilage caused by the comparatively high-energy forces. Extensive destruction of the cartilaginous tissue will then necessitate arthrodesis. When the cartilage is damaged, it is much more susceptible to the effects of malalignment. Unilateral erosions and the development of posttraumatic arthrosis rapidly ensue. Following pilon fractures, seven patterns of malunion are observed:

1. Articular incongruence (steps in the joint line, widening or narrowing of the ankle mortise)
2. Talipes equinus
3. Varus deformity
4. Valgus deformity
5. Antecurvature
6. Recurvation
7. Malrotation

In addition, combinations of the various deformities occur.

Corrective osteotomies are hardly dealt with in the literature [71, 114]. The problems involved are referred to in only a few cases from the large series reported [94, 161, 171, 211]. Before an osteotomy is carried out, various questions must be answered:

Has the osteotomy a chance, or should arthrodesis of the ankle joint be performed? This is probably one of the most difficult questions, and any solution must be individually tailored to fit the expectations and needs of the patient.

Which type of osteotomy is indicated?

Which type of implant shall be employed? Would the use of an external fixator be appropriate?

Is the corrective osteotomy feasible? Or will it rather induce segmental necrosis of bone?

Articular Incongruence

These malalignments are often difficult to correct. Preoperative planning is greatly facilitated by a CT scan. The medial malleolus is probably best suited for osteotomy, provided that blood flow is adequate. Usually, a wedge-resection osteotomy is indicated. But first a careful examination is done to determine if malrotation is the cause of the articular incongruence. If major steps have formed in the sagittal joint line, correction will be more challenging. A Volkmann-like triangle gliding upward may induce posterior subluxation of the talus, or proximal shifting of a large anterior fragment may have occurred. To perform selective osteotomy of this fragment, which has drifted upward, is difficult since the ligamentous attachments of the syndesmosis must be taken into account (Fig. 208). Finally, the trimming of an anterior exostosis at the tibia or the talus should be mentioned (Fig. 206). The main purpose of this procedure is to improve dorsiflexion.

Anterior and Posterior Angulation

In most cases, they occur in combination with valgus or varus deformities or malrotations. When an isolated antecurvature or recurvation requires correction, tension band fixation is recommended.

Text continued on page 265

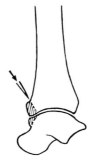

Figure 206. The resection of osteophytes using a chisel.

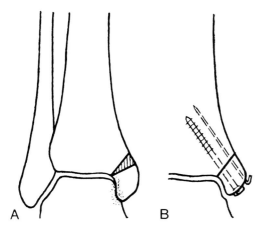

Figure 207. Osteotomy of the medial malleolus. **A.** Wedge-resection osteotomy to cure pressure erosions. The "impingement" at the talus is caused by the medial malleolus. **B.** The osteotomy is fixed with a screw and a Kirschner wire.

A   B

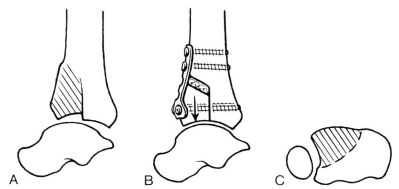

Figure 208. Osteotomy to correct a persisting articular incongruence in the frontal plane. **A.** The incongruence on the lateral radiograph, here being anterior. **B.** Shifting osteotomy: the defect is packed with a corticocancellous bone chip, and the osteotomy is fixed with a small T-plate. **C.** The dislocated area as shown on the CT scan.

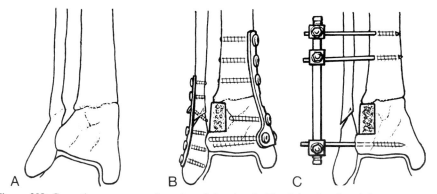

Figure 209. Corrective osteotomy of a valgus deformity. **A.** The deformity viewed from the anterior side. **B.** Oblique osteotomy of the fibula and lateral osteotomy of the tibia. A corticocancellous block is inserted into the slot. The fibula is stabilized with a one-third tubular plate and an interfragmentary lag screw, the tibia with a T-plate. **C.** An alternative solution would be to restrict stabilization to the lateral side using an external fixator.

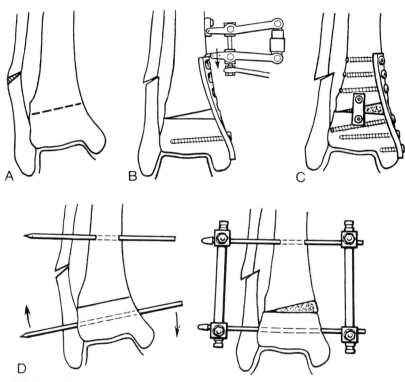

Figure 210. Corrective osteotomy of a varus deformity. **A.** Anterior view of the original position. The resection wedge is indicated at the diaphysis of the fibula, the line of the osteotomy at the proximal tibial metaphysis. **B.** The tibia is realigned from a medial approach and a corticocancellous chip is slotted into the defect. **C.** Paired plates are used to fix the osteotomy. **D.** An alternative solution would be to apply external fixation as a frame construction.

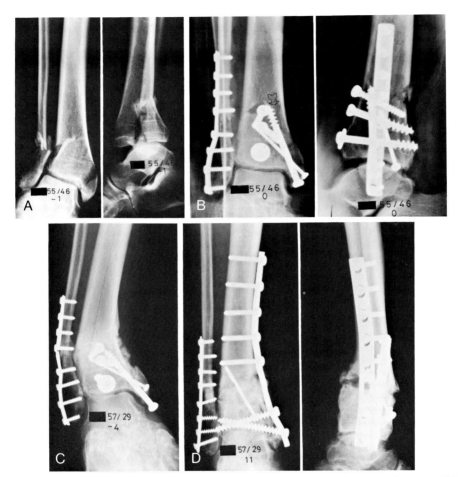

Figure 211. Pseudarthrosis in the tibial metaphysis. **A.** Partial pilon fracture with preserved anteromedial wall. Area of multifragmentation in the posterior metaphysis (partial impaction with subluxation of the talus); valgus position; typical, multifragmented fracture of the fibula above the syndesmosis; vertical fracture of the medial malleolus. Because the fracture occurred only recently, it is not yet included in the case data of the AO documentation center analyzed for this study. Correct classification would be B1.3. This type of fracture is rare. The secondary deviation (into varus position) is different from the initial axial displacement (into valgus position). **B.** Internal fixation of the fibula was carried out with an eight-hole, one-third tubular plate; the tibia was fixed with large screws through an anterior approach. The medial malleolus was stabilized with a large cancellous screw oriented anterior and proximal. This produced a mechanically unfavorable accumulation of gross foreign bodies within the narrow intact metaphysis. Because stability was questionable, the leg was immobilized in plaster for 4 weeks. **C.** Secondary displacement into varus position following a collapse anteriorly and a defect posteriorly. Fracture of the fibular plate. **D.** Revision internal fixation was performed at 9 months for established pseudarthrosis. A medial DCP was attached to the tibia, and the fibula was again stabilized with a one-third tubular plate.

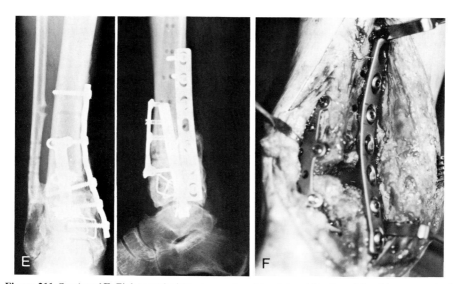

Figure 211 *Continued* **E.** Eight months later, a second revision internal fixation of the tibia was required for persistent pseudarthrosis; this time, a medial titanium DCP was used. In addition, a specially designed cervical plate was applied anteriorly with hollow screws; above the malleolus, two titanium staples were attached medially. Radiograph was taken after fracture union had occurred. **F.** This intraoperative picture shows the arrangement of the two plates at the second intervention for the pseudarthrosis.

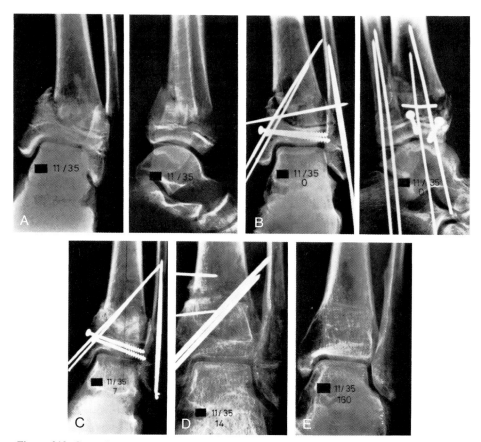

Figure 212. Corrective osteotomy of a varus deformity following partial impaction of an epiphyseal closed fracture in a 14-year-old after a fall during a mountain tour. (The osteotomy and the follow-up were performed in another country.) **A.** Complete articular fracture showing an oblique and principally sagittal split and partial impaction of the medial metaphysis. Varus position and slight antecurvature. Typical, oblique fracture of the fibula above the malleoli. Single case of a complete fracture with an unfused epiphyseal plate. In Figure 124, the same case is shown to illustrate the classification. **B.** Internal fixation of the epiphyseal split with two small horizontal cancellous screws. Stabilization between the proximal and distal parts of the fracture was accomplished with three Kirschner wires. Because the physiological curvature of the fibula had not been taken adequately into account when stabilizing the fracture with Kirschner wires, some varus angulation remained. Uncomplicated postoperative course and plaster immobilization for 6 weeks. **C.** Follow-up at 7 weeks when the plaster cast was removed. The fracture had healed in increased varus position resulting from the defect in the metaphysis. **D.** Corrective osteotomy at the proximal metaphysis with insertion of a cancellous bone graft (14 weeks later). Uncomplicated fracture union. **E.** Follow-up 3 years later (160 weeks). Growth was completed and realignment achieved; the articular lines appeared normal, and the patient had full function. *Comment:* An extremely rare injury. Management of the fibula and the cancellous defect in the metaphysis were the crucial factors accounting for the secondary, increasing drift into varus angulation.

Talipes Equinus

This occurs in association with antecurvature of the tibia, but in most cases it results from chronic pain and compromised aftercare. The posttraumatic footdrop tends to be refractory to therapy, and often the only management is arthrodesis of the ankle (or tibiotalar) joint, if previous soft tissue interventions have failed.

Varus and Valgus Deformities

Before these deformities are corrected, it is mandatory to obtain an x-ray film of the normal side. Because the ankle joint as well as the tibiotalar joint tolerates valgus deformities better than varus deformities, correction of a drift into varus position will be more often indicated. Both corrections also involve osteotomy of the fibula. A single plate is generally insufficient to provide adequate stability. Even the tibia must be stabilized with two different implants in most cases. In a wedge-resection osteotomy, the use of an external fixator should be considered (Figs. 209, 210), and interposition of a corticocancellous chip is often advantageous.

Malrotation

The degree of tibial rotation or torsion is extremely difficult to assess by clinical and radiologic means. In most cases, one has no alternative other than to correct the malrotation during operation, thereby attempting an optimal return of the ankle mortise into place. As above, it holds true here that external malrotation is better tolerated than internal malrotation.

General Advice on Osteotomies

1. A radiograph of the normal side should be obtained before any corrective osteotomy.

2. In the case of articular incongruence, a CT scan of the ankle joint is recommended. At the level of the ankle joint, stratification should be very narrow. The CT scan, usually also obtained from the normal side, allows assessment of incongruences caused by malrotation.

3. In osteotomies, special consideration of blood flow conditions is essential.

4. In wedge-resection osteotomies, the use of corticocancellous chips with additional cancellous bone grafting is recommended.

5. The majority of osteotomies also require osteotomy of the fibula.

6. Optimal stability must be secured by the implants. The tibia will often require two implants (e.g., medial and lateral plating). This in turn poses problems in terms of the soft tissue. The use of an external fixator is indicated for precarious skin and soft tissue conditions.

8.4. Arthrodesis of the Ankle Joint

Arthrodesis is by far the most common secondary operation performed on the ankle joint. In most cases, it is not severely disabling, and the associated handicap is in no way comparable to that after ankylosis of the hip or knee joint. This is why arthroplasty has so far failed to replace it [15, 53].

Primary or late primary arthrodesis may occasionally be indicated. It has the advantage that definitive surgical management is accomplished by one intervention. But to sacrifice the joint at an early stage is only justified in patients with irreversible bony destruction, an associated fracture of the talus, or otherwise unmanageable soft tissue injuries. The more experienced the surgeon, the greater his or her inclination to attempt articular reconstruction, even if the joint is badly destroyed. The patient will thus be given the chances of functional recovery, even though the latter may remain incomplete in some cases. Another fact to be taken into account is that arthrodesis is a technically extremely difficult procedure if carried out at an early stage; it may be more difficult than a demanding reconstruction [78, 186]. A real alternative to early arthrodesis consists in reduction with an external fixator while traction is applied. In combination with the technique of minimal, percutaneous reduction of individual fragments, amazing functional results may be achieved [11, 103]. This can be done without immobilizing the patient, as was previously required when calcaneal traction according to Jahna et al. [84] was applied. Instead of the conventional arthrodesis, Muhr and Breitfuss [126] and Trentz and Friedl [194] recently recommended impaction of the metaphysis into the talus. The shortening will considerably relieve the soft tissues around the fracture site. Lengthening procedures according to Ilizarov and as needed are subsequently initiated by proximal distraction of the callus.

Arthrodesis as a secondary intervention, however, prevails. It is indicated either for longstanding articular infection, i.e., in chronic osteoarthritis where functional recovery is unlikely to occur, or in painful posttraumatic arthrosis.

In chronic infection, cartilage resection and the broad contact of cancellous areas held under compression will induce healing of the infection. The number of arthrodeses indicated for infection is high in hospitals frequently admitting patients with established complications from other hospitals [21, 75–77, 127, 184]. Hospitals in which the complications are managed at the institution itself convey a less pessimistic picture. Unfortunately, most data fail to differentiate whether an arthrodesis was performed because of infection or because of arthrosis (see section 5.3.2).

The course of arthrosis varies considerably. Early arthrosis during the first months may indicate iatrogenic fragment necrosis. An example is given in Figure 190. In most cases, the future of the joint may be assessed toward the end of the first year following the internal fixation. In the boxes in section 3 of the Appendix, we have listed all incidences of prearthrosis and manifest arthrosis at 1 year occurring in the various groups. We also refer the reader to the discussion in section 5.4.7 above.

Among the patients on file at the AO documentation center, four primary or early arthrodeses were carried out in fractures of the B3 and C3 types. During the first year, another three arthrodeses followed. These concerned groups C2 and C3 (see Table 5). The number of arthroses evident on the radiograph at 1 year increased with the severity of the fracture. For details, we refer to the summary in section 5.4.7 and to Tables 3 to 6.

Conclusions regarding functional performance as well as signs and symptoms cannot be drawn from our data. In the majority of cases with painful arthrosis, more than 1 year elapses before arthrodesis is indicated. Our figures are therefore in no way representative of the further course in our patients. The final outcome of arthrodesis may be definitively assessed only after several years [84]. Often, we then observe significant discrepancies between severe radiologic findings and only moderate discomfort with fairly satisfying functional performance [170].

Arthrodesis should only be carried out if the patient demands it because of pain and hindrance when walking. Under these conditions, satisfactory results may be obtained by the operation.

The planning of a secondary arthrodesis requires consideration of many questions and problems, and solutions must be tailored individually. Controversy exists on numerous items, including adequate positioning of the foot [52]. The discussion of technical details is therefore beyond the scope of this book, which is dedicated to the traumatologist.

It should be noted, however, that if arthrodesis is indicated for arthrosis, compression arthrodesis according to Charnley [26] has been largely abandoned and screw fixation has taken its place [78, 81, 89, 114, 187, 191] (Fig. 213).

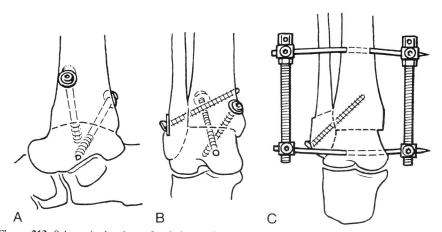

Figure 213. Schematic drawings of techniques of arthrodesis. **A, B.** Techniques of screw arthrodesis. **C.** Classic arthrodesis according to Charnley [26] with two Steinmann pins and bars is preferred in infection.

■ *Appendix*

The Case Material Filed at the AO Documentation Center and Its Classification According to the ABC Principle of the AO-ASIF

1. METHODS AND MATERIALS

In an attempt to evaluate and classify fractures of the distal tibia according to the ABC system, we evaluated the case data compiled at the AO documentation center in Bern. This documentation is, almost without exception, confined to operatively treated cases.

1.1. Selection and Criteria

The review comprised all fractures that were referred to as ''distal tibia'' and that had been filed since the introduction of the ''1980 documentation system'' up to the year 1985. In addition, a certain number of unselected cases taken from the earlier documentation system were included. As previously outlined, a considerable number of patient records had to be excluded from the study. If the definitions had been accurately applied, they would have been classified as diaphyseal or malleolar fracture instead of ''distal tibia.'' But there existed no clear definition of the segments before the publication of Heim [61] in 1987.

When these cases were eliminated together with data files unsuitable for evaluation for technical reasons (e.g., missing radiographs or postinjury radiographs of poor quality), a total of 1077 fractures was left that were consistent with the classification as ''distal tibia'' according to the criteria outlined in Chapter 1, section 2. This number includes fractures of the epiphyseal growth plate, the majority occurring in adolescent patients. The classifying criteria are described in Chapter 2, section 1.1. With one exception, these presented as A- and B-type injuries. The fact that the material analyzed mainly includes cases operated on implies that the series more or less lacks simple fractures amenable to successful conservative management. This precludes making any statements with respect to the special features or incidence of the latter. This does compromise our objective, however, for the problems inherent in the classification predominantly arise with complicated fracture patterns.

To include patients treated by myself in the Kreuzspital Chur from 1961 to 1980, a documentation comprising 221 fractures, appeared to be of little value. Because the majority resulted from skiing accidents, they display quite uniform morphologic and prognostic characteristics. They were dealt with in two doctoral theses in the years 1973 [140] and 1981 [30]. Only the first series was published [67]. Where individual examples are taken from these case records, reference to this is made. In the classification and statistical computations, these data were ignored.

The case material of the AO documentation center comprises 1077 fractures of the distal tibial segment; 397 of these presented as extraarticular fractures of the metaphysis (type A); 680 fractures were intraarticular (B- and C-type pilon fractures). Fractures involving the medial malleolus were excluded or disregarded in the classification (see Chapter 2, section 1).

All records reveal whether the fracture was open or closed. Further details regarding the severity of the soft tissue damage could, as needed, be retrieved from the data file storing the patient's history. Follow-ups of at least 1 year were available in a total of 601 cases (55%). A 1-year follow-up was available in 215 (54%) of the extraarticular A-type fractures, in 173 (60%) of the B-type fractures, and in 213 (53%) of the C-type fractures. Considering fractures of the tibial pilon together (i.e., group B plus group C), a late follow-up is found in 386 (56%) cases. This proportion is higher than is the case with any other fracture of a different site stored at the AO documentation center (about 40%). Moreover, documents at 4 months are available in about one fifth of the cases for which the 1-year follow-up is missing. At this time, complications of fracture union have already manifested themselves; conclusions, however, regarding the final outcome cannot be made. Even though the late follow-ups remain incomplete, the case material analyzed does, to a certain extent, allow prognostic statements. Prognosis is a principal target of the AO classification and of great concern to the AO-ASIF group.

Radiographic data are stored as 35-mm films, and generally no more than postinjury radiographs in two projections are available. Most clinics also obtain additional oblique films of such fractures; occasionally tomograms or CT scans are made. While they enhance preoperative diagnosis, for practical reasons we are unable to include all films in the documentation. Thus each case had to be evaluated and classified from a limited number of documents. This is a problem encountered by other large-scale studies as well [32]. Moreover, the conventional radiograph continues to be the mainstay for any retrospective analysis [7, 43]. On the other hand, our task of classification was facilitated by the fact that a postoperative radiograph was always available. Comparison with the preoperative films reveals important details, including, e.g., the size and position of fragments, the course of fracture lines, the type and position of the implants, and in some cases whether cancellous bone grafting was performed. With these data, inference about the type of injury becomes possible. In the rare case of doubt, the follow-ups were used as an aid to classification.

1.2. The Classifying Procedure

Classification was done in stages. As a first step, the case material was divided into groups according to the main characteristics. Already at this point, the first adjustments had to be made. Extraarticular impacted fractures had initially been classified as A3.1; it became evident that in these fractures, some contact between the main fragments was always preserved, so that allocation to group A2 became necessary. Accordingly, fractures with both a simple wedge and a multifragmented wedge had to be assigned to one subgroup. When the remaining characteristics were taken into account, this proved to be acceptable.

Next those cases were sorted out in which further subdivisions appeared to be justified. For an example, we observed that small depressions of the articular surface sometimes occurred in fractures with metaphyseal impaction or multifragmentation (C2.1 and C2.2). This feature alone was insufficient to make up a discrete subgroup, but when the relevant case records underwent separate analysis, it became evident that these cases were associated with a less favorable outcome compared to the remaining fractures in this subgroup (cf. Group C.2 in section 3.4).

Subsequently, special cases were identified. Reference to them is made in the detailed analysis of the subgroups.

At another stage, axial malalignment and concomitant injuries (fibula, medial malleolus) were reviewed and compared. Then the open fractures (gross soft tissue damage) were sorted out, and their morphologic features were compared with those of the closed fractures in the respective subgroups. The sex and age distribution was also worked out as this was thought to be indispensable for comparison.

To this serial analysis, we owe a growing confidence regarding our general evaluative capacity. The detection of certain correlations has been referred to in the preceding chapters. One example is the typical morphology of the fibular fracture in cases with axial malalignment (see Chapter 2, section 1.3). Analysis of the late follow-ups proved to be of special value, in particular when failures with delayed or impaired fracture union were examined. Finally, characteristic illustrative radiographs were selected. To make reproduction feasible, good phototechnical quality was mandatory.

2. STATISTICAL REVIEW

Like any other long bone, the distal tibia segment is divided into types. Type A = extraarticular fractures, type B = partial intraarticular fractures, and type C = intraarticular, circumferential, or complete fractures (see Fig. 36). The further arrangement into groups and subgroups and their characteristics are dealt with in Chapter 2, sections 5 and 6.

Table 2 enables one to compare the individual fracture patterns and to appreciate their frequencies. Next to the figures indicating the various groups and subgroups, a separate column indicates the number of open fractures. This shows their proportion among the various morphologic patterns.

Table 2

SYNOPSIS OF THE CASE MATERIAL AND THE PROPORTION OF OPEN FRACTURES

Statistical Synopsis	Number of Cases		Open Fractures
Extraarticular Fractures: A	397		
A1: Simple fractures	193		18
.1 spiral	37	0	
.2 oblique	127	16	
.3 transverse	29	2	
A2: Impaction and wedge fractures	150		32
.1 impaction	26	2	
.2 simple and fragmented wedge	73	21	
.3 extending into the diaphysis	51	9	
A3: Complex fractures	54		19
.1 reducible fragments	11	4	
.2 multiple fragments	10	5	
.3 extending into the diaphysis	33	10	
Partial Articular Fractures: B	289		
B1: Split fractures	216		4
.1 frontal split	84	1	
.2 sagittal split	107	2	
.3 multifragmentary in the metaphysis	25	1	
B2: Depression fracture	57		4
.1 frontal depression	12	2	
.2 sagittal depression	23	1	
.3 multifragmentary in the metaphysis	22	1	
B3: Complex articular fracture	16		5
.1 frontal articular	10	3	
.2 sagittal articular	5	2	
.3 multifragmentary in the metaphysis	1	—	
Complete Articular Fractures: C	391		
C1: simple articular and simple metaphyseal fracture	126		8
.1 articular split + simple metaphyseal	55	4	
.2 articular depression + simple metaphyseal	26	1	
.3 extending into the diaphysis	45	3	
C2: Simple articular fracture, multifragmentary in the metaphysis	220		51
.1 metaphyseal impaction	117	6	
.2 metaphyseal multifragmentation	86	39	
.3 extending into the diaphysis	17	6	
C3: Complex articular and complex metaphyseal fracture	45		12
.1 confined to the distal metaphysis	16	4	
.2 multifragmented area extends into proximal metaphysis	19	5	
.3 multifragmented area extends into the diaphysis	10	3	
Total = 1077, A = 397, B = 289, C = 391.			

3. SYSTEMATIC ANALYSIS

3.1. Concomitant Injuries and Axial Malalignment

The significance of axial malalignment was described in full in Chapter 2, section 3. Malrotation cannot be adequately assessed from the postinjury radiograph. It is diagnosed basically on clinical signs. Postoperative radiographs do not disclose malrotation.

Axial malalignment and secondary deformities are dealt with in the systematic analysis of the individual subgroups and subdivisions. The following abbreviations were used: *VL,* valgus; *VR,* varus; *RC,* recurvation; *AC,* antecurvature. The fact that the various positions frequently occur in combination has been mentioned. The most prominent dislocation is indicated.

Fibular Lesions

In the AO classification of fractures [132, 134], lesions of the fibula are recorded by so-called supplementary code numbers. These may be noted after the designation of the respective subgroup, and allow computer storage and retrieval. Accordingly, they are referred to by numbers. The following findings may be recorded: *1,* fibula intact; *2,* simple fibular fracture; *3,* multifragmentary fibular fracture; *4,* segmental fibular fracture; *5,* fibular impaction in the area of the syndesmosis. When the case material is analyzed in detail, a review of the level of the fibular fracture shows that segmental fractures are rare. Special reference to this fact is made when the corresponding subgroups are dealt with. The typical supramalleolar impaction of the fibula in fractures with dislocation into valgus position may easily be overlooked on the postinjury radiograph. Examples are depicted in Figures 40 and 51. To avoid confusion with the reading of the statistical tables, we thought it was more appropriate to use letters to indicate the various fibular lesions, since these will always be listed side by side with numbers. Our differentiation is as follows: *U,* unbroken, intact; *S,* simple fracture; *Mf,* multifragmentary fracture (segmental fractures are included, but special reference to this is made); *H,* high, subcapital fibular fracture; *D,* diaphyseal fracture; *Me,* supraligamentous, metaphyseal fracture; *L,* ligamentous fracture at the level of the syndesmotic ligaments; *B,* fracture below the ligaments. The selection of these letters has the advantage of applying both to German and the English terms alike. The letter *i* was not used to avoid confusion with the number *1.*

Medial Malleolus

Injuries to the medial malleolus and their significance are discussed in Chapter 2, section 1. The arrangement into groups and subgroups provides no opportunity to specify these fractures in further detail. We therefore thought it appropriate to tabulate them first, before the injuries of the tibia are analyzed in a systematic fashion.

Fractures of the medial malleolus in the various groups and subgroups

Number of fractures = 276 (25%) of a total of 1077 fractures of the distal tibia
A-type fractures = 48 (12% of 397 fractures)
A1 = 11; A2 = 25; A3 = 12
B-type fractures = 74 (25% of 289 fractures)
B1 = 22; B2 = 39; B3 = 13
C-type fractures = 154 (39% of 391 fractures) C1 = 41; C2 = 75; C3 = 38

The distribution of the 17 distal fractures of the medial malleolus (transverse fractures and small avulsions) among the various groups

A1 = 2; A2 = 1; A3 = 2
B1 = 3, B2 = 2; B3 = 1
C1 = 2; C2 = 2; C3 = 2

The distribution of the various patterns among the individual groups (*V*, vertical, *Ob*, oblique, *T*, transverse)

A1 =	V 7	Ob 4	T 2
A2 =	V 13	Ob 11	T 1
A3 =	V 10	Ob 0	T 2
B1 =	V 9	Ob 10	T 3
B2 =	V 16	Ob 21	T 2
B3 =	V 5	Ob 7	T 1
C1 =	V 14	Ob 25	T 2
C2 =	V 34	Ob 39	T 2
C3 =	V 14	Ob 22	T 2

Abbreviations

Axial Malalignment

VL = valgus
VR = varus
RC = recurvation
AC = antecurvature

Fibula

U = unbroken
S = simple fracture

Medial Malleolus

V = vertical
Ob = oblique
T = transverse
Mf = multifragmentary
H = high subcapital fracture
D = diaphyseal fracture
Me = metaphyseal fracture
L = ligamentary, at the level of the syndesmotic ligaments
B = deep fracture

A1: simple fracture
A2: multifragmentary fracture in which, after reduction, some contact between the main fragments is preserved
A3: complex fracture in which there is no contact between the main fragments

3.2. Extraarticular Fractures (Type A)

To include the extraarticular fractures of the distal tibial segment in our studies has proved to be of great value, as both the extraarticular and the articular fractures result from an identical mechanism. Also, numerous parallels and close relations exist in terms of morphologic aspects. By analyzing the extraarticular fractures, we greatly facilitate our understanding of the true articular pilon fracture.

Differentiation from the neighboring segment (tibial diaphysis, segment 42): the center of the fracture must be within the metaphysis (see Fig. 28B, 31). Differentiation from articular fractures (B and C): the weightbearing articular surface shows no fracture lines with the exception of pure fissures devoid of any therapeutic or prognostic significance. Fractures of the medial malleolus are disregarded (see Chapter 2, section 1.1).

Like any other fracture of a terminal long bone segment, the extraarticular fractures are divided into three groups:

Group A1

Group A1 comprises all simple extraarticular fractures. The division into subgroups is determined by the type and location of the fracture area: spiral fractures are contained in subgroup A1.1, oblique fractures in subgroup A1.2, and transverse fractures in subgroup A1.3.

Criteria for Subgroup Differentiation

Subgroup A1.1 contains only fractures that show a twisted fracture area. This is bound to be quite short when the center of the fracture is located in the metaphysis. Spiral fractures are rare before fusion of the epiphyses (two cases).

Subgroup A1.2 comprises all oblique fractures. The angle between the fracture plane and the perpendicular onto the diaphyseal axis must exceed 30 degrees on at least one projection. Fractures of the epiphyseal growth plate are common in this subgroup. Then the fracture shows two components: the fracture line which runs upward—often almost vertically—and the traumatic epiphysiolysis. A few patients exhibit an oblique fracture of the metaphysis above the epiphyseal growth plate (five cases). Subgroup A1.3 contains the transverse fractures. All projections must show the angle between the fracture plane and the perpendicular to the diaphyseal axis to be below 30 degrees. In addition to transverse fractures in adults and individual adolescents with incomplete epiphyseal growth, this subgroup also contains the purely traumatic epiphysiolyses.

Subgroup A1.1

Definition: Simple spiral fracture of the metaphysis

No. of Cases: 37

Subdivision: None

Special Patterns: None

Special Cases: Epiphyseal growth plate: 2

Open Fractures: None

Axial Malalignment: Hardly pronounced: ten cases, VL 6, VR 3, RC 1, AC 0

Concomitant Injuries: Fibula: U 18, S 16, Mf 3, H 2, D 4, Me 7, L 6, B 0; 2 remarkable, subcapital fractures of the fibula without disruption of the mortise (see Fig. 60); medial malleolus: V 3, Ob 1, T 2

Operative Technique—Tibia: 33 plate fixations; 4 screw fixations

Late Follow-up: 24; findings: no complications

Assessment: Less serious, closed injury

Figures: For schematics, see Figure 59A; for illustrative radiographs, see Figure 60.

Subgroup A1.2

Definition: simple oblique fracture of the metaphysis

No. of Cases: 127

Subdivision 1: Adults and adolescents with a fracture above the epiphyseal plate: 43 cases

Subdivision 2: Epiphyseal fracture; oblique fracture with partial, traumatic epiphysiolysis: 84 cases

A1.2: SUBDIVISION 1

No. of Cases: 43 (38 adults)

Open Fractures: 7

Special Patterns: 5 cases before closure of the epiphysis (fracture above the plate); 3 cases with an additional, separate fracture of the proximal tibial diaphysis (in segment 42)

Axial Malalignment: 27 cases: VL 20, VR 4, RC 1, AC 2

Concomitant Injuries: Fibula: U 9, S 21, Mf 13, H 0, D 20, Me 14, L 0, B 0; medial malleolus: V4, Ob 3, T 0

Operative Technique—Tibia: 31 fixations with plates, 7 with screws, 3 with Kirschner wires; 2 nonoperative

Late Follow-up: 26; findings: uncomplicated fracture union, no arthrosis

Assessment: Clearly more serious than the spiral fracture; simple operative conditions, uneventful postoperative course

Figures: For schematic, see Figure 59B; for illustrative radiographs, see Figure 61.

A1.2: SUBDIVISION 2

No. of Cases: 84

Open Fractures: 9 (5 of these show an intact fibula)

Special Patterns: 6 cases with split of the medial malleolus in the frontal plane (triplane fracture); not assigned to the medial malleolar fractures, fibula intact in all

Axial Malalignment: 34 cases: VL 29, VR 2, RC 0, AC 3

Concomitant Injuries: Fibula: U 39, S 38, Mf 7, H 0, D 23, Me 21, L 0, B 1 (fibular epiphysiolysis); medial malleolus: V 0, Ob 0, T 0

Operative Technique—Tibia: Fixation mostly with screws, less often Kirschner wires; some nonoperative cases; a few plates

Late Follow-up: 45; findings: the series prevents any statements on premature closure of the epiphyseal plate; no axial deviations at late follow-up

Assessment: The situation resembles that found in oblique fractures of the adult; an intact fibula, however, is more frequently found, but in valgus position, there is always a fibular fracture with typical morphology (see Fig. 45).

Figures: For schematics, see Figures 58C, E; for illustrative radiographs, see Figure 62.

Subgroup A1.3

Definition: Simple transverse fracture of the metaphysis

No. of Cases: 29

Subdivision: None

Special Patterns: Transverse fracture in adults: 11; transverse fracture above the epiphyseal growth plate: 5; purely traumatic epiphysiolysis without fracture: 13

Open Fractures: 2 (in adolescents)

Axial Malalignment: 12 (all affecting patients before natural closure of the epiphysis) VL 12, VR 0, RC 0, AC 0; dislocations toward the axis occur only in fractures of the epiphyseal growth plate.

Concomitant Injuries: Differences within the various subdivisions of this subgroup were not observed; fibula: U 7, S 18, Mf 4, H 0, D 7, Me 13, L 1, B 1 (traumatic epiphysiolysis of the fibula?); medial malleolus: V 0, Ob 0, T 0

Operative Technique—Tibia: Nonoperative or with Kirschner wire in fractures of the epiphyseal growth plate; plate fixation in the adult; 1 external fixator

Late Follow-up: 15; findings: no disturbances of fracture union; strikingly, many young adults are seen; valgus position is frequent after traumatic epiphysiolysis; in adults, only closed fractures were observed.

Figures: For schematics, see Figures 58D, 59C; for illustrative radiographs, see Figure 63.

Summary of Group A1

Total no. of cases: 193. In 109 patients, before epiphyseal maturity: 13 traumatic epiphysiolyses, 84 extraarticular epiphyseal fractures, 12 metaphyseal fractures without involvement of the epiphyseal plate (2 spiral, 4 oblique, 5 transverse)

No. of adult patients: 84. The most serious lesion of the distal tibial metaphysis is the oblique fracture, which is in contrast to the conditions encountered at the diaphysis. The injury is associated with the largest proportion of open fractures, deformities, and concomitant injuries. No differences are observed in terms of severity when the injuries of children and adolescents are compared to those of adult patients. The results obtained in 110 late follow-ups (57%) show that fractures in this group generally have a favorable outcome.

Group A1
No. of cases 193
Open fractures 18
Late follow-up 110
Delayed union, malunion, nonunion 0
Prearthrosis/arthrosis 0

Group A2

In this group of multifragmentary fractures of the metaphysis some contact between the main fragments is preserved after reduction. At the metaphyses of other long bones, this contact is the basic criterion for the further classification into subgroups, which is based either on the way the wedge fragments have split, or on the site and position of the contact areas. The cylindrical shape of the tibial metaphysis precludes defining planes. Sites of contact are spread over the entire circumference. One difference may consist in the technical difficulty at operation: the readily accessible fractures with anteromedial contact are easier to manage than fractures with posterolateral contact.

Here we encounter for the first time the impaction of the metaphysis, characteristic of the distal tibial segment (see Chapter 2, section 5.2.2). While it is often associated with dislocation toward the axis, lateral deviations are rarely found. Considering the number of open fractures, we also find that damage to soft tissues is of little consequence. Concomitant injuries correspond to what is found in wedge fractures. We therefore assigned metaphyseal impaction to subgroup A2.1.

Subgroup A2.2 comprises all wedge fractures. Differences to be noted are those between the simple and the multifragmented wedge, and differences in the basic morphologic patterns, as a wedge may occur in spiral as well as oblique fractures. As we have seen in group A1, these two fracture types vary considerably in terms of severity. The same holds true for wedge fractures, even though the short fracture lines of a metaphyseal fracture may occasionally prevent clear differentiation between the spiral and the oblique forms. Inconsistent results were obtained after repeated counting. This is why differentiation between the two morphologic patterns was not used as a criterion for the further classification of A2 into subgroups.

When we examine the differences between the simple and the multifragmented wedge, it becomes obvious that both forms show the same proportion of open fractures (which prevail in the ''oblique'' morphology). Likewise, there was an even distribution of axial malalignment. The differences found, however, concern fracture of the fibula: when the tibial wedge is multifragmented, multiple fractures of the fibular diaphysis are more frequent.

The technical difficulties encountered at operation are another aspect to be considered, since they are increased when the wedge is multifragmented. Delayed consolidation seen at late follow-up is slightly more common with multifragmentation of the wedge. The evidence appeared to justify assigning fractures with a simple and a multifragmented wedge to the same subgroup.

When one part of a wedge fracture extends with its major portion into the diaphysis, this is considered a metaphyseal-diaphyseal fracture and is classified as subgroup A2.3. These long fractures then allow a better differentiation between spiral and oblique morphologic patterns than is the case with group A2.2. Surprisingly, they are less often associated with open fracture or axial malalignment than the purely metaphyseal fractures.

Subgroup A2.1

Definition: Metaphyseal fracture with impaction; some contact between main fragments preserved

No. of Cases: 26

Subdivision: None

Special Patterns: None

Special Cases: None

Sex and Age Distribution: 16 female, 10 male; mean age: 57 years (range: 35–79 years)

Open Fractures: 2 (automobile accidents with the foot in valgus position)

Axial Malalignment: 16; combinations are common: VL 7, VR 3, RC 4, AC 2

Concomitant Injuries: Fibula: U 2, S 12, Mf 12, H 0, D 8, Me 13, L 3, B 0; the 2 cases with an intact fibula show neither disruption of the mortise nor upward impaction of the articular surface; medial malleolus: V 4, Ob 2, T 0,

Operative Technique—Tibia: 24 plate fixations (plating in pairs in 6 of these, and 1 composite internal fixation); 1 Kirschner wire; 1 external fixator device

Late Follow-up: 12; findings: 2 secondary valgus deformities after failure to buttress a fibular fracture; 1 prearthrosis; 1 osteitis

Assessment: Typical extraarticular fracture of the skier; fracture of the fibula is common, but often simple; close relationship exists with the articular split with impaction (subgroup C2.1; see below).

Figures: For schematics, see Figure 64A; for illustrative radiograph, see Figure 66.

Subgroup A2.2

Definition: Metaphyseal fracture with a simple or multifragmented wedge; contact between the main fragments preserved

No. of Cases: 73

Subdivision: Subdivision 1: simple wedge (34 cases); subdivision 2: multifragmented wedge (39 cases)

A2.2: SUBDIVISION 1 (SIMPLE WEDGE)

No. of Cases: 34

Sex and Age Distribution: 20 male, 14 female; mean age: 55 years (range: 13–87 years)

Special Patterns: Morphologically resembling a spiral fracture: 10 cases; resembling an oblique fracture: 24 cases; short fracture lines make differentiation unreliable.

Special Cases: 1 fracture before epiphyseal maturity (open)

Open Fractures: 10, 8 in the oblique fracture pattern (VL 6, VR 1)

Axial Malalignment: 16 cases: VL 11, VR 4, RC 0, AC 1; axial deviations are less frequent with the spiral morphology.

Concomitant Injuries: Fibula: U 8, S 16, Mf 10, H 0, D 13, Me 12, L 1, B 0; an intact fibula is more common with the spiral type; medial malleolus: V 2, Ob 4, T 1

Operative Technique—Tibia: 29 plate fixations (none in pairs), 4 external fixators, 1 screw fixation

Late Follow-up: 14; findings: 2 delayed consolidations, 1 secondary valgus deformity following external fixator, 1 early drift into varus angulation following premature medial closure of the growth plate, 1 osteitis

Assessment: Despite the frequency of open fractures, the preponderance of plate fixations have a favorable outcome

Figures: For schematics, see Figure 64B; for illustrative radiograph, see Figure 67.

A2.2: SUBDIVISION 2 (MULTIFRAGMENTED WEDGE)

No. of Cases: 39

Sex and Age Distribution: 25 male, 14 female; mean age: 44 years (range: 13–72 years)

Special Patterns: The differentiation between oblique and spiral forms is uncertain with the multifragmented wedge; the appearance of open fractures resembles the oblique form.

Special Cases: 1 fracture before epiphyseal maturity; 1 fracture with an additional, separate fracture of the tibial shaft (segment 42)

Open Fractures: 11: VL 4, VR 3, AC 1

Axial Malalignment: 17 cases: VL 9, VR 4, RC 3 (scarcely distinct), AC 1

Concomitant Injuries: Fibula: U 1, S 18, Mf 20, H 0, D 27 (2 segmental fractures), Me 11, B 0; the fibular fracture, almost always present in the case of a multifragmented wedge, is found in the diaphysis in most cases; medial malleolus: V 2, Ob 3, T 0.

Operative Technique—Tibia: 37 plate fixations (5 in pairs), 2 external fixator devices

Late Follow-up: 20; findings: 6 delayed consolidations; 1 prearthrosis

Assessment: Delayed consolidation is increasing with this type (devitalization of small fragments, lack of cancellous bone graft); 1 valgus deformity following failure to stabilize the fibula.

Figures: For an illustrative radiograph, see Figure 68.

Subgroup A2.3

Definition: Metaphyseal fracture with a simple or multifragmented wedge; 1 wedge fragment extends with its major portion into the diaphysis; some contact is preserved between the main fragments; these long fractures allow a better differentiation between the two morphologic patterns ''oblique'' and ''spiral.''

No. of Cases: 51

Sex and Age Distribution: 30 male; 21 female; mean age: 46 years (range: 16–81 years)

Subdivision: None

Special Patterns: None

Special Cases: 33 spiral, 18 oblique; 25 fractures with a simple wedge, 26 with a multifragmented wedge; the diaphyseal wedge fragment attains twice the height of the metaphysis in 27 cases; the diaphyseal fragment is less than twice the metaphyseal height in 24 cases.

Open Fractures: 9 (6 oblique)

Axial Malalignment: 23 cases, less pronounced than in subgroups A2.1 and A2.2: VL 8, VR 10, RC 3, AC 2

Concomitant Injury: Fibula: U 15, S 20, Mf 16, H 1, D 17, Me 14, L 4, B 0; when the fracture is of the spiral type, we find 12 cases of an intact fibula; there is no upward impaction of the articular surface, nor any signs indicating disruption of the mortise or tears of the syndesmotic ligaments; the intact syndesmosis pulls the tibia into varus position (see Fig. 44A); medial malleolus: V 5; Ob 2; T 0

Operative Technique—Fibula: 43 plate fixations (none in pairs), 4 external fixator devices; screws alone, 2; nonoperative, 2

Late Follow-up: 26; findings: no arthrosis, 1 valgus deformity with synostosis after failure to stabilize a multifragmented fibular metaphysis

Assessment: Fewer open fractures, more intact fibulas indicate an indirect causative mechanism; the same peculiarity is observed in group A3- and C-type fractures

Figures: For schematic, see Figure 64C; for illustrative radiograph, see Figure 69.

Summary of Group A2

Total no. of cases: 150. The main differences are between the impacted fracture, which is almost always closed, and the wedge fracture. The severity of the latter is clearly increased. A multifragmented wedge carries a more unfavorable prognosis than a simple wedge. The metaphyseal-diaphyseal fractures are less serious than the A2.2-type fractures. An intact fibula is more common with the spiral form and in cases with only slight axial displacement. The operative management relies on the plate, even for open fractures. This indicates the less serious nature of the soft tissue damage.

Late follow-ups are available in 72 of 150 cases (48%). There are no cases of arthrosis. In subgroups A2.2 and A2.3, several cases are seen with delayed consolidation, some combined with angulation.

> **Group A2**
>
> No. of cases 150
> Open fractures 21
> Late follow-up 72
> Delayed union, malunion, nonunion 13
> Prearthrosis/arthrosis 2

Group A3

This group comprises complex fractures of the metaphysis in which, after reduction, there is no contact between the main fragments. These injuries look dramatic, but they are not very common. All of the patients are adults. The division into subgroups takes into account the extent of fragmentation as well as the extension of the fracture to the diaphysis: fractures with only a few large fragments readily distinguishable are assigned to subgroup A3.1. When the fracture consists of multiple fragments difficult to tell apart, and anatomic restoration is doubtful, it is classified as A3.2. With subgroup A3.3, problems may arise in differentiating the injury from diaphyseal fractures of segment 42. In a metaphyseal fracture, the center lies in that segment with a large, and purely metaphyseal, distal main fragment. The area of multifragmentation may approach the border of the segment or lie further proximal; some wedge fragments may be located within the diaphysis. For borderline cases, see Figures 32 to 35.

Subgroup A3.1

Definition: Complex metaphyseal fracture (no contact between main fragments) with large fragments easily identifiable (basically, a four-fragment-fracture)

No. of Cases: 11

Subdivision: None

Special Patterns: None

Special Cases: None

Sex and Age Distribution: 6 male, 5 female; mean age: 42 years (range: 18–60 years)

Open Fractures: 4, 2 in valgus position

Axial Malalignment: 6: VL 2, VR 2, RC 1, AC 1

Concomitant Injuries: Fibula: U 0, S 5, Mf 6, H 0, D 8, Me 2, L 1, B 0; medial malleolus: no fractures

Operative Technique—Tibia: 8 plate fixations (2 in pairs); 3 external fixators

Late Follow-up: 6; findings: no disturbances of fracture union; no articular changes

Assessment: Only a few late follow-ups are available. The outcome is surprisingly good despite the high number of open fractures. The evidence implies that the major fragments are not devitalized. This is a remarkable difference in terms of the final results when compared to subgroups A2.2 (10 of 34 cases with delayed consolidation) and A3.2 (3 late deformities in 10 cases).

Figures: For schematics, see Figure 70A; for illustrative radiographs, see Figure 71.

Subgroup A3.2

Definition: Complex metaphyseal fracture (no contact between main fragments); multiple and uncountable small fragments (irreducible)

No. of Cases: 10

Sex and Age Distribution: 7 male, 3 female; mean age: 50 years (range: 21–79 years)

Subdivision: None

Special Patterns: None

Special Cases: None

Open Fractures: 5: VL 3, VR 1

Axial Malalignment: 9: VL 6, VR 3, RC 0, AC 0

Concomitant Injuries: Fibula: U 0, S 4, Mf 6, H 0, D 5, Me 5, L 0, B 0; medial malleolus: V 2, Ob 0, T 1

Operative Technique—Tibia: 9 plate fixations (3 in pairs), 1 external fixator, 2 recognizable cancellous bone grafts, 1 composite fixation with bone cement

Late Follow-up: 9; findings: 3 deformities (2 VL, 1 VR) after delayed consolidation (1 following external fixator, 1 after simple plating, 1 after plates in pairs), 2 synostoses above the malleoli

Assessment: There are marked differences in terms of severity and outcome when compared to subgroup A3.1; delayed consolidation with secondary deformity is increasing in number. The effects of the soft tissue damage on secondary complications cannot be assessed owing to the limited number of case records.

Figures: For schematics, see Figure 70B; for illustrative radiograph, see Figure 72.

Subgroup A3.3

Definition: Complex metaphyseal fracture containing the basic morphologic patterns of groups A3.1 and A3.2; at least one fracture element extends with its major portion in the metaphysis

No. of Cases: 33

Sex and Age Distribution: 20 male, 13 female; mean age: 45 years (range: 18–77 years)

Subdivision: None

Special Patterns: None

Special Cases: None

Open Fractures: 10

Axial Malalignment: 13 cases, less pronounced than in the shorter fractures of subgroups A3.1 and A3.2: VL 6, VR 5, RC 2, AC 0

Concomitant Injuries: Fibula: U 4, S 19, Mf 10, H 0, D 15 (1 segmental fracture), Me 11, L 3, B 0; the 4 cases with an intact fibula show no signs of disruption of the mortise or impaction of the tibial articular surface; only slight dislocation or varus angulation (Fig. 39) is present; medial malleolus: V 8, Ob 0, T 1.

Operative Technique—Tibia: 29 plate fixations (some following previous application of traction), no plates in pairs, 4 external fixators

Late Follow-up: 18; findings: 3 deformities (VL 2 after failure to stabilize the fibula; VR 1). 1 arthrosis resulting from intraarticular screw position; 1 osteitis; 1 supramalleolar synostosis

Assessment: Similar to subgroup A2.3, axial malalignment is less pronounced than in the shorter fractures; also, the fibula may remain intact. The proportion of open fractures tends to be smaller; plate fixation prevails; good results are obtained in most of cases.

Figures: For schematics, see Figure 70C; for illustrative radiographs, see Figures 73 and 74.

Summary of Group A3

Total no. of cases: 54. The increasing severity of complex extraarticular fractures manifests itself by the proportion of open fractures and the increase in secondary deformities as a result of delayed consolidation. In most cases, however, it is still possible to carry out the typical plate fixation attached medially or anteriorly.

The number of concomitant injuries is considerably higher when compared to groups A1 and A2. An intact fibula is rare, and multiple fibular fractures predominantly of the shaft are common. The degree of axial malalignment is generally modest. Late follow-ups are available in 33 of the 54 cases (61%). The good prognosis of A3.1-type fractures is noteworthy. In subgroups A3.2 and A3.3, deformities occurred following delayed consolidation, two after failure to stabilize the fibular fracture. The 1 case of arthrosis resulted from a technical fault (screw placed intraarticularly).

Group A3

No. of cases 54
Open fractures 19
Late follow-up 33
Delayed union, malunion, nonunion 6
Prearthrosis/arthrosis 1

3.3. Partial Articular Fractures (Type B)

The B-type fractures comprised those injuries in which one part of the articular surface has remained intact, and has thereby maintained its morphologic and structural continuity with the metaphysis and diaphysis.

There is no doubt that, in comparison to the less stable, circular C-type fractures, these injuries constitute a separate entity in that their intact articular portion, even if small, is of paramount importance both as an aid to reconstruction and a buttress for stabilization.

Axial malalignment is rare in partial articular fractures (see Chapter 2, section 3). The angulation may become relevant only in circular fractures involving the whole circumference of the bone (A and C types). The morphology of some splits and numerous depressions indicate that the foot was positioned in valgus or varus position at the moment of impact. But with depressions affecting only a small area, the talus will glide back into its original position so that on the radiograph, the skeletal axis will have regained its normal position. Simple partial fractures are relatively common; complex fractures are becoming less frequent. Group assignment is done according to the criteria given in Chapter 2, section 6.3. Split fractures are classified as B1, depression fractures as B2, and fractures with disintegration of the articular surface as B3. These injuries allow further classification into subgroups by considering the plane of the fracture which, in simple fractures, is exhibited both by the fragment and the intact articular portion. In complex fractures, identification is generally based on the intact portion.

Group B1

Group B1 comprises all types of pure articular splits occurring in partial fractures with the exception of depressions (B2) and complex articular injuries (B3). Subgroups are categorized according to the plane of the split—its site or where it is best demonstrated on the x-ray film. Problems may arise if the split takes an oblique or kinked course (Fig. 100). In ambiguous cases, classification may be easier by taking into account the intact part of the joint. Without a tomogram, it may be difficult to decide whether there is only a simple split or whether there are multiple splits in the joint.

Subgroup B1.1 contains split fractures in the frontal plane (posteriorly or anteriorly), which are better evident on the lateral film. In some of them, additional independent fractures exist in the diaphysis, i.e., in segment 42. These require a second, distinct classification.

Subgroup B1.2 comprises all partial splits in the sagittal plane (medially or laterally) which are better evident on the AP film. In this group, we find many fractures passing through an epiphyseal growth plate.

Subgroup B1.3 denotes all those fractures in which multiple splits may be recognized in the metaphysis. They are assumed to go along with multiple splits of the articular surface. Such circumstances may also prevent the clear differentiation of the various planes. Extension into the diaphysis is rare, and not a marker for differentiation. Differentiation from depression (B2) or disintegration of the articular surface (B3) is quite straightforward.

Subgroup B1.1

Definition: Partial articular split in the frontal plane (posteriorly or anteriorly); better demonstrable on the lateral view

No. of Cases: 84

Subdivision: Subdivision 1: injury confined to the ankle joint, 36 cases; subdivision 2: articular split plus fracture of the tibial diaphysis in segment 42, 48 cases

B1.1: Subdivision 1 (Injuries Confined to the Ankle)

No. of Cases: 36

Sex and Age Distribution: 29 male, 7 female; mean age: 41 years (range: 14–75 years)

Special Patterns: 21 posterior splits; 15 anterior splits

Special Case: 1 open fracture through an epiphyseal growth plate (anterior split)

Open Fractures: 1

Axial Malalignment: None

Concomitant Injuries: Fibula: U 23, S 8, Mf 5, H 0, D 2, Me 6, L 5, B 0; with anterior splits, the fibula is intact in most cases; medial malleolus: V 3, Ob 5, T 2

Operative Technique—Tibia: 29 screw fixations, 6 plate fixations, 1 nonoperative

Late Follow-up: 30; findings: following faults of technique, 3 cases of prearthrosis, 1 varus deformity; 1 synostosis after complex fracture of the fibula above the syndesmotic ligaments; 1 osteitis

Assessment: In some cases the differentiation of a posterior B1.1-type fracture from a Volkmann's triangle in a malleolar fracture becomes difficult (cf. Chapter 2, section 1.2). A posterolateral position of the fragment was found once, in combination with a complex, supraligamentous fracture of the fibula. B1.1-type fractures have a good prognosis and with meticulous operative technique, they heal without sequelae.

Figures: For schematics, see Figure 98A; for illustrative radiographs, see Figures 99 and 100.

B1.1: Subdivision 2 (Combination of Partial Articular Split in the Frontal Plane with Diaphyseal Fracture of the Tibia in Segment 42)

No. of Cases: 48

Sex and Age Distribution: 18 male, 30 female; mean age: 42 years (range: 16–69 years); 9 patients less than 25 years old

Special Patterns: Posterior split: 24 with morphologic continuity (distal extension) with the spiral fracture of the diaphysis (13 with fracture of the fibula, 11 with intact fibula); posterior split: 22 without morphologic continuity with the diaphyseal fracture (11 with fracture of the fibula, 11 with intact fibula); anterior split: 2 with no morphologic connection with the diaphyseal fracture (both with intact fibula)

Open Fractures: None

Axial Malalignment: None

Concomitant Injuries: Fibula: U 24, fractured at the level of the tibial shaft; medial malleolus: V 5, Ob 0, T 0

Operative Technique—Tibia: 39 screw fixations; 1 plate; 8 nonoperative

Late Follow-up: 31; findings: 1 case of prearthrosis in valgus position after failure to operate the articular fragment

Assessment: This combination injury shows a strikingly high proportion of female and juvenile patients. Obviously, the diagnosis is made in the majority of cases. All but 1 case were treated successfully after internal fixation.

Figures: For schematics, see Figure 42B, C; for illustrative radiograph, see Figure 101.

Subgroup B1.2

Definition: Partial articular fracture with split in the sagittal plane, better evident on the AP view

No. of Cases: 107

Subdivision, Special Patterns, Special Cases: Subdivision 1: fractures crossing the epiphyseal growth plate, 75; subdivision 2: fractures in adults, 28; subdivision 3: sagittal splits combined with fracture of the tibial diaphysis, 4

B1.2: Subdivision 1 (Fractures Passing
Through the Epiphyseal Growth Plate)

No. of Cases: 75

Special Patterns: Laterally shifting, epiphyseal separation, 30; lateral shift with extension to the metaphysis, 17; medially shifting, epiphyseal separation, 8; medial shift with extension to the metaphysis, 20

Open Fractures: 1

Axial Malalignment: 1, slight varus angulation

Concomitant Injuries: Fibula: U 67, S 8, Mf 0, H 0, D 0, Me 8, L 0, B 0; fibular fractures are only present in combination with fractures of the tibia extending into the proximal metaphysis; medial malleolus: V 0, Ob 0, T 0

Operative Technique—Tibia: 71 screw fixations, 4 with Kirschner wires

Late Follow-up: 40; some patients were followed for years with no evidence of secondary angulation, no disturbances of fracture union

Assessment: This is the fracture of the adolescent patient. Premature closure of the epiphyseal plate is unlikely to cause asymmetric growth with deformity.

Figures: For schematics, see Figure 58F, G, H; for illustrative radiographs, see Figures 105 and 106.

B1.2: SUBDIVISION 2 (SAGITTAL SPLIT IN THE ADULT)

No. of Cases: 28

Sex and Age Distribution: 22 male, 6 female; mean age: 39 years (range: 16–77 years)

Open Fractures: 1

Axial Malalignment: None

Concomitant Injuries: Fibula: U 24, S 2, Mf 2, H 0, D 1, Me 2, L 1, B 0; medial malleolus: V 0, Ob 2, T 1

Operative Technique—Tibia: 24 screw fixations, 2 plate fixations, 1 tension band fixation, 1 nonoperative

Late Follow-up: 15; findings: 3 cases of prearthrosis (following inadequate reduction)

Assessment: comparatively minor injury with good prognostic outcome

Figures: For schematics, see Figure 98B; for illustrative radiographs, see Figures 102 and 103.

B1.2: SUBDIVISION 3 (SAGITTAL SPLIT COMBINED WITH DIAPHYSEAL FRACTURE OF THE TIBIA IN SEGMENT 42)

No. of Cases: 4

Sex and Age Distribution: 2 male, 2 female; mean age: 26 years (range: 15–40 years)

Open Fractures: 2 (diaphysis)

Special Patterns: 2 medial, 2 lateral splits (1 before epiphyseal maturity); no morphologic connection with the diaphyseal fracture: 3

Axial Malalignment: None

Concomitant Injuries: Fibula: U 0, S 4, Mf 0, H 0, D 4, Me 0, L 0, B 0; medial malleolus: V 0, Ob 0, T 0

Operative Technique—Articular Split: 4 screw fixations

Late Follow-up: 4; findings uneventful

Assessment: A rare injury; after diagnosis and stabilization, it heals without sequelae

Figures: For illustrative radiograph, see Figure 104.

Subgroup B1.3

Definition: Articular split fracture with multiple splits in the metaphysis

No. of Cases: 25

Sex and Age Distribution: 12 male, 13 female; mean age: 48 years (range: 22–78 years)

Open Fractures: 1

Subdivision, Special Patterns: Split predominantly in the frontal plane (lateral view), 13; split predominantly in the sagittal plane (AP view), 12; extension into the diaphysis, 10

Special Case: Marginal fragment of the talus additionally sheared off (flake); after screwing, complete healing (Fig. 56)

Axial Malalignment: 1 varus angulation

Concomitant Injuries: Fibula: U 11, S 7, Mf 7, H 0, D 5, Me 4, L 5, B 0; the findings on the fibula are uniform in the various subdivisions; medial malleolus: V 1, Ob 3, T 0

Operative Technique—Tibia: 17 plate fixations, 8 screw fixations

Late Follow-up: 18; findings: 3 cases of prearthrosis (2 following inadequate reduction)

Assessment: Multiple splits in the metaphysis only occur in the adult; the preponderance of plating in this subgroup points to an additional instability. A similar constellation is found in group B2.3.

Figures: For schematics, see Figure 117A; for illustrative radiograph, see Figure 119.

Summary of Group B1

Total no. of cases: 216, 139 in adults, 77 in adolescents before epiphyseal maturity; 4 open fractures. This large group displays the complete spectrum of splits in the ankle joint. All age groups are affected. The split affects every plane. There are isolated injuries to the joint as well as combinations with proximally located fractures of the diaphysis. The problem of differentiation from the malleolar fracture is discussed in Chapter 2, section 1.4.

In this subgroup, we do not find serious soft tissue lesions (only four open fractures). This makes operative technique simple. Screw fixation alone dominates with the simple split; it is replaced by plate fixation in cases where multiple metaphyseal splits are present (subgroup B1.3).

A late follow-up is available in 128 cases (59%). The ten cases of prearthrosis, the one valgus and the one varus deformity all appear to result from primary errors in technique. After meticulous reduction, no pathologic changes in the joint are evident at late follow-up.

Group B1

No. of cases 216
Open fractures 4
Late controls 128
Delayed union, malunion, nonunion (metaphysis) 1
Prearthrosis/arthrosis 10

Group B 2

Group B2 comprises all partial fractures showing simple articular depression. They occur only in adults. The differentiation from pure split fractures tends to be unambiguous, but problems often arise with the correct interpretation of some details. The arrangement into subgroups is, as in group B1, based on the plane where the depression and the concomitant split are best visualized on the radiograph.

Subgroup B2.1 comprises the fractures with depression and split in the frontal plane, better evident on the lateral view. The anterior or posterior aspect of the joint is intact. With regard to problems with posterior depressions, the reader is referred to the explanations given in Chapter 2, section 1.2. Subgroup B2.2 comprises fractures with depression and a split in the sagittal plane (better evident on the AP view). The depression, which principally is located on the anterior side, affects either the lateral or the medial aspect of the joint facing the intact part of the articulation on the opposite side. Subgroup B2.3 contains all fractures with multiple fracture lines in the metaphysis. This subgroup combines the basic morphologic patterns of subgroups B2.1 and B2.2. Because of the multiplicity of metaphyseal fracture lines, the articular elements may be visualized equally well in both projections. Differentiation of these details is therefore of minor significance in this last subgroup.

Subgroup B2.1

Definition: Depression and split in the frontal plane (better evident on the lateral view); intact part of the joint anteriorly or posteriorly

No. of Cases: 12

Sex and Age Distribution: 8 male, 4 female; mean age: 38 years (range: 23–61 years)

Open Fractures: 2

Special Patterns: Anterior depression, 10 (3 of these of the pestle form); posterior depression, 2

Special Case: Posterior depression combined with tibial shaft fracture (medullary nail)

Axial Malalignment: None

Concomitant Injuries: Fibula: U 7, S 4, Mf 1, H 0, D 0, Me 2, L 3, B 0; medial malleolus: V 1, Ob 9, T 0. An intact fibula is surprisingly often combined with an oblique fracture of the medial malleolus. In these cases the depressed area is not directly adjacent to the malleolus. Rotatory mechanisms may play a role.

Operative Technique—Tibia: 10 screw fixations, 2 plate fixations

Late Follow-up: 6; findings: 2 cases of prearthrosis following pestle-form depressions (inadequate reduction)

Assessment: Owing to its accessibility, the predominantly anterior depression has a good prognosis.

Figures: For schematics, see Figure 111A; for illustrative radiographs, see Figures 113 and 114.

Subgroup B2.2

Definition: Depression with split in the frontal plane (better evident on the AP view); intact portion of the articular surface medially or laterally

No. of Cases: 23

Sex and Age Distribution: 14 male, 9 female; mean age: 37 years (range: 17–62 years)

Open Fractures: 1

Special Patterns: Depression and lateral split, 4; a tibial fragment always remains attached to the syndesmosis; the depression does not extend to the fibular notch; 19 medial depressions; in some fractures, the medial split is located at a clear distance from the medial malleolus.

Special Case: Shear of the talus, the so-called flake fragment; questionable tear of the deltoid ligament (Fig. 52)

Axial Malalignment: 2 slight varus angulations

Concomitant Injuries: Fibula: U 11, S 12, Mf 0, H 0, D 0, Me 0, L 10, B 2; medial malleolus: V 8, Ob 8, T 0

Operative Technique—Tibia: 11 screw fixations, 1 with plate, 1 with Kirschner wire and screw

Late Follow-up: 17; findings: 1 severe arthrosis (inadequate reduction), 3 cases of prearthrosis (inadequate reduction, fibular deformity)

Assessment: When compared to subgroup B2.1, there is a striking frequency of plate fixations; the proportion of patients developing arthrosis is about equal for medial and lateral depressions

Figures: For schematics, see Figure 111B; for illustrative radiographs, see Figures 52, 115, and 176.

Subgroup B2.3

Definition: Multiple fracture lines in the metaphysis combined with split and depression of the articular surface

No. of Cases: 22

Sex and Age Distribution: 15 male, 7 female; mean age: 39 years (range: 17–77 years)

Open Fractures: 1

Special Patterns: Depression with anterior split, 7; with posterior split, 2; depression with medial fracture, 10; with lateral fracture, 3

Special Case: 1 extension into the diaphysis

Axial Malalignment: 6: VL 2, VR 4, RC 0, AC 0

Concomitant Injuries: Fibula: U 9, S 10, Mf 3, H 0, D 2, Me 3, L 5, B 3; medial malleolus: V 7, Ob 4, T 2

Operative Technique—Tibia: 10 screw fixations, 11 plate fixations, 1 by fibular plating alone; internal fixations are more complex than those in subgroups B2.1 and B2.2.

Late Follow-up: 16; findings: 1 severe arthrosis, 7 prearthrosis (inadequate reduction); 4 subchondral scleroses (devitalization ?)

Assessment: As in group B1, we also find that multiple splits in the metaphysis characterize the more complex injury, which is evidenced by the type of treatment and the prognosis.

Figures: For schematics, see Figure 117B; for illustrative radiograph, see Figure 120.

Summary of Group B2

Total no. of cases: 57. There are only four open fractures (8%). Thus depression is not associated with soft tissue damage any more serious than that found in pure splits. With regard to operative technique, it becomes evident that depressions require greater interfragmental compression in order to stabilize and hold the reduction. While screws are used for the simpler cases, plates are increasingly being used in subgroups B2.2 and B2.3.

There are 39 late follow-ups available (68%). These include 12 patients with prearthrosis and 2 with arthrosis resulting from technical shortcomings or inadequate reduction.

Depression fractures are clearly more serious than pure splits. The most favorable prognosis is found with anterior depression and one fragment split off. Lateral and medial trap-door depressions have a less favorable prognosis, and management is more difficult. The worst prognosis is definitely associated with fractures showing multiple splits in the metaphysis: instability is greater, and operative technique more complicated.

Group B2

No. of cases 57
Open fractures 4
Late follow-up 39
Delayed union, malunion, nonunion (metaphysis) 0
Prearthrosis/arthrosis 14

Group B3

This group comprises all injuries in which some part of the articular surface is preserved, while the various elements of the fractured area have disintegrated. The term *disintegration* is defined in Chapter 2, section 6.3.4. The fractured area covers most of the articular surface. Changes resulting from multiple splits, impactions, or depressions are so pronounced as to prevent recognition of any continuity or details. Such findings are, of course, rare in partial fractures. The intact part of the articular surface, which maintains continuity with the diaphysis, is always small.

The arrangement according to planes is not as clear-cut as with simple splits and depressions. Orientation is most reliable when based on the uninjured wall. In doing so, it could be shown that the anterior wall is always fractured. Intact portions of the articular wall are found posteriorly, posterolaterally, posteromedially, and anteromedially, but they are never exclusively confined to the anterior wall. In these fractures, we always observe multiple splits in the metaphysis.

Differentiation from simpler fractures (B1 and B2) may give rise to problems when there are superimpositions and the radiograph takes on a dramatic appearance. If a second projection fails to aid in the clarification, then additional radiologic investigations (tomogram, CT scan) are required. Differentiation in our analysis became possible by use of the postoperative radiographs. Subgroup B3.1 comprises all fractures with disintegration of the articular surface in which no more than the posterior wall has been preserved. They are better evident on the lateral view.

Subgroup B3.2 contains the fractures in which either the lateral or the medial wall has remained intact. They are better evident on the AP view.

Subgroup B3.3 comprises fractures with the rare finding of extension into the diaphysis.

Subgroup B3.1

Definition: Disintegration of the articular surface with preservation of the posterior wall (better evident on the lateral view)

No. of Cases: 10

Sex and Age Distribution: 9 male, 1 female; mean age: 33 years (range: 21–71 years)

Open Fractures: 3

Special Patterns: 7 cases with the anterolateral tubercle (Tillaux-Chaput) broken off

Axial Malalignment: None

Concomitant Injuries: Fibula: U 6, S 3, Mf 1, H 0, D 1, Me 0, L 2, B 1; the fibula is intact in most cases; attached to the posterior syndesmotic ligament, it maintains its continuity via the intact tibial wall; medial malleolus: V 3, Ob 4, T 1

Operative Technique—Tibia: 7 plate fixations, 3 with screws alone

Late Follow-up: 6; findings: 1 severe arthrosis with subluxation; 2 cases of prearthrosis, 3 cases with satisfying joint outcome; 1 osteitis

Assessment: Striking findings in this subgroup are the preponderance of men and the low average age of the patients. Operative techniques rely on plate fixation, even for open fractures. This allows the conclusion that soft tissue damage is not serious in these cases.

Figures: For schematics, see Figure 130A; for illustrative radiographs, see Figures 132 and 186.

Subgroup B3.2

Definition: Disintegration of the articular surface with preservation of the lateral or medial wall; better evident on the AP view

No. of Cases: 5

Sex and Age Distribution: 4 male, 1 female; mean age: 37 years (range: 22–50 years)

Open Fractures: 2

Subdivision: In 2 cases, we find the intact wall on the posteromedial side, in 2 on the anterolateral side, and in 1 on the posterolateral side.

Axial Malalignment: 4; VL 2, VR 2, RC 0, AC 0

Concomitant Injuries: Fibula: U 0, S 2, Mf 3, H 0, D 2, Me 2, L 1, B 0; medial malleolus: V 2, Ob 3, T 0

Operative Technique—Tibia: 1 plate fixation, 2 with screws, 1 Kirschner wire (open), 1 external fixator (open)

Late Follow-up: 3; findings: 2 cases of arthrosis after inadequate reduction, 1 secondary arthrodesis, 2 osteitides.

Assessment: This subgroup carries a significantly worse prognosis than subgroup B3.1; possibly because of the problems with fracture exposure (the intact portions of the articular surface and wall are less favorably situated than in subgroup B3.1).

Figures: For schematics, see Figure 130B; for illustrative radiograph, see Figure 133.

Subgroup B3.3

Definition: Disintegration of the articular surface in partial fractures; extension into the diaphysis. This extremely rare morphologic pattern was found in only one patient. The fracture is closed. The intact parts of the joint and articular wall are on the lateral side. The fibula is intact. Internal fixation was carried out with a long plate in pairs. Significant arthrosis was found at late follow-up.

Summary of Group B3

Total no. of cases: 16, including 5 open fractures (almost one third.) In contrast to groups B1 and B2, there is more soft tissue damage in this subgroup. Despite the disintegration of the articular surface, the fibula remained intact in 7 patients.

Subgroup B3.1 is the only one containing some cases with a favorable prognosis. Late follow-up: 10. In general, the results are unsatisfactory, showing prearthrosis or arthrosis. Injuries in this group must be considered as severe as the C3-type fractures (see below).

Group B3

No. of cases 16
Open fractures 5
Late follow-up 10
Delayed union, malunion, nonunion (metaphysis) 0
Prearthrosis/arthrosis 6
Arthrodesis 1

3.4. Complete Articular Fractures (Type C)

C-type fractures comprise all those injuries where the mechanical link between the articulation and the diaphysis has been completely lost. They are more unstable than partial fractures of the B type. Differentiation on the basis of planes is precluded, since an intact wall, which would serve as a guide, is missing.

The articular surface presents with the same injuries as partial fractures: the simple split prevails, but split-depressions are also frequently observed. These two patterns of simple articular lesion make up group C1.

As outlined in Chapter 2, section 6.3.2, depressions are seen even in young adults. The average age of patients with depressions does not exceed that of patients with splits, a finding observed in groups B1 and B2. Similarly, when these patients are followed, we find less favorable late results after depression. Combinations of simple articular injuries with the metaphyseal morphologic findings characteristic of the distal tibia are common. The typical patterns are impaction and multifragmentation in the metaphysis. Those of the A-type underwent a special analysis (see Chapter 2, section 5.2.2). Fractures with the combination are assigned to group C2.

Fractures showing complex injury of the articular surface (disintegration) are classified as group C3. The morphologic findings are spectacular and characteristic, but rare.

Complete fractures are injuries of the adult patient (only in C.2.1, 1 case in an epiphyseal growth plate in varus position; see Fig. 124).

Group C1

This group contains all fractures in which a simple split or split-depression is recognized at the joint (analogous to B1- and B2-type fractures), but which in the metaphysis or distal diaphysis presents as a complete, i.e., circular, fracture.

The split shows the simple Y or T shape. Multiple splits may occur in the metaphysis. The presence of impactions or multifragmentation, however, dictates a classification as C2.

An important morphologic appearance in these injuries is the spiral fractures extending into the joint, as was pointed out by Böhler [13] and Gay and Evrard [46]. The fractures are closed, and often, they result from a less serious mechanism of accident. As in diaphyseal fractures, the operative management is not particularly difficult, and the prognosis tends to be good.

Subgroup C1.1: comprises all complete articular splits.
Subgroup C1.2: comprises all complete articular split-depressions.
Subgroup C1.3: comprises all complete fractures which show simple splits or depressions of the articular surface, and a fracture line extending into the diaphysis.

Subgroup C1.1

Definition: Articular split becoming circular in the metaphysis

No. of Cases: 55

Sex and Age Distribution: 30 male, 25 female; mean age: 43 years (range: 18–83 years)

Subdivision: None

Special Patterns: 30 cases of spiral morphology

Open Fractures: 4

Axial Malalignment: 17, slightly pronounced; VL 5, VR 8, RC 1, AC 3

Concomitant Injuries: Fibula: U 25, S 21, Mf 9, H 1, D 12 (1 segmental), Me 11, L 5, B 1; medial malleolus: V 4, Ob 8, T 0

Operative Technique—Tibia: 44 plate fixations, 10 screw fixations, 1 external fixator

Late Follow-up: 30; findings: 4 delayed consolidations, 1 in varus, 2 in valgus position; 2 synostoses above the malleoli; 1 arthrosis

Assessment: In this group, problems are found with consolidation in the metaphysis as a manifestation of circular instability. Similar findings were noted in A2- and A3-type fractures.

Figures: For schematics, see Figure 98C; for illustrative radiograph, see Figure 107.

Subgroup C1.2

Definition: Articular split depression in a simple, circular fracture of the metaphysis

No. of Cases: 26

Sex and Age Distribution: 17 male, 9 female; mean age: 41 years (range: 20–70 years)

Subdivision: None

Special Patterns: Shorter fractures than in C1.1; marked spiral morphologies are found in only 4 cases; morphology of the depression: 14 triangular and trap-door depressions, 8 pestle-shaped, 4 trough-shaped depressions; 11 in the frontal plane (lateral view), 15 in the sagittal plane (AP view); 7 lateral, 15 medial

Special Case: 1 case with an additional fracture of the diaphysis in segment 42 (plate fixation)

Open Fractures: 1 (important dislocation)

Axial Malalignment: 6, slightly pronounced; VL 1, VR 5, RC 0, AC 0

Concomitant Injuries: Fibula: U 14, S 7, Mf 5, H 0, D 4, Me 2, L 6, B 0; medial malleolus: V 4, Ob 1, T 0

Operative Technique—Tibia: 24 plate fixations, 2 screw fixations

Late Follow-up: 13; findings: 3 cases of severe arthrosis, 6 of prearthrosis after incomplete reduction

Assessment: The late results give further proof of the greater severity of depression when compared to the split alone. Although the associated soft tissue damage here is certainly less grave, the overall prognosis is worse.

Figures: For schematics, see Figure 111C; for illustrative radiograph, see Figure 116.

Subgroup C1.3

Definition: Split or depression of the articular surface in a circular fracture; extension into the diaphysis

No. of Cases: 45

Sex and Age Distribution: 30 male, 15 female; mean age: 42 years (range: 20–75 years); mean age is 38 years in patients with depression

Subdivision: None

Special Patterns: Dominance of spiral morphologies, in particular with depressions; 10 depressions, 3 of these of the pestle-type, 3 trough-shaped; 5 split fractures branching off and becoming circular at the diaphysis (young patients).

A few patients in this subgroup present borderline cases to be differentiated from subgroups B1.1 (subdivision 2) and B1.2 (subdivision 3). But the articular split in the C1.3-type fracture takes a course along the axis passing through the metaphysis into the diaphysis where it becomes circular. In B1-type fractures, the split is short and marginal terminating at the metaphysis. Thus a second, independent center in the diaphysis can be clearly distinguished from the articular part (see Figs. 101, 104, and 118).

Open Fractures: 3

Axial Malalignment: 10; VL 3, VR 7, RC 0, AC 0

Concomitant Injuries: Fibula: U 23, S 13, Mf 9, H 0, D 14, Me 8, L 0, B 0; medial malleolus: V 6, Ob 6, T 2

Operative Technique—Tibia: 39 plate fixations, 5 by screws alone; 1 external fixator

Late Follow-up: 28; findings: 2 severe arthroses in depression; the remaining cases include 1 prearthrosis and 1 arthrosis due to incongruence; 1 secondary varus deviation

Assessment: These long fractures show comparatively minor degrees of dislocation. Consequently, there are few open fractures, and an intact fibula is common. Except for the cases with depression, the prognosis is favorable.

Figures: For schematics, see Figure 117E; for illustrative radiographs, see Figures 127, 178, and 179.

Summary of Group C1

Total no. of fractures: 126. There are only 8 (6%) open fractures. Spiral morphologies are often found. There is only a slight degree of axial dislocation, predominantly into varus position. The intact fibula and the intact medial malleolus are noteworthy.

In almost half of the cases (62 out of 126), there is no fracture of the fibula. This is why group C1 is especially suited for study of tears of the syndesmotic ligaments (see section 1.3). A review of the operation reports in this group was made. In 21 cases, we found evidence on the postoperative radiographs for an additional lateral incision from which the lateral ligamentous complex could have been repaired. Rupture of the syndesmotic ligament was reported in only 1 of these 21 cases, and a torn anterior fibulotalar ligament was indicated in another case. In the remaining operative reports, the ligamentous complex is passed over in silence.

Operative management relies on plate fixations.

Late follow-up: 71 (56%). An unsatisfactory outcome is mainly due to arthrosis, and almost without exception, a consequence of depression. A few patients developed problems with consolidation in the metaphyses.

Group C1

No. of cases 126
Open fractures 8
Late follow-up 71
Delayed union, malunion, nonunion (metaphysis)* 5
Prearthrosis/arthrosis 14

---

*In C-type fractures, problems with fracture union in the metaphysis are only specified when they are not combined with arthrosis.

Group C2

This is by far the largest group in our series, especially in the framework of complete articular fractures. It comprises all fractures with the combination of a simple articular component (split or split-depression) and a principal finding in the metaphysis, the latter consisting either of impaction or multifragmentation. Thus, the metaphyseal morphology is the outstanding feature. Except for the articular component, classification corresponds to that of A2-type fractures.

We do not always know for certain whether the articular split is simple. The fracture lines may occasionally take an oblique or kinked course arousing doubts on examination of the radiographs, and preventing the exclusion of a double split formation. At least on one projection, it must be possible to evaluate the articular contours. This enables us to safely distinguish the finding from articular disintegration, which must be classified as C3.

Subgroup C2.1 comprises fractures with metaphyseal impaction and an articular split (an additional small articular depression is possible). This large subgroup characterizes the typical pilon fracture of the skier (Chapter 2, section 6.2; Fig. 87). Except for the injuries in valgus position, where some of the fractures are open, there is only minor soft tissue damage.

Subgroup C2.2 comprises fractures with metaphyseal multifragmentation and articular split (articular depressions may also be present). This group is characterized by the large number of open fractures and the increasing severity of the concomitant injuries, a finding similar to the situation with the extraarticular subgroup A2.2.

Patients in subgroups C2.1 and C2.2, in whom depression of the articular surface exists in addition to the split, undergo a separate analysis.

Subgroup C2.3 also comprises fractures extending into the diaphysis (C2.3). It combines the basic morphologic patterns of the previous two subgroups, i.e., metaphyseal impaction and multifragmentation. Both require separate analysis. We also find two cases in which an additional depression is suspected.

Subgroup C2.1

Definition: Metaphyseal impaction with articular split (possibly combined with simple depression)

No. of Cases: 117

Sex: 65 male, 52 female

Open Fractures: 6 (4 with split and valgus deviation, 2 with depression and valgus position)

Subdivision: None

Special Patterns: To facilitate the understanding of the ample case material, a subdivision considering the direction of axial dislocation has proved to be useful; combinations are frequent. The classification is based on the most prominent dislocation. Subdivision 1: impaction with valgus position, 33 cases; subdivision 2: impaction with varus position, 21 cases; subdivision 3: impaction with recurvation, 28 cases; subdivision 4: impaction with antecurvation, 6 cases; subdivision 5: impaction without angulation, 15 cases; subdivision 6: additional articular depression, 14 (4 of these in valgus, 2 in varus position; 3 with recurvation; 3 without angulation).

C2.1: Subdivision 1 (33 Cases with Dominance
of Valgus Position)

Age: Mean age: 53 years (range: 29–76 years)

Open Fractures: 4

Concomitant Injuries: Fibula: U 0, S 8, Mf 25, H 0, D 7, Me 12, L 11, B 3; medial malleolus: V 0, Ob 0, T 2

Operative Technique—Tibia: 28 plate fixations, 2 with screws alone, 1 with screws plus traction, 1 external fixator, 1 nonoperative

Late Follow-up: 20; findings: 2 cases of severe arthrosis with recurrent drift into valgus position; 1 arthrodesis; 6 prearthroses, 3 of these presenting as recurrent valgus deformities due to absent or inadequate fibular stabilization; 3 osteitides, 10 good results

Figures: For schematics, see Figure 117C; for illustrative radiographs, see Figures 121, 122, and 181.

C2.1: Subdivision 2 (21 Cases with Dominance
of Varus Position)

Age: Mean age: 40 years (range: 14–86 years)

Special Case: 1 fracture with an epiphyseal growth plate (Fig. 124)

Open Fractures: None

Concomitant Injuries: Fibula: U 0, S 13, Mf 8, D 6 (1 segmental), Me 14, L 1, B 0; medial malleolus: V 10, Ob 6, T 0

Operative Technique—Tibia: 20 plate fixations, 1 traction

Late Follow-up: 10; findings: 1 arthrosis (traction), 3 prearthroses, 6 good results

Figures: For schematics, see Figure 117C; for illustrative radiograph, see Figure 123.

C2.1: SUBDIVISION 3 (28 CASES IN RECURVATION;
THE DEGREE OF AXIAL DEVIATION IS
COMPARATIVELY SMALL, THE IMPACTION ONLY
PARTIAL [POSTERIOR] AND COMBINED WITH
ADDITIONAL, ANTERIOR SPLITS)

Age: Mean age: 40 years (range: 19–69 years)

Open Fractures: None

Concomitant Injuries: Fibula: U 7, S 12, Mf 9, H 0, D 8, Me 13, L 0, B 0; medial malleolus: V 4, Ob 4, T 0

Operative Technique—Tibia: 26 plate fixations, 2 screw fixations

Late Follow-up: 15; findings: 3 prearthroses, 1 of these with recurrent recurvation, 12 good results

Assessment: Recurvation fractures show the best late results among all types of axial malalignment.

Figures: For schematics, see Figure 117C; for illustrative radiograph, see Figure 182.

C2.1: SUBDIVISION 4 (6 CASES IN ANTECURVATION;
ONLY SLIGHT DEGREE OF DISLOCATION)

Age: Mean age: 40 years (range: 36–51 years)

Open Fractures: None

Concomitant Injuries: Fibula: U 0, S 2, Mf 4, H 0, D 3, Me 2, L 1, B 0; medial malleolus: V 0, Ob 3, T 0

Operative Technique—Tibia: 6 plate fixations

Late Follow-up: 4; findings: 1 arthrosis, 1 prearthrosis with synostosis, 2 good results

C2.1: Subdivision 5 (15 Cases Without Axial
Deviation; On Morphologic Grounds, in
Particular with Regard to the Fibular Injury,
It Is Assumed That Before Taking the
Postinjury Radiograph, Angulation in the
Following Directions Was Present: VR 3, RC 1,
VL 11)

Age: Mean age: 35 years (range: 19–56 years)

Open Fractures: None

Concomitant Injuries: Fibula: U 3, S 8, Mf 4, H 0, D 3, Me 8, L 1, B 0; medial malleolus: V 1, Ob 4, T 0

Operative Technique—Tibia: 15 plate fixations

Late Follow-up: 11; findings: 5 cases of prearthrosis, 6 good results

C2.1: Subdivision 6 (14 Cases with Additional
Depression of the Articular Surface; the
Depressions Are Found at Different Sites,
Which Corresponds to the Situation in
Subgroup C1.2: 2 Are of the Pestle-form, and
11 Occur with Axial Malalignment: VL 4, VR
4, RC 3; the Articular Surface Is not Severely
Displaced [Mitigating Effect of the
Metaphyseal Impaction?])

Age: Mean age: 40 years (range: 21–65 years)

Open Fractures: 2 (in valgus)

Concomitant Injuries: Fibula: U 3, S 8, Mf 3, H 0, D 4, Me 4, L 3, B 0; medial malleolus: V 4, Ob 5, T 0

Operative Technique—Tibia: 12 plate fixations, 2 primary arthrodeses

Late Follow-up: 8; findings: 5 prearthroses (1 with valgus and 1 with varus deformity), 1 secondary arthrodesis, 2 fairly satisfactory results, 1 osteitis

Assessment: When depression is combined with metaphyseal impaction, this certainly entails deterioration of local perfusion conditions, and complicates operative reduction.

Figures: For illustrative radiographs, see Figures 51 and 125.

Summary of Subgroup C2.1

The main feature of this very large subgroup is in impaction of the metaphysis. In most illustrations, it is depicted in recurvation, which means that it is viewed from the lateral side [132]. Our analysis shows that the injury occurs most frequently in valgus position, which is also the most serious form, because all of the 6 open fractures observed occurred in this position (2 of these in the group combined with depression). Dislocation into valgus position is always associated with (predominantly multifragmentary) fractures of the fibula. Valgus fractures also have a less favorable outcome than is the case after other forms of angulation.

There is no doubt, however, that the prognosis is worst in cases where impaction is combined with articular depression. Six out of eight cases for which follow-ups are available show arthrosis or significant prearthrosis, and in two cases arthrodesis has already been carried out. So this type presents the most adverse situation encountered in terms of biological and operative conditions.

When the group is considered as a whole, the overall prognosis is fairly good. Among the 68 late results, we observe 38 good outcomes with respect to the articular surface. Secondary, and correctable, metaphyseal deformities occasionally occur. The best results are found after recurvation, the pattern in which we also most often find an intact fibula.

Subgroup C2.2

Definition: Metaphyseal multifragmentation with articular split (possibly combined with depression)

No. of Cases: 86

Sex and Age Distribution: 50 male, 36 female; mean age: 45 years (range: 18–73 years)

Special Patterns: 10 fractures with additional depression of the articular surface, 4 of these open; 4 trap-door depressions; 4 pestle- and 2 trough-shaped depressions

Open Fractures: 39; VL 19, VR 0, RC 1, AC 1 (14 in neutral position, 4 with depression)

Axial Malalignment: 56: VL 37, VR 11, RC 4, AC 3

Concomitant Injuries: Fibula: U 3, S 34, Mf 49, H 0, D 56 (6 segmental fractures), Me 29, L 1, B 0; compared with subgroup C2.1, the large number of multiple, diaphyseal fractures of the fibula is striking; medial malleolus: V 12, Ob 16, T 0.

Operative Technique—Tibia: 75 plate fixations, 8 external fixators (3 as primary arthrodesis), 3 screw fixations (1 combined with traction)

Late Follow-up: 42; findings: the 6 cases with depression showed 3 arthroses, 2 prearthroses, and 1 good outcome; the prognostic outcome of the remaining cases does not depend on the original position of the axis: 12 prearthroses, 8 arthroses; 5 valgus deformities following delayed consolidation in the metaphysis (1 pseudarthrosis), 11 good outcomes; 4 osteitides.

Assessment: In relation to impaction, this injury is clearly more critical; almost 50% of the fractures are open. The poorest results are obtained in the 10 cases with articular depression. We also find an increase of delayed consolidation with deformity.

Figures: For schematics, see Figure 117D; for illustrative radiographs, see Figures 126 and 181.

Subgroup C2.3

Definition: Articular split with metaphyseal impaction or multifragmentation; the fracture extends into the diaphysis (double metaphyseal height)

No. of Cases: 17

Sex and Age Distribution: 11 male, 6 female; mean age: 45 years (range: 23–68 years)

Subdivision: None

Special Patterns, Special Cases: 5 cases of the impacted type (all closed), 12 cases of the multifragmentary type as in subgroup C2.2 (6 open), 2 questionable cases of articular depression (out of focus)

Open Fractures: 6 (all of the multifragmentary metaphyseal type)

Axial Malalignment: 8, slightly pronounced: VL 2, VR 2, RC 2, AC 1

Concomitant Injuries: Fibula: U 1, S 11, M 5, H 2, D 8 (2 segmental), Me 5, L 1, B 0; medial malleolus: V 3, Ob 1, T 0

Operative Technique—Tibia: 11 plate fixations, 3 by screws and traction; 2 external fixators, 1 with screws alone

Late Follow-up: 9; findings: 1 prearthrosis after impaction; after metaphyseal multifragmentation: 3 prearthroses, 1 arthrosis with arthrodesis, 1 valgus deformity; 2 osteitides

Assessment: The degree of axial malalignment is less when the fracture extends into the diaphysis. In general, the results correspond to those found in the respective morphologic types of the basic injury classified as C2.1 and C2.2.

Figures: For schematics, see Figure 117F; for illustrative radiograph, see Figure 129.

Summary of Group C2

Total no. of cases: 220. This is the largest group in our case material. The main characteristic is complex injury of the metaphysis combined with an articular split. The comparison with extraarticular fractures with the same morphologic appearance is justified. The only significant difference is that the average age is higher in patients in subgroup A2.1 (see above).

With the complete fracture with impaction (C2.1), a further subdivision with separate analysis of the various subgroups has proved to be advantageous. Even though the approach does not improve the structural organization of the classification, it helps to recognize the individuality of both the valgus deviation and the additional depression of the articular surface.

Impactions combined with an articular split rarely present as an open fracture (less than 10%), but because of the articular component, the late results are clearly poorer than after the extraarticular forms. When the fracture shows multifragmentation of the metaphysis (C2.2), a further subdivision will not reveal more differences. Here we find the highest proportion of soft tissue injuries in the series, namely, in the form of open fractures (39 of 87 cases, or 45%). We also find that valgus deviation prevails, and that the concomitant fibular fracture is predominantly in the diaphysis.

The subgroup characterized by diaphyseal extension (C2.3) does not differ from the first two subgroups as far as the details of the injury are concerned. As in other fractures with important extensions, the insignificance of the axial malalignment is striking.

There are 119 follow-ups available (54%). When compared with group C1, important differences are found with respect to arthrosis and secondary deviation. The most unsatisfactory prognoses attend, firstly, fractures with additional articular depression, and secondly, fractures with valgus deviation. The poor results may be considered a manifestation of the difficulties encountered during the reduction of these complex fractures with significant involvement of the metaphysis. The outcome varies greatly between fractures with impaction and those with metaphyseal multifragmentation; in C2.1 fractures, we find 38 good results out of 68 late controls (55%). In C2.2-type fractures, we find 11 good results out of 42 late controls (26%).

Group C2

No. of cases 220
Open fractures 51
Late follow-up 119
Delayed union, malunion, nonunion* 16
Prearthrosis/arthrosis 54
Arthrodesis 2

---

*In C-type fractures, problems with fracture union in the metaphysis are only specified when not combined with arthrosis.

Group C3

Group C3 comprises all fractures with disintegration of the articular surface. Terms and definitions are explained in Chapter 2, section 6.3.4. The recognition of articular depressions as such requires that they remain attached to major articular fragments. When the elements have disintegrated, identification of details of the depression is often impossible.

The arrangement into subgroups takes into account the extension of multifragmentation along the tibial axis. Subgroup C3.1 comprises fractures confined to the epiphysis and distal metaphysis. Subgroup C3.2 comprises fractures extending up to the proximal metaphysis, and subgroup C3.3 comprises fractures reaching the diaphysis. The diaphyseal extension is mainly composed of large individual fragments which may be recognized as such. This is different from the situation found around the metaphysis and epiphysis. In subgroup C3.1, where we have a localized area of disintegration, we often observe that the elements are too badly damaged to allow surgical restoration. By contrast, fractures extending into the upper metaphysis often show a less severely disintegrated articular surface (mitigating effect?). This may complicate the differentiation between subgroups C3.2 and C2.2. In C2-type fractures, only splits of the articular surface are present, in some cases combined with simple depressions. When the fracture is displaced, superimposing effects in one projection may produce the impression of articular disintegration, but this disappears when the radiograph taken in the second projection is studied. The clinical classification of such cases depends on the results of further radiologic studies. In our series, an unambiguous differentiation was made possible by postoperative radiographs.

Subgroup C3.1

Definition: Disintegration of the articular surface with limited extension (confined to the distal metaphysis)

No. of Cases: 16

Sex and Age Distribution: 12 male, 4 female; mean age: 42 years (range: 22–73 years)

Open Fractures: 4

Axial Malalignment: VL 1, slightly pronounced

Concomitant Injuries: Fibula: U 1, S 7, Mf 8, H 0, D 4, Me 4, L 6, B 1; medial malleolus: the medial malleolus is always fractured: V 4, Ob 12, T 0

Operative Technique—Tibia: Open fractures: 2 by external fixator, 1 by stabilizing the fibula alone, 1 by screws alone; closed fractures: 7 plate fixations, 4 by screwing only, 1 by traction

Late Follow-up: 7; findings: 2 arthroses, 4 apparently progressing cases of prearthrosis, 1 fairly satisfactory articular result

Assessment: Within group C3, the localized disintegration of the articular surface appears to account for the greatest difficulties encountered at operation, and is associated with the poorest prognosis.

Figures: For schematics, see Figure 131A; for illustrative radiograph, see Figure 134.

Subgroup C3.2

Definition: Disintegration of the articular surface; extension of the multifragmented area to the upper metaphysis

No. of Cases: 19

Sex and Age Distribution: 14 male, 5 female; mean age: 39 years (range: 23–61 years)

Special Case: Combined with sagittal fracture of the talar trochlea (Fig. 135)

Open Fractures: 5 (no differences in morphology between open and closed fractures)

Axial Malalignment: Evaluation is hampered by the great number of fragments; 11 in total: VL 3, VR 6, RC 2, AC 0.

Concomitant Injuries: Fibula: U 4, S 6, Mf 9, H 0, D 7, Me 7, L 1, B 0; the fibular fracture is generally more proximal than in subgroup C3.1; medial malleolus: V 6, Ob 7, T 1

Operative Technique—Tibia: No differences in management between open and closed fractures; 16 plate fixations, 2 primary arthrodeses, 1 external fixator (subsequently plated)

Late Follow-up: 10; findings: 1 arthrosis, 2 prearthroses, 1 secondary arthrodesis, 6 satisfactory articular results, 2 osteitides

Assessment: There is a noteworthy difference when the late results are compared with those of C3.1. Fractures extending far proximally carry a better prognosis than fractures in which the multifragmentation is confined to the epiphysis and distal metaphysis.

Figures: For schematics, see Figure 131B; for illustrative radiographs, see Figures 135 and 136.

Subgroup C3.3

Definition: Articular disintegration with extension into the diaphysis (twice the metaphyseal height)

No. of Cases: 10

Sex and Age Distribution: 7 male, 3 female; mean age: 39 years (range: 22–55 years)

Open Fractures: 3

Axial Malalignment: The more extensive the fracture, the less pronounced the degree of axial malalignment; 5 in total: VL 2, VR 3, RC 0, AC 0.

Concomitant Injuries: Fibula: U 1, S 7, Mf 2, H 0, D 8 (1 segmental), Me 1, L 0, B 0; medial malleolus: V 4, Ob 3, T 1

Operative Technique—Tibia: No differences in technique between open and closed fractures; 9 plate fixations, 1 primary arthrodesis

Late Follow-up: 6; findings: 3 arthroses, 2 arthrodeses, 1 satisfactory articular result, 2 osteitides, 1 case of pseudarthrosis with arthrosis; despite reintervention, redevelopment of valgus deformity

Assessment: The implant material frequently used in this subgroup is the long straight plate. The results are in no way satisfactory, in particular when compared to subgroup C3.2.

Figures: For schematics, see Figure 131C; for illustrative radiographs, see Figures 49 and 137.

Summary of Group C3

Total no. of cases: 45. Group C3 comprises those fractures of the distal tibial joint which display the most severe morphologic features. What surprises, however, is that the proportion of open fractures, i.e., of severe soft tissue injuries, is lower than in subgroup C2.2. An intact fibula is rare (6 cases), and fracture of the medial malleolus very common (38 cases).

Late Follow-up: 23 (51%). As expected, the most unsatisfactory results in the series are contained in group C3. They are concentrated in subgroups C3.1 and C3.3. With the latter fracture, a negative effect may be attributed to the choice of osteosynthetic material. We would draw attention to the fact that the number of available late follow-up studies is restricted, and there is a tendency to overestimate the frequency of these spectacular injuries.

Group C3

No. of cases 45
Open fractures 12
Late follow-up 23
Delayed union, malunion, nonunion (metaphysis)*
Arthrosis/prearthrosis 12
Arthrodesis 3

---

*In C-type fractures, problems with fracture union in the metaphysis are only specified when not combined with arthrosis. See Table 5.

Table 3

LONG-TERM RESULTS OF EXTRAARTICULAR FRACTURES (TYPE A)

Subgroup, Subdivisions, Definition		Total	No. of Late Follow-ups	Delayed Union, Nonunion/ Malunion (Metaphysis)	No. of Prearthroses, Arthroses	No. of Arthrodeses
A1.1	Simple spiral fracture of the metaphysis	37	24			
A1.2	Simple oblique fracture of the metaphysis	127				
	Subdivision 1: adults (37) Fracture proximal to an epiphyseal growth plate (6)	43	26			
	Subdivision 2: epiphyseal fracture	84	45			
A1.3	Simple transverse fracture of the metaphysis (incl. traumatic epiphyseolysis)	29	15			
A1	Total	193	110			
A2.1	Metaphyseal impaction	26	12	2	1	
A2.2	Metaphyseal wedge fracture	73				
	Subdivision 1: simple wedge	34	14	4		
	Subdivision 2: multifragmented wedge	39	20	6	1[a]	
A2.3	Extension of the wedge into the diaphysis	51	26	1		
A2	Total	150	72	13	2	
A3.1	Complex fracture of the metaphysis, individual fragments	11	6			
A3.2	Complex fracture, multiple fragments	10	9	3		
A3.3	Complex fracture, extending into the diaphysis	33	18	3	1	
A3	Total	54	33	6	1	

[a]Technical mistake.

Table 4

LONG-TERM RESULTS OF PARTIAL ARTICULAR FRACTURES (TYPE B)

Subgroup, Subdivisions, Definition	Total	No. of Late Follow-ups	Delayed Union, Nonunion/ Malunion (Metaphysis)	No. of Prearthroses, Arthroses	No. of Arthrodeses
B1.1 Partial split in the frontal plane (lateral view)	84				
Subdivision 1: simple split	36	30	1	3	
Subdivision 2: additional and independent fracture of the diaphysis (segment 42)	48	31		1	
B1.2 Partial split in the sagittal plane (AP view)	107				
Subdivision 1: fracture of an epiphyseal plate	75	40			
Subdivision 2: adults	28	15		3	
Subdivision 3: additional and independent fracture of the diaphysis (segment 42)	4	4			
B1.3 Articular split, multiple in the metaphysis	25	18		3	
B1 Total	216	138	1	10	
B.2.1 Depression with a frontal split (lateral view)	12	6		2	
B2.2 Depression with a sagittal split (AP view)	23	17		4	
B2.3 Articular split-depression, multiple in the metaphysis	22	16		8	
B2 Total	57	39		14	
B3.1 Complex partial articular fracture, intact posterior wall	10	6		3	
B3.2 Complex partial articular fracture, intact lateral or medial wall	5	3		2	1
B3.3 Complex partial articular fracture, metaphyseal-diaphyseal	1	1		1	
B3 Total	16	10		6	1

Table 5

LONG-TERM RESULTS OF COMPLETE ARTICULAR FRACTURES (TYPE C)

Subgroup, Subdivisions, Definition	Total	No. of Late Follow-ups	Delayed Union, Nonunion/Malunion (Metaphysis)	No. of Prearthroses, Arthroses	No. of Arthrodeses
C1.1 Simple articular split, circular in the metaphysis	55	30	4	1	
C1.2 Articular split depression, circular in the metaphysis	26	13	a	9	
C1.3 Split or depression of the articular surface, extension into the diaphysis	45				
Subdivision 1: pure split	35	22	1	2	
Subdivision 2: additional articular depression	35	6	a	2	
C1 Total	126	71	5a	14	
C2.1 Articular split, metaphyseal impaction	117				
Subdivision 1: valgus angulation	33	20	3	8	1
Subdivision 2: varus angulation	21	10	a	4	
Subdivision 3: recurvation	28	15	a	3	
Subdivision 4: antecurvature	6	4	a	2	
Subdivision 5: no angulation	15	11	a	5	
Subdivision 6: additional depression of the articular surface	14	8	a	5	1
C2.2 Articular split, metaphyseal multifragmentation	86				
Subdivision 1: pure articular split	76	36	5	20	
Subdivision 2: additional articular depression	10	6	a	5	
C2.3 Articular split with impaction or multifragmentation of the metaphysis; additional extension to the diaphysis	17				
Subdivision 1: impacted type	5	1	a	1	1
Subdivision 2: multifragmentary type	12	8	1	3	
C2 Total	220	119	9a	56	3
C3.1 Complex at the articular surface, distal metaphysis	16	7	a	6	
C3.2 Complex at the articular surface, extending to the proximal metaphysis	19	10	a	3	1
C3.3 Complex at the articular surface, extending to the diaphysis	10	6	a	3	2
C3 Total	45	23		12	3

aIn C-type fractures, delayed union, nonunion, or malunion in the metaphysis is only specified when they are not combined with arthrosis. Details are noted each time in the systematic analysis of the various subgroups (see section 3).

Table 6

OSTEITIS AMONG THE CASE DATA COMPILED AT THE AO DOCUMENTATION CENTER[a]

Groups with Osteitis	Osteitis Cases	Following Open Fractures	Following Closed Fractures	Late Follow-up	No. of Internal Fixations
A2	2	1	1	72	150
A3	1	1	—	33	54
B1.1	1	—	1	61	84
B3	3	3	—	10	16
C2.1	4	1	3	68	117
C2.2	4	1	3	42	86
C2.3	2	2	—	9	17
C3.2	2	1	1	10	19
C3.3	2	1	1	6	0
Total	21	11	10	311	552
Cases of osteitis not found in groups A1, B1.2, B1.3, B2, C1, and C3.1				304	524
Total				615	1077

[a]The groups showing the highest frequency of osteitis are B3, C2, and C3: they contain 17 cases of osteitis out of 152 late follow-ups after 281 internal fixations. This corresponds to about 12% of osseous infections in severe pilon fractures. By contrast, after also including the less complicated fractures, we find a total number of osteitides of 21 out of 615 cases, about 3.4%. These are evenly distributed among open and closed fractures, thereby confirming the available literature.

Bibliography

Because it was necessary to list the most recent publications, the references from the German edition of this book had to be completely rearranged and updated. During the review of the literature for the English edition, I realized—to my surprise—that I had also missed some earlier papers of value in the German version. I have now read them all carefully, introduced them into the new list, and refer to them at the appropriate place in the text. The oversight was partly due to difficulties with the term "pilon," as I explained on pages 49 and 90. Even an extensive literature search with the help of the modern data banks did not bring a complete overview, because many papers about pilon fractures are concealed under the major topic "ankle injuries," which are devoted mainly to malleolar fractures. The literature on these injuries is enormous. Looking for the distal tibia fractures, it is impossible to collect and read everything written about the ankle joint.

In spite of my efforts it is possible that I still missed some papers. I apologize and assure the startled author that his work has not been left out on purpose and that I am quite willing to introduce it if a further edition should take place.

Another problem in this same matter is the perceptible language barrier between English versus French and German, French versus German, and German versus French. I feel that the pilon fracture is a prime example of these difficulties, which induce misunderstandings and cannot be avoided with the use of our electronic data tools. A personal effort by the younger generation in this area would be helpful.

Urs Heim

1. Allgöwer M (1963). Unterschenkelfrakturen. In Müller ME, Allgöwer M, Willenegger H (eds): *Technik der operativen Frakturenbehandlung*. Heidelberg, Springer.
2. Aubry P, Fiévé G (1984). Vascularisation osseuse et cutanée du quart inférieur de jambe. *Rev Chir Orthop* 70:589–597.
3. Ayeni JP (1988). Pilon fractures of the tibia: a study based on 19 cases. *Injury* 19:109–114.
4. Bandi W (1970). Zur Mechanik der supramalleolären intraartikulären Schienbeinbrüche des Ski-fahrers. Presented at Congress of SITEMSH, Nebel Garmisch-Partenkirchen.
5. Bandi W (1974). Die distalen intraartikulären Schienbeinbrüche des Skifahrers. *Aktuel Traumatol* 4:1–6.
6. Bauer G, Zenkl M, Kurz H, et al (1992). Die OSG-Arthrodese bei posttraumatischen Fehlstellun-gen. In Rahmanzadeh R, Meissner A (eds): *Fortschritte in der Unfallchirurgie*. Heidelberg, Springer, pp 366–370.
7. Beck E (1993). Results of operative treatment of pilon fractures. In Tscherne H, Schatzker J (eds): *Major Fractures of the Pilon, the Talus, and the Calcaneus*. Heidelberg, Springer, pp 49–51.
8. Benz G, Schmid H, Daum R (1988). Vaskularitätsstörungen nach kindlichen Sprungge-lenksfrak-turen. *Kinderchirurgie* 43:183–185.
9. Berchtold R, Hamelmann H, Peiper H-J (1990). *Chirurgie*, ed 2. Munich, Urban-Schwarzenberg.
10. Biga N, Richter D (1984). Résultats à long terme du traitement des fractures de la pince malléo-laire. *Ann Orthop Ouest* 16:95–151.
11. Biga N, Laurent M, Alain J, Thomine JM (1992). Facteurs pronostiques, évolutivité, corrélation radio-clinique et tolérance des cals vicieux. In Copin G, Nérot C (eds): *Les fractures récentes du pilon tibial de l'adulte. Rev Chir Orthop* 78(suppl)1:76–79
12. Bloom, Fawcett DW (1962). *A Textbook of Histology*. Philadelphia, WB Saunders.
13. Böhler L (1951). *Die Technik der Knochenbruchbehandlung*, eds. 12, 13. Vienna, Maudrich.
14. Börner M (1982). Einteilung, Behandlung und Ergebnisse der Frakturen des Pilon tibial. *Unfall-chirurgie* 8:230–235.
15. Bolton-Maggs BG, Sudlow RA, Freeman MA (1985). Total ankle arthroplasty. A long-term review of the London Hospital experience. *J Bone Joint Surg [Br]* 67:785–790.
16. Bone LB (1987). Fractures of the tibial plafond. *Orthop Clin North Am* 18:95–104.
17. Bone L, Stegemann P, McNamara K, et al (1993). External fixation of severely comminuted and open pilon fractures. In Tscherne H, Schatzker J (eds): *Major Fractures of the Pilon, the Talus, and the Calcaneus*. Heidelberg, Springer, pp 53–58.
18. Bonnel F, Lesire M, Gomis R, et al (1981). Arterial vascularization of the fibula microsurgical transplant techniques. *Anat Clin* 3:13–22.
19. Bourne RB (1989). Pilon fractures of the distal tibia. *Clin Orthop* 240:42–46.
20. Bourne RB, Rorabeck CH, Macnab J (1983). Intraarticular fractures of the distal tibia: the pilon fracture. *J Trauma* 23:591–596.
21. Breitfuss H, Muhr G, Neumann K, et al (1988). Prognose und Therapie geschlossener, distaler, intraartikulärer Unterschenkelbrüche. *Unfallchirurg* 91:557–564.
22. Brunelli G (1960). Le gravi fratture comminute chiuse del piatto tibiale distale. *Minerva Ortop* 11:597–599.
23. Brunner CF, Weber BG (1981). *Besondere Osteosynthesetechniken*. Heidelberg, Springer.
24. Caffinière de la JY, Fauroux L, Haas JL (1990). La fracture séparation-enfoncement, postérieure dans les fractures bimalléolaires. *Rev Chir Orthop* 76:568–578.
25. Cauchoix J, Duparc J, Vayre P (1961). Les fractures malléolaires consécutives aux accidents de ski. *Rev Prat* 11:3287–3308.
26. Charnley J (1951). Compression arthrodesis of the ankle and shoulder. *J Bone Joint Surg [Br]* 33:180–191.
27. Childress HM (1976). Vertical transarticular pin fixation for unstable ankle fractures. *Clin Orthop* 120:164–171.
28. Close JR (1956). Some applications of the functional anatomy of the ankle joint. *J Bone Joint Surg [Am]* 38:761–781.
29. Colton C (1982). Injuries of the ankle. In Watson-Jones R (ed): *Fractures and Joint Injuries*. Edinburgh, Churchill Livingstone, pp 1104–1151.
30. Comminot C (1981). *Die Pilon tibial-Fraktur. Nachkontrolle einer Serie von 136 Patienten des Kreuzspitals Chur,* Inaugural dissertation, Basel.
31. Coonrad RW (1970). Fracture-dislocations of the ankle joint with impaction injury of the lateral weight-bearing surface of the tibia. *J Bone Joint Surg [Am]* 52:1337–1343.

32. Copin G, Nérot G (1992). Les fractures récentes du pilon tibial de l'adulte. *Rev Chir Orthop* 78(suppl)1:34–83.
33. Couvelaire R, Rodier P (1937). Sur une variété de fracture par eclatement du pilon tibial. *Rev Orthop* 24:329–346.
34. Crenshaw AH (1971). Fractures. In Crenshaw AH (ed): *Campbell's Operative Orthopaedics,* vol 1. St Louis, Mosby–Year Book, pp 515–519.
35. Debrunner HU (1985). Biomechanik des Fusses Stuttgart, Enke.
36. Decoulx P, Razemon J-P, Rousselle Y (1961). Fractures du pilon tibial. *Rev Chir Orthop* 47:563–577.
37. Destot E (1911). *Traumatisme du pied et rayons X.* Paris, Masson.
38. Dick W, Schlatter S, Delley A, et al (1984). Bewegungsumfang des oberen Sprunggelenkes bei 1441 erwachsenen Probanden. In Hackenbroch MH, Refior HJ, Jäger M, et al (eds): *Funktionelle Anatomie und Pathomechanik des Sprunggelenkes.* Stuttgart, Thieme, pp 24–51.
39. Dillin L, Slabaugh P (1986). Delayed wound healing, infection, and nonunion following open reduction and internal fixation of tibial plafond fractures. *J Trauma* 26:1116–1119.
40. Draenert K (1984). Neue Beobachtungen zur Anatomie und Funktion des oberen Sprunggelenkes. In Hackenbroch MH, Refior HJ, Jäger M, et al (eds): *Funktionelle Anatomie und Pathomechanik des Sprunggelenkes.* Stuttgart, Thieme, pp 5–9.
41. Durbin F (1992). Posttraumatische Fehlstellungen des Sprunggelenks und ihre Korrektur. In Rahmanzadeh R, Meissner A (eds): *Fortschritte in der Unfallchirurgie.* Heidelberg, Springer, pp 362–365.
42. Dürig M, Zeugin M, Rüedi T (1978). Vergleichende Ergebnisse nach operativer Versorgung von Pilon tibial-Frakturen an zwei verschiedenen Kliniken. *Hefte Unfallheilkd* 131:158–162.
43. Etter C, Ganz R (1991). Long-term results of tibial plafond fractures treated with open reduction and internal fixation. *Arch Orthop Trauma Surg* 110:277–283.
44. Fröhlich H, Gotzen L, Adam U (1984). Experimentelle Untersuchungen zur gehaltenen Aufnahme des oberen Sprunggelenks. In Hackenbroch MH, Refior HJ, Jäger M, et al (eds): *Funktionelle Anatomie und Pathomechanik des Sprunggelenkes.* Stuttgart, Thieme, pp 74–77.
45. Ganzoni N, Jirecek V (1989). Muskellappenplastik bei Frakturen am Pilon tibial. *Helv Chir Acta* 56:255–258.
46. Gay R, Evrard J (1963). Les fractures récentes du pilon tibial chez l'adulte. *Rev Chir Orthop* 49:397–512.
47. Gedeon P, Ficat P (1977). Pilon tibial fractures, indications and results. In *Proceedings of the Austrian Society for Surgery,* Graz, p 643.
48. Giachino AA, Hammond DI (1987). The relationship between oblique fractures of the medial malleolus and concomitant fractures of the anterolateral aspect of the tibial plafond. *J Bone Joint Surg [Am]* 69:381–384.
49. Grete W (1972). *Das Tibialis-Anterior-Syndrom nach Osteosynthese am Unterschenkel,* Inaugural dissertation, Zurich.
50. Hackenbruch W (1977). Die Pilon-Fraktur des Skifahrers. *Fortschr Med* 95:219–227.
51. Hagen RJ (1986). Ankle arthrodesis. Problems and pitfalls. *Clin Orthop* 202:152–162.
52. Hefti F (1981). *Die Stellung des Fusses bei Arthrodesen des oberen Sprunggelenkes,* vol 28: *Bücherei des Orthopäden.* Stuttgart, Enke.
53. Hefti FL, Baumann JU, Morscher EW (1980). Ankle joint fusion—determination of optimal position by gait analysis. *Arch Orthop Trauma Surg* 96:187–195.
54. Heim U (1970). Zur operativen Technik der distalen intraartikulären Tibiaimpressionsfrakturen. Presented at Congress of SITEMSH. Nebel Garmisch-Partenkirchen.
55. Heim U (1972). Le traitement chirurgical des fractures du pilon tibial. *J Chir* 104:307–322.
56. Heim U (1975). Erfahrungen mit der Spaltung der lateralen Fascia cruris bei Tibiaosteosynthesen. *Helv Chir Acta* 42:451–456.
57. Heim U (1983). Malleolarfrakturen. *Unfallheilkunde* 86:248–258.
58. Heim U (1983). Die Risse der Membrana interossea bei Malleolarfrakturen. Ihre Bedeutung für Klassifikation und Operationstechnik. *Hefte Unfallheilkd* 165:247–250.
59. Heim U (1985). Las fracturas intraarticulares de la tibia distal. *Acta Ortop Latinoam* 12:13–16.
60. Heim U (1986). Arthrosehäufigkeit nach Osteosynthesen des Volkmannschen Dreiecks bei Malleolarfrakturen. *Z Unfallchir Versicherungsmed* 79:99–113.
61. Heim U (1987). Die Grenzziehung zwischen Diaphyse und Metaphyse mit Hilfe der Viereckmessung. *Unfallchirurg* 90:274–280.

62. Heim U (1989). Trimalleolar fractures: late results after fixation of the posterior fragment. *Orthopedics* 12:1053–1059.
63. Heim U (1990). Die Bedeutung der Fibula bei der Pilon tibial-Fraktur. *Z Unfallchir* 83:187–195.
64. Heim U (1993). Morphological features for evaluation and classification of pilon tibial fractures. In Tscherne H, Schatzker J (eds): *Major Fractures of the Pilon, the Talus, and the Calcaneus.* Heidelberg, Springer, pp 29–41.
65. Heim U, Damur-Thür F (1977). Spongiosa aus dem Tibiakopf als autologes Transplantationsmaterial. *Arch Orthop Unfallchir* 89:11–217.
66. Heim U, Grete W (1972). Das Tibialis-anterior-Syndrom nach Osteosynthese am Unterschenkel. *Helv Chir Acta* 39:667–677.
67. Heim U, Näser M (1976). Die operative Behandlung der Pilon tibial-Fraktur. Technik der Osteosynthese und Resultate bei 128 Patienten. *Arch Orthop Unfallchir* 86:341–356.
68. Heim U, Näser M (1977). Fracures du pilon tibial. Résultats de 128 ostéosynthéses. *Rev Chir Orthop* 63:5–12.
69. Heim U, Pfeiffer KM (1972). *Periphere Osteosynthesen.* Heidelberg, Springer.
70. Heim U, Pfeiffer KM (1973). *Small Fragment Set Manual.* New York, Springer.
71. Heim U, Pfeiffer KM (1987). *Internal Fixation of Small Fractures,* ed 3. New York, Springer.
72. Heim U, Pfeiffer KM (1988). *Periphere Osteosynthesen,* ed 3. Heidelberg, Springer.
73. Heim U, Pfeiffer KM (1991). *Periphere Osteosynthesen,* ed 4. Heidelberg, Springer.
74. Hille E, Schulitz KP, Perzborn V (1984). Die Druck- und Kontaktverläufe des oberen Sprunggelenkes unter verschiedenen Funktionen. In Hackenbroch H, Refior HJ, Jäger M, et al (eds): *Funktionelle Anatomie und Pathomechanik des Sprunggelenkes.* Stuttgart, Thieme, pp 52–57.
75. Hochstein P, Winkler H, Wentzensen A (1991). Verfahrenswechsel nach primärer Anwendung des Fixateur externe bei Unterschenkelschaftfrakturen—Prophylaxe drohender knöcherner Fehlheilungen? In Rahmanzadeh R, Meissner A (eds): *Störungen der Frakturheilung.* Heidelberg, Springer, pp 224–230.
76. Hochstein P, Aymar M, Winkler H, et al (1992). Zur Verfahrenswahl bei Frakturen des Pilon tibiale. In Berenty J (ed): *Osteosynthese International.* Budapest, pp 459–462.
77. Hochstein P, Heppert V, Wentzensen A (1992). Infektionen im Bereich des oberen Sprunggelenkes—Ursachen und Therapie. In Rahmanzadeh R, Meissner A (eds): *Fortschritte in der Unfallchirurgie.* Heidelberg, Springer, pp 371–376.
78. Holz U (1990). Die Arthrodese des oberen Sprunggelenks mit Zugschrauben. *Operative Orthop Traumatol* 2:131–138.
79. Höntzsch D (1990). Ein- oder zweizeitige (mit Fixateur externe) Versorgung der schweren Pilon-Tibial-Fraktur. *Aktuel Traumatol* 20:199–204.
80. Hourlier H (1981). *Fractures récentes du pilon tibial,* Thesis, Amiens.
81. Hvid I, Rasmussen O, Jensen NC, et al (1985). Trabecular bone strength profiles at the ankle joint. *Clin Orthop* 199:306–312.
82. Inman VT (1976). *The Joints of the Ankle.* Baltimore, Williams & Wilkins.
83. Jahna H (1956). Die intraartikulären Stauchungsbrüche am distalen Schienbeinende und ihre Behandlung. In *Proceedings of the 44th Congress of the German Orthopedic Society,* pp 327–332.
84. Jahna H, Wittich H, Hartenstein H (1979). Der distale Stauchungsbruch der Tibia. *Hefte Unfallheikd* 137.
85. Judet J, Judet R, Letournel E (1967). Un procédé d'osteosynthése pour fracture multifragmentaire du pilon tibial. *Mem Acad Chir* 17–18:547–549.
86. Kapandji IA (1980). *Physiologie articulaire,* ed 5. Paris, Maloine.
87. Kärrholm J, Hansson LI, Selvik G (1985). Mobility of the lateral malleolus. *Acta Orthop Scand* 56:479–483.
88. Kellam JF, Waddell JP (1979). Fractures of the distal tibial metaphysis with intraarticular extension—the distal tibial explosion fracture. *J Trauma* 19:593–601.
89. Kitaoka HB, Anderson PJ, Morrey BF (1992). Revision of ankle arthrodesis with external fixation for non-union. *J Bone Joint Surg [Am]* 74:1191–1200.
90. Koebke J (1983). A biomechanical and morphological analysis of human hand joints. *Adv Anat Embryol Cell Biol* 80:1–85.
91. Küsswetter W, Wirth CJ (1984). Simultane Dehnungsmessungen des Kapselbandapparates am oberen Sprunggelenk unter physiologischen und pathologischen Bedingungen. In Hackenbroch HH, Refior HJ, Jäger M, et al (eds): *Anatomie und Pathomechanik des Sprunggelenkes.* Stuttgart, Thieme, pp 78–92.

92. Laer L von (1985). Classification, diagnosis and treatment of transitional fractures of the distal part of the tibia. *J Bone Joint Surg [Am]* 67:687–698.
93. Lambotte A (1913). *Chirurgie opératoire des fractures.* Paris, Masson.
94. Lamprecht E, Ochsner PE (1984). Spätprobleme nach konservativ und operativ behandelten. ''Pilon tibial'' - Frakturen. *Helv Chir Acta* 51:629–631.
95. Landin LA, Danielsson LG, Jonsson K, et al (1986). Late results in 65 physeal ankle fractures. *Acta Orthop Scand* 57:530–534.
96. Lantz BA, McAndrew M, Scioli M, et al (1991). The effect of concomitant chondral injuries accompanying operatively reduced malleolar fractures. *J Trauma* 5:125–128.
97. Lanz T, Wachsmuth W (1972). *Praktische Anatomie,* Heidelberg, Springer.
98. Lauge-Hansen N (1954). Fractures of the ankle III. Genetic roentgenologic diagnosis of fractures of the Ankle. *AJR* 71:456.
99. Lauge-Hansen N (1963). Die genetische Reposition und Retention. *Zentralbl Chir* 88:545.
100. Leach RE (1983) Fractures of the tibial plafond. In Yablon IG, Segal D, Leach R (eds): *Ankle Injuries.* New York, Churchill Livingstone.
101. Lecestre P, Ramadier JO (1976). Les fractures bimalléolaires et leurs équivalents. *Rev Clin Orthop* 62:71–89.
102. Lecestre P, Lortat-Jacob A, Ramadier JO (1977). Les fractures du pilon tibial. *Ann Chir* 31:665–671.
103. Lechevallier J, Thomine JM, Biga N (1989). Le fixateur externe tibio-calcanéen dans le traitement des fractures du pilon tibial. *Rev Chir Orthop* 74:52–60.
104. de Lestang M, Hourlier H, Warlaumont et al (1985). La voie d'abord antéro-externe pour le traitement des fractures de l'extrémité inférieure de jambe. *Rev Chir Orthop* 71:73–74.
105. Lewis YL (1964). The effect of ankle injury forces. *J Bone Joint Surg [Am]* 46:1380.
106. Lindsjö U (1985). Classification of ankle fractures: the Lauge-Hansen or AO system? *Clin Orthop* 199:12–16.
107. Lippay S (1977). Frühergebnisse operierter distaler intraartikulärer Stauchungsbrüche des Unterschenkels. In *Proceedings of the Austrian Society for Surgery*, Graz, pp 659–661.
108. Ludolph E, Hierholzer G, Gretenkord K (1984). Untersuchungen zur Anatomie und Röntgendiagnostik des fibularen Bandapparates am Sprunggelenk. In Hackenbroch MH, Refior HJ, Jäger M, et al (eds): *Funktionelle Anatomie und Pathomechanik des Sprunggelenkes.* Stuttgart, Thieme, pp 70–73.
109. Lugger LJ, Hölzl H, Oberhammer J (1977). Zur Operationsindikation intraartikulärer Stauchungsbruchformen der distalen Tibia. In *Proceedings of the Austrian Society for Surgery*, Graz, pp 666–669.
110. Macek LJ (1984). *Behandlung und Ergebnisse bei Frakturen des Pilon Tibiale* 1965–1977, Inaugural dissertation, Mainz.
111. Mackinnon AP (1928). Fracture of the lower articular surface of the tibia in fracture dislocation of the ankle. *J Bone Joint Surg* 10:252–262.
112. Macko VW, Matthews LS, Zwirkoski P, et al (1991). The joint-contact area of the ankle. *J Bone Joint Surg [Am]* 73:347–351.
113. Mainwaring BL, Daffner RH, Riemer BL (1988). Pylon fractures of the ankle: a distinct clinical and radiologic entity. *Musculoskeletal Radiol* 168:215–218.
114. Marti R, Raaymakers ELFB (1990). Sekundäreingriffe bei fehlverheilten Frakturen des oberen Sprunggelenks. *Clin Orthop* 19:400–408.
115. Massari L, Martinez Flores D, Traina GC (1992). Fratture del pilone tibiale nell'adulto. In Malerba F, Neri M, Grandi A, et al (eds): *Fratture della Tibio-Tarsica.* Bologna, Aulo Gaggi pp 129–137.
116. Mast JW, Spiegel PG, Pappas JN (1988). Fractures of the tibial pilon. *Clin Orthop* 230:68–82.
117. Mast J, Jakob R, Ganz R (1989). *Planning and Reduction Technique in Fracture Surgery.* Heidelberg, Springer.
118. Mast J (1993). Pilon fractures of the distal tibia: a test of surgical judgment. In Tscherne H, Schatzker J (eds): *Major Fractures of the Pilon, the Talus, and the Calcaneus.* Heidelberg, Springer, pp 7–27.
119. McGuire MR, Kyle RF, Gustilo RB, et al (1988). Comparative analysis of ankle arthroplasty versus ankle arthrodesis. *Clin Orthop* 226:174–181.
120. Meyer GH (1867). Die Architektur der Spongiosa. *Arch Anat Physiol Wiss Med*, pp 615–628.
121. Mischkowsky T, Dichgans M (1980). Behandlung und Spätergebnisse von 33 Frakturen des Pilon tibial. *Unfallchirurgie* 6:253–255.

122. Mittelmeier T, Hertlein H, Lob G, et al (1992). Gelenkerhaltende Therapie der posttraumatischen Arthrose des oberen Sprunggelenks. In Rahmanzadeh R, Meissner A (eds): *Fortschritte in der Unfallchirurgie.* Heidelberg, Springer, pp 347–353.

123. Möller BN, Krebs B (1982). Intra-articular fractures of the distal tibia. *Acta Orthop Scand* 53:991–996.

124. Möllers N, Lehmann K, Koebke J (1986). Die Verteilung des subchondralen Knochenmaterials an der distalen Gelenkfläche des Radius. *Anat Anz* 161:151.

125. Möseneder H (1977). Pilon tibial-Frakturen nach Ski-Unfällen. In *Proceedings of the Austrian Society for Surgery,* Graz, pp 656–668.

126. Muhr G, Breitfuss H (1993). Complications after pilon fractures. In Tscherne H, Schatzker J (eds): *Major Fractures of the Pilon, the Talus and the Calcaneus.* Heidelberg, Springer, pp 65–67.

127. Müller K-H, Prescher W (1978). Posttraumatische Osteomyelitis nach distalen intraarticulären Unterschenkelfrakturen. *Hefte Unfallheilkd* 131:163–183.

128. Müller ME, Engelhardt P (1982). Verletzungen des Halte- und Bewegungsapparates. In Berchtold R, Hamelmann H, Peiper H-J (eds): *Arbeitsbuch Chirurgie.* Munich, Urban & Schwarzenberg, pp 489–561.

129. Müller ME, Allgöwer M, Willenegger H (1963). *Technik der operativen Frakturenbehandlung.* Heidelberg, Springer.

130. Müller ME, Allgöwer M, Schneider R, et al (1977). *Manual der Osteosynthese,* ed 2. Heidelberg, Springer.

131. Müller ME, Allgöwer M, Schneider R, et al (1979). *Manual of Internal Fixation.* New York, Springer.

132. Müller ME, Nazarian S, Koch P (1987). *Classification AO des fractures.* Heidelberg, Springer.

133. Müller ME, Allgöwer M, Schneider R, et al (1990). *Manual of Internal Fixation,* ed 3. Heidelberg, Springer.

134. Müller ME, Nazarian S, Koch P, et al (1990). *The Comprehensive Classification of Fractures of Long Bones.* Heidelberg, Springer.

135. Müller-Gerbl M (1989). Zur Verteilung der subchondralen Mineralisierung in den Sprunggelenken. Kölner Biomechanisches Kolloquium (in press).

136. Müller-Gerbl M, Schulte E, Putz R (1987). The thickness of the calcified layer in different joints of a single individual. *Acta Morphol Neerl Scand* 25:41–49.

137. Müller-Gerbl M, Schulte E, Putz R (1987). The thickness of the calcified layer of articular cartilage: a function of the load supported? *J Anat* 154:103–111.

138. Müller-Gerbl M, Putz R, Hodapp N, et al (1989). Computed tomography-osteoabsorptiometry for assessing the density of subchondral bone as a measure of long-term mechanical adaptation in individual joints. *Skeletal Radiol* 18:507–512.

139. Müller-Gerbl M, Putz R, Hodapp N, et al (1993). Die Darstellung der subchondralen Dichtemuster mittels der CT-Osteoabsorptiometrie (CT-OAM) zur Beurteilung der individuellen Gelenkbeanspruchung am Lebenden. *Z Orthop* 131:10–13.

140. Näser M (1977). *Die Pilon tibial-Frakturen im Krankengut des Kreuzspitals in Chur* 1961–1973, Inaugural dissertation, Zurich.

141. Nordin JY, Perraudin JE (1992). Arthrodèses précoces dans les fractures du pilon tibial. In Copin G, Nérot C (eds): Les fractures récentes du pilon tibial de l'adulte. *Rev Chir Orthop* 78(suppl 1):60–61.

142. Nordin JY, Pagès C, Barba L, et al (1988). Ostéosynthèse par fixateur externe de 35 fractures ouvertes et/ou comminutives de la cheville. *Rev Chir Orthop* 74(suppl 2):230–233.

143. Oestern H-J, Tscherne H (1983). Pathophysiologie und Klassifikation des Weichteilschadens. *Hefte Unfallheilkd* 162:1–9.

144. Orthner E, Reimann R, Anderhuber F, Wagner M (1986). Änderungen des Flächenkontaktes im oberen Sprunggelenk nach schrittweiser Verkürzung der Fibula. *Hefte Unfallheilkd* 181:88–91.

145. Osterwalder A, Ganz M, Harder F (1984). Zur Problematik der Pilon Tibial-Trümmerfraktur mit grossem Defekt. *Z Unfallchir Versicherungsmed* 77/4:227–231.

146. Ovadia DN, Beals RK (1986). Fractures of the tibial plafond. *J Bone Joint Surg [Am]* 68 4:543–551.

147. Perraudin JE, Nordin JY (1992). Ostéosynthèse par fixateur externe des fractures du pilon tibial. In Copin G, Nérot C (eds): Les fractures récentes du pilon tibial de l'adulte. *Rev Chir Orthop* 78(suppl 1):56–58.

148. Pfister A, Milachowski K, Plitz W (1984). Experimentelle Untersuchungen zur Pathomechanik der

isolierten Ruptur der vorderen Syndesmose. In Hackenbroch MH, Refior HJ, Jäger M, et al (eds): *Funktionelle Anatomie und Pathomechanik des Sprunggelenks.* Stuttgart, Thieme, pp 115–125.

149. Pierce RO, Heinrich JH (1979). Comminuted intraarticular fractures of the distal tibia. *J Trauma* 19:828–832.
150. Poigenfürst J (1977). Offene Stauchungsbrüche am distalen Schienbeinende. In *Proceedings of the Austrian Society for Surgery,* Graz, pp 644–650.
151. Raasch WG, Larkin JJ, Draganich LF (1992). Assessment of the posterior malleolus as a restraint to posterior subluxation of the ankle. *J Bone Joint Surg [Am]* 74:1201–1206.
152. Raimbeau G, Toulemonde JL, Albaret P, Pillet J (1979). The anterior tibial artery: interest of profile arteriography. *Anat Clin* 1:325–329.
153. Ratliff AHC (1959). Compression arthrodesis of the ankle. *J Bone Joint Surg [Br]* 41:524–534.
154. Rauber-Kopsch (1911). *Anatomie des Menschen,* vol 3: Muskeln und Gefässe. Leipzig, Thieme.
155. Raymond O (1979). Comminuted intraarticular fractures of the distal tibia. *J Trauma* 19:828.
156. Reihmann R, Anderhuber F (1980). Kompensationsbewegungen der Fibula, die durch die Keilform der Trochlea tali erzwungen werden. *Acta Anat* 108:60–67.
157. Reihmann R, Anderhuber F, Gerold J (1986). Über die Geometrie der menschlichen Sprungbein-rolle. *Acta Anat* 127:271–278.
158. Reihmann R, Anderhuber F, Gerold J (1988). Modelle zur Geometrie der menschlichen Sprung-beinrolle: Zwei Reihen geometricsher Modelle zur Veranschaulichung der Biomechanik des ob-eren Sprunggelenkes. *Gegenbaurs Morphol Jahrb* 134:351–380.
159. Reimers C (1953). Die Brüche des fussnahen Unterschenkelabschnittes. *Langenbecks Arch Chir* 276:260–277.
160. Resch H, Pechlaner S, Benedetto KP (1986). Spätergebnisse nach konservativer und operativer Behandlung von Pilon Tibial-Frakturen. *Aktuel Traumatol* 16:117–123.
161. Resch H, Pechlaner S, Benedetto KP (1986). Die Entwicklung der posttraumatischen Arthrose nach Pilon tibial-Frakturen. *Unfallchirurg* 89:8–15.
162. Riede UN, Schenk RK, Willenegger H (1971). Gelenkmechanische Untersuchungen zum Problem der posttraumatischen Arthrosen im oberen Sprunggelenk. I. Die intraartikuläre Modellfraktur. *Langenbecks Arch Chir* 328:258–271.
163. Riede UN, Müller M, Mihatsch MJ (1973). Biometrische Untersuchungen zum Arthroseproblem am Beispiel des oberen Sprunggelenkes. *Arch Orthop Unfallchir* 77:181–194.
164. Riede UN, Schweizer G, Marti J, et al (1973). Gelenkmechanische Untersuchungen zum Problem der posttraumatischen Arthrosen im oberen Sprunggelenk. III. Funktionell-morphometrische Ana-lyse des Gelenkknorpels. *Langenbecks Arch Chir* 333:911–1107.
165. Rieunau G, Gay R (1956). Enclouage du péroné dans les fractures supra-malléolaires. *Lyon Chir* 51:594–600.
166. Rogge D (1983). Gelenktransfixation bei Gelenkverletzungen mit schwerem Weichteilschaden. *Hefte Unfallheilkd* 162:97–110.
167. Rommens PM, Claes P, De Boodt P, et al (1994). Therapeutisches Vorgehen und Langzeitergeb-nisse bei der Pilonfraktur in Abhängigkeit vom primären Weichteilschaden. *Unfallchirurg* 97:39–46.
168. Rüedi T (1973). Fractures of the lower end of the tibia into the ankle joint: Results 9 years after open reduction and internal fixation. *Injury* 5:2.
169. Rüedi T (1984). Intraarticular fractures of the distal tibia. *Surg Rounds:* Nov: 85–92.
170. Rüedi T (1993). Treatment of pilon tibial fractures: state of the art. In Tscherne H, Schatzker J (eds): *Major Fractures of the Pilon, the Talus, and the Calcaneus.* Heidelberg, Springer, pp 3–5.
171. Rüedi T, Allgöwer M (1978). Spätresultate nach operativer Behandlung der Gelenkbrüche am distalen Tibiaende (sog. Pilon-Frakturen). *Unfallheikunde* 81:319–323.
172. Rüedi T, Allgöwer M (1979). The operative treatment of intraarticular fractures of the lower end of the tibia. *Clin Orthop* 138:105–110.
173. Rüedi T, Matter P, Allgöwer M (1968). Die intraartikulären Frakturen des distalen Unterschenke-lendes. *Helv Chir Acta* 35:556–582.
174. Rüedi Th, Heim U, Zeugin M (1977). Die Behandlungsmöglichkeiten der Pilon tibial-Frakturen aus der Sicht der Spätergebnisse. In *Proceedings of the Austrian Society for Surgery,* Graz, pp 634–638.
175. Rüter A (1978). Einteilung und Behandlung der Frakturen des Pilon tibial. *Hefte Unfallheilkd* 131:143–157.
176. Salter RB, Simmonds DF, Malcolm BW, et al (1980). The biological effects of continuous passive

motion on the healing of full thickness defects in articular cartilage: an experimental investigation in the rabbit. *J Bone Joint Surg [Am]* 62:1232–1251.

177. Schatzker J, Tile M (1987). *The Rationale of Operative Fracture Care.* Heidelberg, Springer.
178. Scheller EE, Meissner A, Rahmanzadeh R (1992). Pilontibialfrakturen—Komplikation, Spätfolgen und Konzept zur Infektreduzierung. In Rahmanzadeh R, Meissner A (eds): *Fortschritte in der Unfallchirurgie.* Heidelberg, Springer, pp 383–386.
179. Schmidt HM (1981). Die Artikulationsflächen der menschlichen Sprunggelenke. *Adv Anat Embryol Cell Biol* 6:1–81.
180. Schmidt HM, Geissler F (1983). Die Artikulationsflächen des proximalen Handgelenkes beim Menschen. *Z Morphol Anthropol* 74:145–172.
181. Schweiberer L, Betz A, Nast-Kolb D, et al (1987). Spezielle Behandlungstaktik am distalen Unterschenkel und bei Pilonfraktur. *Unfallchirurg* 90:253–259.
182. Seiler H (1986). Biomechanik des oberen Sprunggelenkes. *Orthopadie* 15:415–422.
183. Soeur R (1961). La classification des fractures malléolaires. *Acta Orthop Belg* 27:537–583.
184. Songis-Mortreux M (1975). *Les fractures du pilon tibial,* Thesis, Lille.
185. Stampfel O, Mähring M (1977). Komplikationen und Ergebnisse 40 operierter Pilon-tibial-Stauchungsfrakturen. In Proceedings of the Austrian Society for Surgery, Graz, pp 639–692.
186. Stiehl JB, Dollinger B (1988). Primary ankle arthrodesis in trauma: report of three cases. *J Orthop Trauma* 2:277–283.
187. Swärd L, Hughes JS, Howell CJ, et al (1992). Posterior internal compression arthrodesis of the ankle. *J Bone Joint Surg [Br]* 74:752–756.
188. Takechi H, Ito S, Takada T, Nakayama H (1982). Trabecular architecture of the ankle joint. *Anat Clin* 4:227–233.
189. Tassler H (1981). Behandlungsprinzipien bei drittgradig offenen Frakturen des distalen Unterschenkels. *Unfallheilkunde* 84:509–513.
190. Thielemann FW, Holz U (1992). Die Korrektur posttraumatischer intraartikulärer Fehlstellungen am Knie- und Sprunggelenk. In Rahmanzadeh R, Meissner A (eds): *Fortschritte in der Unfallchirurgie.* Heidelberg, Springer, pp 9–12.
191. Thordarson DB, Markolf K, Cracchiolo A (1992). Stability of an ankle arthrodesis fixed by cancellous bone screws compared with that fixed by an external fixator. *J Bone Joint Surg [Am]* 74:1050–1055.
192. Tile M (1987). Fractures of the distal tibial metaphysis involving the ankle joint: the pilon fracture. In Schatzker J, Tile MS (eds): *The Rationale of Operative Fracture Care.* Heidelberg, Springer, pp 343–369.
193. Tillman B, Bartz B, Schleicher A (1985). Stress in the human ankle joint: a brief review. *Arch Orthop Trauma Surg* 103:385–391.
194. Trentz O, Friedl HP (1993). Critical soft tissue conditions and pilon fractures. In Tscherne H, Schatzker J (eds): *Major Fractures of the Pilon, the Talus, and the Calcaneus.* Heidelberg, Springer, pp 59–64.
195. Trojan E (1956). A propos du traitement des fractures articulaires de l'extrémité inférieure de la jambe. *Rev Chir Orthop* 42:382–384.
196. Trojan E, Jahna H (1956). Zur Behandlung der Stauchungsbrüche am distalen Unterschenkelende. *Klin Med* 11:313–317.
197. Trumble TE, Benirschke SK, Bedder NB (1992). Use of radial forearm flaps to treat complications of closed pilon fractures. *J Trauma* 6:358–365.
198. Tscherne H (1983). Management offener Frakturen. *Hefte Unfallheilkd* 162:10–32.
199. Tscherne H, Gotzen L (1984). *Fractures with Soft Tissue Injuries.* Heidelberg, Springer.
200. Tscherne H, Rojczyk M (1983). Behandlung geschlossener Frakturen mit Weichteilschaden. *Hefte Unfallheilkd* 162:39–45.
201. Tscherne H, Schatzker J (1993). *Major Fractures of the Pilon, the Talus and the Calcaneus.* Heidelberg, Springer.
202. Vichard P, Watelet F (1973). Les formes de transition entre les fractures de la malléole interne et les fractures du pilon tibial. *Rev Chir Orthop* 59:657–665.
203. Vivès P, Hourlier H, De Lestang M, et al (1984). Etude de 84 fractures du pilon tibial de l'adulte. *Rev Chir Orthop* 70:129–139.
204. Waddell JP (1993). Tibial plafond fractures. In Tscherne H, Schatzker J (eds): *Major Fractures of the Pilon, the Talus, and the Calcaneus.* Heidelberg, Springer, pp 43–48.
205. Wagner H, Pock HG (1982). Die Verschraubungsarthrodese der Sprunggelenke. *Unfallheilkrunde* 85:280–300.

206. Watson-Jones R (1982). *Fractures and Joint Injuries,* ed 6. Edinburgh, Churchill Livingstone.
207. Weber BG (1967). *Die Verletzungen des oberen Sprunggelenkes.* Bern, Huber.
208. Weber BG (1981). Brüche von Knöcheln und Talus. Bewährtes und Neues in Diagnostik und Therapie. *Langenbecks Arch Chir* 355:421.
209. Weissmann JA, Lazis AK (1978). Das normale Arthrogramm des oberen Sprunggelenks. *Radiol Diagn* 19:733–741.
210. Weissmann JA, Lazis AK (1980). Über die röntgenologischen Symptome der distalen tibiofibularen Syndesmose. *Fortschr Röntgenstr* 133:46–51.
211. Welz K (1982). Besondere Aspekte und Ergebnisse der Behandlung von Pilon-Tibial-Frakturen. *Orthop Traumatol* 29:632–643.
212. Welz K (1992). Verfahrenswahl und Infektminderung bei Osteosynthesen von Pilontibialfrakturen. In Rahmanzadeh R, Meissner A (eds): *Fortschritte in der Unfallchirurgie.* Heidelberg, Springer, pp 377–382.
213. Willenegger H (1961). Die Behandlung der Luxationsfrakturen des oberen Sprunggelenks nach biomechanischen Gesichtspunkten. *Helv Chir Acta* 28:225.
214. Willenegger H (1971). Spätergebnisse nach konservativ und operativ behandelten Malleolar-Frakturen. *Helv Chir Acta* 38:321.
215. Wirth CJ (1978). Biomechanische Aspekte der fibularen Bandplastik. *Hefte Unfallheilkd* 133:148–156.
216. Witt AN (1960). Supramalleoläre Frakturen kombiniert mit Luxationsfrakturen des oberen Sprunggelenks. Ihre Gefahren für die Zirkulation und ihre Behandlung. *Wiederherstellungschir Traumatol* 5:15–60.
217. Yablon IG, Segal D, Leach RE (1983). *Ankle Injuries.* New York, Churchill Livingstone.
218. Ziegelmüller R, Börner M, Schnettler R (1990). Korrektureingriffe nach operative versorgten Pilonfrakturen. In Rahmanzadeh R, Meissner A (eds): *Fortschritte in der Unfallchirurgie.* Heidelberg, Springer, pp 387–389.
219. Zwipp H, Tscherne H (1984). Die Rotationsinstabilität Pathomechanik. Diagnostik und Therapie. In Hackenbroch MH, Refior HJ, Jäger M, et al (eds): *Funktionelle Anatomie und Pathomechanik des Sprunggelenks.* Stuttgart, Thieme, pp 126–130.

Index

Note: Page numbers in *italics* refer to illustrations; page numbers followed by T refer to tables.

ISBN 0-7216-5658-7

90038

9 780721 656588